Dr Raj Persaud is a consultant psychiatrist working in the British National Health Service at the world-famous Maudsley Hospital in south London, and an honorary senior lecturer at the Institute of Psychiatry, University of London. Uniquely for a doctor, he also holds a first-class honours degree in psychology from University College London, which recently awarded him the title of Fellow in recognition of his ground-breaking work in psychiatry. Other medical awards and honours include the prestigious Royal College of Psychiatrists' Research Prize and Medal, the Denis Hill Prize and the Osler Medal.

As well as medicine, psychology and psychiatry, he holds university-level qualifications in statistics, history and philosophy.

Raj Persaud is the author of *Staying Sane* and his work has been published in academic medical journals, including the *British Medical Journal*, the *Lancet* and the *British Journal of Psychiatry*. He writes regularly for the national press and hosts BBC Radio 4's *All in the Mind* – the only broadcast series dedicated specifically to reporting on academic psychology and psychiatry. He also appears regularly on television programmes such as *Question Time*, *Newsnight* and *Tomorrow's World*. In a recent poll of members of the Royal College of Psychiatrists published in the *Independent on Sunday* newspaper, he was voted one of the top ten psychiatrists in the UK.

He is married to an eye surgeon, has a son and a daughter, and lives in London.

www.booksattransworld.co.uk

Also by Raj Persaud

Staying Sane

FROM THE EDGE OF THE COUCH

RAJ PERSAUD

BANTAM PRESS

LONDON · NEW YORK · TORONTO · SYDNEY · AUCKLAND

TRANSWORLD PUBLISHERS
61–63 Uxbridge Road, London W5 5SA
a division of The Random House Group Ltd

RANDOM HOUSE AUSTRALIA (PTY) LTD
20 Alfred Street, Milsons Point, Sydney,
New South Wales 2061, Australia

RANDOM HOUSE NEW ZEALAND LTD
18 Poland Road, Glenfield, Auckland 10, New Zealand

RANDOM HOUSE SOUTH AFRICA (PTY) LTD
Endulini, 5a Jubilee Road, Parktown 2193, South Africa

Published 2003 by Bantam Press
A division of Transworld Publishers

A catalogue record for this book is available from the British Library.
ISBN 0593 04696X

Set in 11/14pt Sabon by Falcon Oast Graphic Art Ltd.

Printed in Great Britain by
by Mackays of Chatham plc, Chatham, Kent

3 5 7 9 10 8 6 4 2

This is for my son Sachin, who, in being born, dragged me back from the edge of the couch.

There are more things in heaven and earth, Horatio,

Than are dreamt of in your philosophy.

Hamlet, I, v 166

CONTENTS

ABBREVIATIONS

ADHD   Attention deficit hyperactivity disorder
AEA   Autoerotic asphyxia
BDD   Body dysmorphic disorder
CAWD   Chronic alternate-world disorder
CD   Capgras delusion
CS   Capgras syndrome
DID   Dissociative identity disorder
DMI   Delusional misidentification
GSM   Genital self-mutilation
IPD   Induced psychotic disorder
MAOI   Monoamine oxidase inhibitors
MHP   Monosymptomatic hypochondriacal psychosis
MPD   Multiple personality disorder
MSBP   Munchausen syndrome by proxy
NVAW   National Violence Against Women Survey
OCB   Obsessive-compulsive behaviour
OCD   Obsessive-compulsive disorder
OMPI   Occupational mass psychogenic illness
ORS   Olfactory reference syndrome
PEA   Phenylethylamine
PTSD   Post-traumatic stress disorder
SPD   Shared psychotic disorder
SRS   Sexual reassignment surgery
TM   Trichotillomania
TS   Tourette's syndrome

ACKNOWLEDGEMENTS

All single-authored books are really the result of collaborations. I must thank all those who made this work possible, in particular my marvellous wife, Francesca, who, as with all my undertakings, was the rock on which this is built. My hard-working agent Maggie Pearlstine provided the thoughtful guidance I have come to depend on, and she introduced me to the marvellous Brenda Kimber, my stalwart editor at Transworld, who, with the help of copy-editor Beth Humphries, sculpted my original manuscript into the shape you now hold. I am also grateful to Patrick Janson-Smith, who was the original inspiration for this book following a very informal discussion with him, and to Emma Dowson, my tennis doubles partner and PR manager at Transworld, who has never let me down either on or off the tennis court.

My thanks also to my secretary at the Maudsley Hospital, Sheila Banks, the paragon of efficiency who enables me to work part-time in the NHS and at the University and do other things as well. I am also supported ably by my team of community nurses, Asha Tait, Iqbal Surfaz, Pauline Laforge and Sandra Binney. I am particularly indebted to Professor Robin Murray, Dean George Szmuckler and Chief Executive Stewart Bell, the senior figures at the Institute of Psychiatry and the Maudsley Hospital whose support has made this large task possible.

But above all else I am indebted to all the discoverers of the case histories that appear in abridged form in this book; a list of their names follows, and I take this opportunity to record my grateful thanks for their permission for these cases to appear here.

Elsebet Steno Hansen, Tom G. Bolwig, Atsush Ichimura, Isao Nakajima, Hiroshi Juzoji, Richard O'Reilly, Ladi Malhotra, Anna Cantagallo, Luigi Grassi, Sergio Della Sala, Thomas N. Wise, Ram

Chandran Kalyanam, Nicholas Broughton, Paul Chesterman, James Briscoe, Alan Anderson, Jakob Camp, Christopher M. Filley, Frank J. Jarrett, R. D. Goldman, P. Schacter, M. Katz, R. Bilik, I. Avigad, Srikala Bharath, Mehendra Neupane, Somnath Chatterjee, Roger Byard, Phillip D. Jaffe, Frank DiCataldo, Paul Mullen, Brian Spitz, Jordi Serra-Mestres, Mary M. Robertson, Anne-Marie O'Dwyer, Isaac Marks, H. Tei, M. Iwata, Y. Miura, Elke Richartz, Henning Wormstall, Tamara L. Hartl, Randy O. Frost, N. Beecroft, L. Bach, N. Tunstall, R. Howard, S. Scheftel, Amy S. Nathan, Andrew M. Razin, Peter Mezan, M. L. Bourgeois, P. Duhamel, H. Verdoux, Dan J. Stein, Leon Le Roux, Colin Bouwer, Ben Van Heerden, E. Sobanski, M. H. Schmidt, Marjorie L. Hatch, C. S. Attila Kovács, T. H. Péter, Eliezer Witztum, Yuly Bersudsky, Hanoch Mayodovnik, Moshe Kotle, Claire Draucker, Padmal De Silva, Amanda Pernet, Kerry O. Ferris, Judy T. Okimura, Scott A. Norton, Dr J. Arturo Silva, Gregory B. Leong, Tara O'Reilly, William Hirstein, V. S. Ramachandran, S. Tucker Landrum, Thomas P. Cornwall, S. J. Kiraly, D. H. Ropschitz, Harvey A. Rosenstock, Kenneth R. Vincent, John E. Rhodes, Simon Jakes, Rachel Forsyth, Yair Bar-el, Glenn Catalano, Hakan Ay, Dr Lewis, Ferdinand Buonanno, Thomas Wenzel, J. Modestin, G. Ebner, Walter Everaerd, David Ames, Arnold Waugh, Robin Powell, Neil Boast, Edi-Osagie, J. Patrick, Marc Feldman, Charles Ford, Elke Richartz, Henning Workstall, Sharon Zeitlin, Martin Goldstein, Missagh Ghadirian, Baak Yücel, Robert Cavanaugh, Srikala Bharath, Marc L. Bourgeois, B. D. Kelly, Anthony Samuels, Albert Roberts, Sophia Dziegielewski, Adriana Neagoe, Raj Shiwach, John Prosser, Richard Bryant, Mary Seeman, Atul Pande, L. B. Raschka, Ratnin Dewaraja, Richard Caplan, Judith Komaromi, Mike Rhodes, Brian McGuire, George L. Choon, Parva Nayer, Julia Sanders, Jo Johnstone, Rhodri Huws, K. M. Beier, Michael Heap, Paula H. Salmons, David J. Clarke, Eric Schendel, Ronald-Frederick C. Kourany, T. R. Dening, A. West, Aaron Kulick, Kiran Rao, Thomas O'Reilly, Robin Dunbar, Richard Bentall, Daniel E. Jacome, A. Kelly Forrest, Yukio Uchinuma, Yoshio Sekine, Laura Weiss Roberts, Michael Hollifield, Teresita McCarty, Claire L. Templeman, S. Paige Hertweck, K. R. Nicholls, T. S. Ananthanarayanan, Marianne Regard, Theodor Landis, John Money, Russell Jobaris, Gregg Furth, D. L. Gordon, Irene Bates, Michael Prendergast Lampert, A. Ernst Van Woerkom, Thomas E. Joiner Jr, Natalie Sachs-Ericsson, A. R. Tomison, W. M. Donovan.

INTRODUCTION

It is a far, far better thing to have a firm anchor in nonsense than to put out on the troubled seas of thought.

J. K. Galbraith

In my experience, both inside and outside my consulting rooms, practically everyone suffers from one of two basic delusions, and quite frequently both. The first is the delusion that we are extraordinarily wonderful in some way and it is peculiar and puzzling to us that the rest of the world hasn't realized this and accorded us due respect. The second is that we are a much more frightful and depraved individual than anyone realizes and sooner or later we are going to be found out.

The latter delusion even has a name — Impostor Syndrome – and relates to the belief that in daily life we are merely masquerading impostors and our veneer of social acceptability will soon be penetrated. When this happens it is inevitable that everyone will finally understand just how truly terrible we are. It is only by some minor miracle that we have managed to hide the truth from the rest of the world for so long!

But if delusions are at the core of the modern psychiatric understanding of what differentiates the seriously mentally ill from the rest of us – and if, indeed, most of us harbour delusions – this strikes

1

at the heart of clinical practice and theory.

My reason for writing this book is to argue that delusions are more common than is generally supposed and they represent a vital key to understanding how the normal brain and mind work. However, the current scientific view is that delusions as observed in the clinical arena are nothing but the random outpourings of disturbed brain biochemistry and, therefore, should not be taken seriously, other than to establish which psychiatric diagnosis is warranted.

But what if delusions are more common than psychiatrists realize – indeed, suppose they are practically universal? What then differentiates those who end up receiving treatment from the rest of us becomes an even more subtle and fascinating question.

I wrote extensively about the mental-health benefits of positive illusions in my previous book, *Staying Sane: How to Make Your Mind Work for You*. In that work I focused on why it might be necessary to make the effort to see the positive in dire circumstances – even when this isn't an immediately natural thing to do. The worthwhile goal was to maintain your grip on sanity in the face of extreme provocation to lose it.

However, the argument in this book is an importantly different one. Here, instead, I want to discuss delusions that we tend to naturally hold, but don't realize that we do.

One reason for maintaining a delusion is that it might have surprisingly positive benefits. An example of a commonly held and even pragmatically useful delusion was recently uncovered by Dr Sandra Murray and psychologist colleagues at the State University of New York; it is a delusion that might lie at the heart of all successful long-running marriages.[1]

Dr Murray's research was an attempt to discover whether we stay with our spouses because we tend to perceive them in a more positive light than fits with strict reality. In other words, being relatively blind to our partners' faults and vices helps us to live with them and keeps marriages going for much longer than if we were more dispassionately aware of their faults.

In their research the psychologists compared what happily married spouses thought of each other with the opinions of very close friends and others who knew the couples well.

Few decisions have higher stakes than the decision to commit to one particular romantic partner and in perhaps no other context do we voluntarily tie the satisfaction of our hopes and goals to the good will of another. To feel happy and secure in the face of such vulnerability we need to believe that our relationship really is strong. We need to feel that our partner will always be caring and supportive, however tough life may get.

The psychologists in this research study argued that perhaps those of us involved in apparently satisfying, stable relationships resolve the tension between the doubts we experience and our desire for certainty and closure by seeing our partners in the best possible light; what underpins the successful long-running marriage is a largely delusionally positive perception of a partner. This theory was supported by much of the evidence that came to light during this and other studies.

Dr Murray concludes that we are happier in our relationships when we perceive virtues in our partners that are not necessarily apparent to others (or even to the partners themselves). The reason these delusions about partners are so common is that to be happy we need to believe we are in the right relationship with the right person, someone who will be there for us come what may. However, sustaining this belief with a partner who sometimes disappoints us seems to require a protective buffer, one that is afforded by the perception of special virtues in the partner. Once achieved, argues Dr Murray, this positive perceptual bias allows satisfied, secure intimates to dispel potential doubts or reservations almost in advance of their occurrence.

In other words, we need to be delusion-prone when it comes to our views about our partner for a marriage to work and give us satisfaction. This is an example of how delusions seem to serve a positive function. But delusions are not always so obviously helpful.

This book is a collection of accounts of the most extraordinary states of mind it is possible for human beings to experience. Newspaper and magazine cartoons depicting the mentally ill in a humorous fashion often use caricatures to portray psychosis. The patient is usually shown as someone who believes himself to be Napoleon, complete with Napoleonic hat and arm tucked into jacket, and it is easy to see how one might consider this person to be mentally ill. But what of the patient's wondrous thoughts and experiences? What if these same experiences could be shared, or viewed from the psychotic's perspective? Then delusions such as this might not seem quite so ridiculous.

The link between insanity and grandeur is rendered even closer and more complex by the increasing realization that many famous figures like Napoleon were probably suffering from psychological disturbance. Similarly, some psychotic patients believe they are the Messiah, but it is worth remembering that in ancient times religious prophets actually did suffer from some form of psychosis. The Hebrew word *nabi* means both insanity and those carried away by religious visions, and while the prophets Amos and Jeremiah were then deemed 'insane', the prophet Ezekiel could very easily be diagnosed today as a paranoid schizophrenic.

Indeed, many will assume that in this book I am at last ready to give my account of all those producers, presenters and editors I have encountered in my disturbing journey through the media. That, I am afraid, will have to await another project.

In fact, most of my time is spent working in the obscure conditions of the National Health Service at the Maudsley Hospital in south London, where I wrestle each day with the kind of mental health problems that are presented here. Among the inspirations that motivated me to write this book were accounts by therapists who work entirely in private practice, whose case histories are popularly presented in book form and widely read. These collections of cases of middle-class angst bear so little resemblance to the kind of problems our patients suffer from, that my colleagues at the Maudsley pressed me with increasing urgency to set the record straight about what psychiatry and psychology 'on the front line' is actually about.

The problem has been that public debate about psychiatry is informed by a distorted view of what really goes on in our clinics, because, understandably, our work remains strictly confidential. But given the right safeguards, this does not mean psychiatry and clinical psychology should remain so unknown as to leave a huge vacuum in the public understanding of vital mental health issues.

The reader who is not clinically trained may find these descriptions difficult to give credence to. Yet all have been drawn from reports by doctors who have encountered at first hand the people who experienced these states. In the acknowledgements section I list in detail all my physician colleagues from around the world who have kindly granted me permission to analyse their reports and bring them to a wider audience, beyond the specialized medical and psychological community where they tend to remain.

4

But this raises the natural question of whether chronicles of people suffering from such extreme psychological problems should be brought to a general readership at all. They could remain within the more obscure domain of the academic community from where they originated. Some tendentious critics on a cursory inspection might even level the accusation that this publication is merely a 'freak show', produced with no higher ambition than to titillate and astound.

Obviously there is an immediate issue of patient confidentiality: all the names plus other identifying characteristics of the people within these pages have been changed to protect their privacy. I have also only considered cases for this book that have already been subject to peer review, in that other colleagues have vetted and checked the facts of each illustration, and have agreed that publication does not damage the patient.

Although I have looked after many patients with conditions similar to those described in this book, it must be emphasized that none of the patients mentioned here are mine. To ask my patients to consent to appear in this work would compromise the doctor–patient relationship. I have always worked hard to try to ensure that my patients feel my commitment to their personal care is never threatened by projects I am involved in outside the clinic. Such a large collection of case material could raise the question in a patient's mind of whether I would at some point wish to include them in a similar project. I do not want my patients ever to be troubled by that.

This does not mean that I necessarily condemn other clinicians for publishing their own series of case histories. After all, perhaps the most famous doctor of recent centuries, Sigmund Freud,[2] established his reputation not by research with double-blind randomly assigned clinical trials, but with case reports. His analysis of these had a profound impact on medicine, and indeed culture, which larger sample research still struggles to rival.

The real problem in relation to Freud is that one wonders whether his own developing theories began to overly bias what he looked for, and what he saw, when he was with his own patients. The fact that the theoretician and the person looking for evidence to test the theories were one and the same person, interviewing clients with no-one else to easily check with, became a problematic project in terms of persuading sceptics. This led to much effort being invested in tracking down his original patients so that they could be reinterviewed in attempts to corroborate Freud's reports. It seemed to me one way of avoiding this conundrum was to rely on case reports from other clinicians, particularly doctors from very different parts of the world with contrasting theoretical orientations. For if such disparate groups describe clinical phenomena that begin to converge towards support for certain ideas in brain and mind science, then no-one could suspect the material of originating in a biased concept.

I have stuck religiously to cases already reported in respectable medical journals that follow a strict ethical policy involving case reports. Their policy means the individuals concerned who are written about have themselves read the reports prior to submission and have offered no objection to their publication, following a full discussion of the implications of publication with respect to confidentiality. All the cases assembled here were already in the public domain, but they were scattered across the thousands of academic medical and scientific journals that currently exist.

Those outside the field would be surprised at how generous patients are in giving up their time to assist with medical research in the hope that their own case will help improve doctors' understanding and benefit future patients. It is in this spirit that those who populate this book consented to have their predicaments described.

Case histories remain an important part of medical communication about attempts to understand the human brain and mind because it is only through contact with real life cases that actuality can be properly debated. Psychology and psychiatry are often burdened with a huge amount of theory that can easily divorce these disciplines from the realities they are supposed to explain. All of the phenomenal cases in this book throw down a direct challenge to our current knowledge of human nature.

It is important that the public become aware of the kind of examples in this book. It is precisely these exemplars from which theories are derived. It is the most extreme and unusual states of mind that offer the strongest provocation to our thinking about brain and mind, and these are often indirectly the biggest help in understanding ourselves.

The vast majority of cases reported here, on receiving skilled psychiatric help, made full recoveries, so this book attempts to show that the pessimism over prognosis in psychiatry is unwarranted. The key point is that if these extraordinary experiences and behaviours are amenable to treatment, and even cure, then the stigma surrounding psychological disturbance can be effectively challenged.

The taboo surrounding mental illness is gradually breaking down, as evidenced by the media's growing interest in this area. Consequently there has been a huge explosion of publications attempting to explain the mind and brain to a wider audience, but none dared to include explicit accounts of real human behaviour such as will be found here. This I believe has been their great weakness, because any theory, no matter how refined, must always be tested against the actual world, and the people within these pages show us an incredible reality that few realize exists. Yet because the public is unaware that such extraordinary people live and breathe, they remain unable to properly judge psychiatry and psychology, and what these disciplines are attempting to do. Much of psychological and psychiatric explanation often seems strange to outsiders, as a vital part of the picture – the cases on which the theories are based and tested – usually remains hidden.

But another reason for bringing these cases together in the most comprehensive collection that has ever been attempted in the history of psychiatry is that within the academic community the detailed case report has been falling out of fashion.

I am keen to revive the art.

THE FIGHT AGAINST REDUCTIONISM

Recently there has been a tendency to see medical advances as based mainly on studies where such large numbers of patients are incorporated into the research that complex statistics have to be employed to glean findings. In this kind of work the person is reduced to a subject, and then a mere number, and vital individual variability is lost from view. Psychiatry, ever desperate to gain prestige by hanging on for grim death to the coat tails of medicine, has blindly followed this trend. Before considering a research submission, academic journal editors appear to be interested only in the number of subjects one has recruited for the trial, and the more the better. The publication of individual detailed case reports is gradually dying out in academic psychiatry.

This I believe is a fundamental error, and is due to a basic misapprehension amongst doctors of the vital difference between the mind and the body. It is true that when a physician encounters patients with something wrong with their kidneys, the difference in basic biology between clients with the same renal disorder is usually negligible. However, the contrast between people with the same psychiatric diagnosis is often huge, due to differences in, amongst other areas, background and personality.

Another problem is that the current domination of reductionism in psychiatry means we don't talk about whole people any more when we try to understand them: instead we break them down into receptors or defence mechanisms. The properly detailed case report puts the correct object of study back into the frame – the whole person.

To me, the attraction of psychiatry and psychology as a choice of career was always that these disciplines were supposed to confront the most consequential issues in life, like what our response could or should be to catastrophe and despair, or what reality is, given that it appears so easy to lose one's grip on it. Yet when I arrived in the field it seemed the academics were elegantly waltzing around the difficult issues, instead embracing anything that might produce a publishable though irrelevant result. There is currently an obsession with the measurable and with data, so that the vital controversies are not even addressed by our current reductionist approaches.

As a result of my strong opposition to reductionism I went about studying a wide variety of subjects at university level, including the history of medicine, statistics and economics. It was probably due to my paying too much attention to Sociology of Law at University College London, plus Life Drawing at the adjoining Slade School of Art, that I came to fail anatomy in my first year at medical school . . . so the reductionists had the last laugh. In order to pass medical finals and the rigorous postgraduate exams required to become a Member of the Royal College of Psychiatrists, I had to feign a belief in reductionism for a long while.

According to hard-core scientific reductionists everything that happens, including mental events, only occurs as a result of the interaction of the four forces currently recognized by physics to exist – strong and weak nuclear forces, gravity and electromagnetism. Reductionists would logically have us all ultimately become physicists in order to help our patients and make discoveries about the mind. We should not be too hasty to abandon reductionism because it did give us the Human Genome and space travel, amongst many other modern wonders. But its current hold on science means that all explanation has to be attempted in terms of ever more minute entities. Yet the major methodological triumph of recent years has been the demonstration that the unit of classical heredity, the gene, is a macromolecule.

The first reductionist thinker and the first Western philosopher was Thales, a Greek born around 636 BC in Turkey. Although his reductionism led to some real howlers – such as his belief that water was the fundamental substance of which all matter was constituted – he also successfully predicted there would be an eclipse of the sun in 585 BC. This is arguably the first example of successful prediction based on scientific principles – though some claim it was just a lucky guess. How little has changed over the millennia . . .[3]

The trouble is that as all reduction is about simplification, there is always the risk of oversimplification. Sometimes, by reducing something we are merely eliminating it from our description of the world: if a mental state is explained simply as a combination of neurotransmitter actions, have we removed the personal sensations involved in that experience, by dropping down to the level of molecules?

It was Thales who first conceived the principle of explaining a multitude of phenomena by a small number of hypotheses. For example, he apparently explained earthquakes on the basis of his mistaken belief that the Earth floats on water. But the real importance of Thales' idea is that he is the first recorded person who tried to explain such phenomena by rational rather than by supernatural means. This can be seen as the very first attempt to establish laws of nature – something that scientists are still trying to do today.

Plato tells us that one night Thales was gazing at the sky as he walked, and so fell into a ditch. A pretty servant girl lifted him out and said, 'How do you expect to understand what is going on up in the sky if you do not even see what is at your feet?' Perhaps this is the first absent-minded professor joke in the West!

What I find inspiring about Thales is the scale of his ambition given how few resources he had compared to us today, and this continues to encourage me whenever a colleague gets a big research grant and I don't. But his struggles raise the issue of whether the attempt to come up with laws in psychology and psychiatry is fundamentally misguided. Unlike the remainder of the natural world, our subject matter – human minds – constantly changes in essence. The kind of person born today possesses a mind very different from someone alive just a hundred years ago, so laws of behaviour or mind are likely to be merely transient and constantly need revising or updating. Perhaps the first and only law of human behaviour is that there is no fixed human nature.

It is vital, I believe, in any attempt to scientifically understand the human condition, to study whole individuals, and especially their experiences, in depth. In writing this book I hope to revive the art of the in-depth case report by showing my colleagues how much can be learned from them. In particular I should like this work to be useful to junior doctors and to training psychiatrists who are attempting to recognize conditions they read about as a cluster of symptoms in textbooks. Junior psychiatrists struggle in preparation for their exams because they usually do not have ready access to the exceptional case studies on which so much dry theory is based.

This book is not a comprehensive account of the range of psychiatric cases. I have consciously omitted the body of cases which would come under the remit of forensic psychiatry – in other words those people whose behaviour involves violence or threat to others. Although there is a need for a book that includes such cases, I decided to leave that for a later project. Instead I was anxious to ensure that my readers understood that the vast majority of mental health problems do not involve aggression to others – an unfortunately stigmatizing misconception that the popular press has in part been responsible for fostering.

Finally I didn't want fear of the people who populate these pages to obscure a proper appreciation of what it must be like for them to go through what they have.

Many, on reading about the extraordinary delusions I have collected here, will wonder how any of this applies to them. Indeed many have already commented on how these bizarre stories have helped them to feel more normal. What I hope will emerge is how at the core of all convictions is a breakdown of the healthy mechanism of doubt. Doubt drives the collection of evidence and internal debate before we arrive at conclusions. Yet we need to suspend doubt when the time comes for us to act, otherwise we would be impeded by indecision. In fact the study of delusion leads to more questions about how we come to think logically and apparently correctly most of the time, rather than why we are occasionally prone to delusion. Asking this question leads to the surprising conclusion that delusions are more an established part of our mental life than we might realize. So might delusions serve some function?

10

WHY OUR TROUBLES ARE CAUSED BY OUR DELUSIONS

One major consequence of our tendency to reason in ways suscepti-
ble to delusional errors is that we are rather prone to come into
conflict with each other. It seems that politicians and generals
involved in fighting wars might be destined by evolutionary biology
to make the kind of delusional mistakes that appear to be the
inevitable consequence of war. This is the startling conclusion of the
study of the long history of battles in human and animal societies.
We seem to be the only species which battles with its own kind, with
the possible exception of ants, a battle being defined as aggression
where both sides willingly go to war rather than use other options,
like withdrawing. Although we like to think of nature as 'red in
tooth and claw' in fact there is relatively little violent conflict
between animals of the same species. Instead there is much more
threat display, during which animals decide whether it is in their
interest to take on the adversary, with one opponent usually opting
to withdraw in the face of evidence that they are unlikely to win a
fight.[4,5]

Animals use their weapons more often for ritualized contests
within species than for inflicting real damage on their own kind.[6] For
example, deer use their antlers to interlock in a pushing contest
where victory goes to the larger, stronger and healthier individual,
but the structure of antlers and the behaviour of contestants are
adapted to prevent serious injury to the other animal.[7]

Since it appears there is evolutionary pressure for animals to
assess accurately when it is not worth fighting, and these rituals help
determine this, why do humans so frequently go to war when any
rational assessment should indicate a low probability of victory, or
little advantage to fighting? Inaccurate prior assessment of the
enemy results in more damage and lower chances of future survival
than if a judicious withdrawal had been selected.[8]

Most wars start between two parties who are unequal, or where
the final result of losing for one side could have been anticipated
long before the bitter end.[9] The losing side, by continuing to fight,
sustains much more damage than if it had dispassionately assessed
the likelihood of victory from the time it first began to lose.[10] While
anthropologists have found that 95 per cent of primitive human
societies regularly engage in war, battle is almost unknown in the
rest of nature. Most animals are acutely sensitive to any initial
asymmetry between contestants before a fight begins, and will

usually rapidly concede to the animal displaying any advantage.

Raids, in the form of a surprise attack by one side on another, which thus has no choice to avoid the conflict, are also rare in nature, but much more common than battles. Interestingly, the only other mammals besides ourselves which raid are our closest genetic relatives, chimpanzees. Within 21 primitive human societies recently studied, raids accounted for 0.5 per cent of deaths each year – equivalent to more than a billion war deaths if raiding occurred at similar rates in the twentieth century world-wide – and in raiding cultures up to 30 per cent of male deaths occur because of violence.[11] This high level of mortality in our primitive past means raiding must have played a vital role in determining who passed on their genes to the next generation.

Raiding occurs only when one side appraises its enemy as likely to suffer more from a surprise attack.[12] There must be an evolutionary pressure to get this assessment right, otherwise raiding would be of little benefit. The likelihood is that raiding evolved in the common ancestor we share with chimpanzees,[13] which means it has been subject to continuous selection in our ancestors and us for 5–6 million years, which must mean, some anthropologists argue, that our brains are evolved to raid. The cerebral lobes must be genetically designed to impose violence on vulnerable neighbours and to assess accurately the outcome of an attack before we plan one.[14]

Battles, on the other hand – where both sides willingly go to war and believe they are going to win, no matter what a dispassionate assessment might suggest – have no known analogy in chimpanzees or other primates.[15] Indeed, chimpanzees are observed to be hugely influenced in their decision to raid by whether they have a numerical advantage over the enemy.[16] The fact that battles are so specific to our species suggests there may be some evolutionary reason, linked to a proneness of the brains on both sides to believe each is going to win, no matter how unlikely victory might be.[17]

One possible explanation is linked to the prevalence of deception in war. Deception is associated with war from the Greek legend of the Trojan horse,[18] to the modern examples of Normandy in 1944 where the Germans were deceived as to where the D-Day landing would take place. Sun Tzu declared 'all warfare is based on deception' and Churchill is reported to have said that 'in time of war, the truth is so precious it must be attended by a bodyguard of lies'. Victory in human fights, unlike nature in general, is often linked not simply to superior resources, but to ingenuity in fooling the enemy.[19]

Indeed many evolutionary biologists now argue that the whole reason why intelligence evolved in humans was more to assist us in deceiving each other, and to detect deception, than for any real practical benefit for solving physical problems. This is based on observations of great apes[20] and bushmen, who seem to spend much more time using their brain power to manipulate each other rather than the environment.[21]

But might there come a point, in the continuing evolution of our improved ability to mislead others, when we get so good at deception that we start to deceive ourselves?[22]

The anthropological argument is that a tendency towards self-deception has been wired into our brains by evolution so that we tend to overestimate our own abilities, while we underestimate and belittle the strengths and capacities of our opponents. This probably carries an evolutionary advantage: favouring your own side enhances the cohesiveness and cooperation of our group; and believing you are going to win, no matter the odds, has been shown experimentally to divert attention from anxiety, pain and fatigue when in competition – it enhances performance.[23]

Positive self-illusions may also be good for your mental health.[24] The clinically depressed are more accurate in their assessment of their abilities than the non-depressed, who suffer from an overconfidence bias. These illusions may be helpful because they reduce internal conflicts within both the person and the group.[25] A side that is dithering and divided will prove more vulnerable than one united in the conviction they are better than anyone else.[26] The other benefit of deceiving yourself that you will win a battle is that you might also mislead the enemy, whose assessment of you could determine whether they bother to fight. Bluffing that you are superior might secure a cheap victory.[27]

Bluffing certainly seems common in nature. Many animals as part of their threat display pretend to be bigger than they are: dogs raise their neck hair, lions use their manes, fish raise fins and birds fluff out their feathers.[28] The difference between humans and animals is that the rest of nature does not usually have the mental capacity to dwell on the issue of whether they are being deceived by a threat display, to consider a counter-deception in turn. Responses to threats are usually acted on more rapidly and often with the judicious aim of living to fight another day.[29]

But once the capacity to consider the possibility of deception in your enemy evolves, this creates an arms race in which each opponent attempts to bluff the other. The self-deception involved in really believing you are superior, when you might not be, assists in the achievement of a successful bluff. Evolutionarily, it appears that those suffering from positive self-deceptions succeed sufficiently often for it to pay to suffer from such illusions.[30]

If our brains are designed by our violent evolutionary past to be prone to battle, this suggests peacemakers need to emphasize (particularly to the side most likely to lose but still bent on fighting) the personal advantages of peace. Our tendency to assume the other side's insistence on continuing to fight, despite impossible odds, is down to their fanaticism, stupidity or mental instability prevents us from understanding how to produce peace.[31,32]

At a time like this disaster can best be avoided if those taking the ultimate decisions are advised by people not psychologically committed to the outcome.[33] Unfortunately, as hostilities escalate, it becomes dangerous for anyone close to the leaders to disagree with the rising excitement at the prospect of a battle.[34] If the theoretically uncommitted advise that battle may not be wise, they risk being treated as hostile agents by our battle-hardened brains.[35]

So one possibility as to why we are prone to delusion is that it served an evolutionary benefit by helping us to intimidate others by falsely but successfully promoting ourselves.[36]

You don't have to be mad to work here but it helps

Perhaps there are other advantages to psychosis or deranged thinking. Researchers have suggested that there might be an association between psychotic traits and creativity. The idea of a continuum between psychotic traits and normal functioning may help resolve one of the most puzzling aspects of psychosis, namely the persistence of psychotic traits within populations over many generations.[37] Studies of clinical communities indicate that psychosis has grim implications for survival and reproduction. Patients often have difficulty maintaining employment, are frequently impoverished, often socially isolated, face a high risk of early death from suicide, and enjoy less reproductive success than normal individuals.

Unless these social and reproductive disadvantages of psychosis are balanced by advantages, genes that confer vulnerability to psychiatric disorder should theoretically never get passed on to successive generations.

Some argue that the behaviour associated with psychosis might in itself confer advantages. Perhaps the genes for paranoia encourage a healthy defensiveness in threatening environments; and maybe schizophrenia genes, with their tendency to social isolation, facilitate the splitting of over-large groups in primitive societies. These hypotheses are highly speculative and the only substantial research exploring the possible benefits of madness has focused on creativity.

Associations between madness and creative genius have been noted by observers from ancient Greek times. This has been fostered partly by a notion of creativity as involving divine intervention or diktat, i.e. some kind of mystical, mysterious and inchoate eruption from the sea of unconsciousness from which madness was also, popularly, thought to emerge. More recently the famous late Professor of Psychology at the Maudsley Hospital, Hans Eysenck, proposed that intellectual characteristics associated with psychotic thinking tends to facilitate originality and creativity.[38]

Biographical studies designed to discover the extent to which historically important creative individuals have experienced psychotic or related disorders, have been one of the most popular tests of the association between creativity and psychopathology. These studies have generally demonstrated a closer relationship between creative achievement and mood disorders as opposed to creative achievement and schizophrenia. One study of 47 British writers and artists found that 38 per cent had been treated for mood disorders.[39] A 1995 survey of 1,004 people judged to be influential in the twentieth century observed high rates of alcoholism, schizophrenia and mood disorders.[40] A 1996 investigation of 291 eminent British and American achievers found that episodic psychiatric conditions had occurred in the majority, although mood disorders were more evident than psychosis. This study also found that the majority of those studied had close relatives with a history of severe psychiatric conditions, which included mood disorder and psychosis.[41]

A 1987 study of members of the University of Iowa's writers' workshop and their families found a very high rate of mood disorder compared with controls.[42] A 1993 investigation of award-winning European writers, poets, painters, sculptors and blues musicians found that approximately half had suffered from a major depressive episode, and that nearly two-thirds exhibited recurrent severe mood swing tendencies.[43]

Taking a different approach, some researchers have attempted to find evidence of abnormal creativity in psychiatric patients and their relatives. These studies have demonstrated an association between creativity and both schizophrenia and mood disorder. A comparison of schizophrenic patients with psychiatric and normal controls on several measures of creativity found that the non-paranoid schizophrenic patients scored higher than the other groups in an 'unusual uses' test which required participants to think of novel uses for familiar objects.[44] Also an examination of the occupational status of relatives of schizophrenia patients admitted to hospital in Iceland between 1851 and 1940, using available records to enable a comparison with the general population, showed that the closest relatives of the patients significantly entered creative occupations more often.[45]

The evolutionary hypothesis linking madness to creativity implies that the benefit from psychosis genes will be felt most by those who have the genes but do not become overtly psychotic. For this reason, studies of the relationship between a spectrum of psychotic traits and creativity are likely to be especially revealing. In other words the key point might be that it is those who lie a little further away from the spectrum of psychosis than the extreme of the frankly clinically ill who might receive some benefit from their position. It may be that the severely mentally unwell are individuals in whom a group of psychosis genes have come together which normally are more thinly spread in the population. In too high a concentration these genes are not good for you, but in smaller doses they could be beneficial in loosening your thinking so you come up with ideas the rest of us could never conceive.

There are many different pathways that might link psychosis with different measures of creativity. For example frank psychotic symptoms may be provoked by the frustrations involved when people with creative ambitions have those ambitions thwarted.

As we shall see, there are many roads to delusion – almost as many as the individuals involved – which means that coming up with theories to explain delusions is one of the most challenging tasks of science.

To the actors in these stories their conviction was so great that they persistently ignored the disbelief of all those around them, despite the fact that peer pressure and the influence of others are usually so powerful in human affairs. Amidst the tragedy produced by these disordered ideas, there is still something awe-inspiring about this. How many of us can claim to be driven by beliefs that rise above the mundane and the agreeable?

We still don't know where delusions come from, but certainly one possible reason, as you will see, for sticking to your delusion is that if the belief is so engaging or absorbing, it is worth it.

In other words if you are going to suffer from a delusion, you might as well make it a grand one.

1

WEREWOLVES, VAMPIRES AND WITCHES: WHEN THE PAST COMES BACK TO HAUNT US

There is also, concerning witches who copulate with devils, much difficulty in considering the methods by which such abominations are consummated . . . the Inquisitor of Como in the County of Burbia, who in the space of one year, which was the year of grace 1485, caused forty-one witches to be burned; who all publicly affirmed, as it is said, that they had practised these abominations with devils.

Malleus Maleficarum, 1486

THE WEREWOLF DELUSION

Today werewolves might seem merely the stuff of legend and awful Hollywood films but there have been at least 24 separate cases described in the medical literature in the past 20 years. The experience of being changed into a wolf or other animal is referred to within psychiatry as lycanthropy and the accompanying sensations as lycanthropic feelings.

Carl Gustav Jung, the Swiss psychiatrist, a close associate of Freud's, described in 1928 a woman who later 'became insane and would exhibit a sort of lycanthropy in which she crawled on all fours and imitated the grunting of pigs, the barking of dogs and the growling of bears'. Another psychiatrist of this time described a girl with schizophrenia who bought a dog and decided to imitate it in order to know how to act.[1]

In one of the most famous recent research studies on modern werewolves, collected by a group of Harvard psychiatrists, six patients apparently believed themselves to be, or acted like, wolves or dogs; two believed themselves to be cats; one patient believed himself to be a gerbil (he had raised gerbils as a hobby for six years) and one a bird. In the other two cases in this series the psychiatrists decided the werewolf beliefs were in fact consciously manufactured, under voluntary control, and basically a pretence, in order for the patient to gain some conscious or unconscious personal advantage. The werewolf 'delusion' in these two cases rapidly disappeared following confrontation over their theatrical nature by the medical staff.[2]

The history of medical reports of lycanthropy shows that these mostly responded well to anti-psychotic medication. This leads most psychiatrists to conclude that, although curious and colourful, the delusion of being transformed into an animal actually bodes no more ill than any other psychiatric delusion. This view is controversial, as even in the small number of cases described by doctors there are a few where extreme danger to others was an associated outcome – though again it must be emphasized that the vast majority of cases of mental illness are not linked with violence.[3]

A review of werewolf cases reported in the medical literature concludes that the following psychiatric diagnoses are the most likely underlying causes: (1) schizophrenia, (2) biological organic brain lesion with psychosis, (3) psychotic depressive reaction, (4) hysterical neurosis, (5) manic-depressive psychosis, and (6) epilepsy. Certainly the conclusion must be that while lycanthropy is a rare phenomenon, it does exist. It should be regarded as a symptom cluster and not a diagnosis in itself – rather as anaemia is not a diagnosis but a pointer that something pathological is occurring in the body. So the term 'lycanthropy' probably obscures more than it reveals. Although it may generally be an expression of an underlying schizophrenic condition, at least five other differential diagnostic entities must be considered.[4]

But it cannot be understood purely as a medical diagnosis, for delusions of being a wolf or some other feared animal are universal and, although rare in the industrialized countries, still occur in

China, India, Africa, and Central and South America. The animals in the delusional transformation include leopards, lions, elephants, crocodiles, sharks, buffaloes, eagles and serpents.[5]

Not infrequently, bizarre and chaotic sexuality is expressed in a primitive way through lycanthropic symptoms. Patients whose internal fears exceed their coping capabilities may externalize them via projection and constitute a serious threat to others. So the aggressive behaviour of someone who considers himself a wolf is really about internal hostility projected on the outside world. Whatever the final conclusion about their particular behaviour, throughout the ages such individuals have been feared because of their tendency to commit bestial acts and have therefore been hunted and killed by the community. Many of these individuals were probably paranoid schizophrenics.[6]

Lycanthropy's history stretches back to classical times, but it is uncommon in the present era. It attracted attention from several nineteenth-century psychiatrists but these also commented on the scarcity of the symptom, suggesting that social trends were the cause of this change. In particular, epidemics of lycanthropy, possibly a form of collective hysteria, had become rare, leaving only sporadic cases.[7]

In medieval Europe the wolf was the most abhorred and dreaded natural enemy, a sly opponent who would be the consummate accomplice for the Devil or his demons. Hence the wolf became an embodiment of the community's worse apprehensions, and it was widely believed that the Devil could make a person behave like a wolf.[8]

In 1765 Denis Diderot and Jean d'Alembert, in the famous *Encyclopédie*, distinguished two kinds of werewolf:[9]

1   'Those whom the devil covers with a wolf's skin and are made to ramble aimlessly in the cities and in the country, howling and causing havoc.'
2   'This half savage sect of men, who think they have become a wolf after a disease and consequently, imitate all their actions . . . a sort of melancholia in which humans believe they have been transformed into a wolf . . .'

So while transformation into a wolf constitutes one of the most ancient and universal beliefs, for quite a long time in history it was associated with mental illness. Today the belief or sensation that you are being transformed into a wolf or other animal would be seen as a symptom of psychosis – the form of mental disorder characterized by delusions and hallucinations.[10]

The medieval counterpart for much of the strange behaviour we class today as psychiatric disorder would come under the rubric of witchcraft, and the fear of strange behaviour led to the publication of *Malleus Maleficarum*, or 'The Witches' Hammer', an infamous fifteenth-century manual for 'diagnosing' (in fact persecuting) witchcraft. It was this book's advice and exhortation that led to the burning of several hundred thousand people accused of witchcraft during the Middle Ages. The monks who wrote this book believed that a physical body could not be transformed, but that evil charms or spirits could create a delusion so that a person could appear to himself or others as a wolf. So the emphasis in this ancient text was on a shift in perception rather than in actual shape. Oddly enough, as we shall see, this parallels the modern debate on what is really going on in those who believe themselves to be transformed into a wolf.[11]

Dr Paul Keck[12] and colleagues from Harvard Medical School conducted a review of all psychiatric cases admitted to a 250-bed teaching hospital over 12 years in suburban Boston, and from a baseline of over 5,000 psychotic patients uncovered 12 cases of lycanthropy. Meanwhile in the 1980s a French psychiatrist, Dr Michael Benzech,[13] conducted a survey of 320 psychiatrists working in the south-western public hospitals of France and found amongst their patients two cases of wolf delusions, plus three other cases of pathological animal behaviour.

The widespread belief in werewolves across the world in times past contrasts with the rarity of its reports in the modern West. Yet the belief of human transformation into animal form is common to the folklore of most cultures. For example the Malaysians believed that the ghosts of deceased soothsayers entered the bodies of tigers, and the Maori are convinced the souls of the betrayed dead enter the bodies of lizards to exact revenge.[14]

Since the werewolf syndrome may be the first account of mental illness we have in recorded history, it becomes a more important phenomenon than its current prevalence in modern urban society might suggest.

In perhaps one of the earliest recorded examples of mental illness, the biblical Book of Daniel records that the Babylonian King Nebuchadnezzar (605–562 BC) was transformed into an ox for seven years as divine punishment and that he was '... banished from the society of men and ate grass like oxen; his body was drenched by the dew of heaven until his hair grew long like goat's hair and his nails like eagle's talons' (Daniel 4: 33). Eventually God took pity and restored him to human form. This is the very first case report of lycanthropy.[15]

Because it remains an obscure area of psychology, confusion surrounds the term 'lycanthropy'. Does it specifically refer to the delusion of transformation into a wolf, or will any animal do? The belief in personal transformation into other animals has been reported even in modern times and includes gerbils, birds, rabbits and pussy cats (as we shall see later). Technically some specialists use the term 'therianthropy' or 'shape-shifting' to refer to changing into any sort of animal, but lycanthropy is now generally used in the literature. 'Therianthropy' is regarded now as rather old-fashioned.[16]

Separated from the case of King Nebuchadnezzar by a gap of around 2,500 years, psychiatrists Dening and West while working at St Crispin Hospital in Northampton recently reported the following strange case. This is the case of a 43-year-old housewife married to a gamekeeper, who was referred to the psychiatric services as an emergency after 18 hours of increasingly agitated and bizarre behaviour.[17]

The woman who changed into several different animals

The general practitioner rang the psychiatrists from the patient's house. Over the telephone the patient could be heard shouting and screaming until eventually an assault on the GP by the patient was heard by the duty psychiatrists.

The woman had a turbulent family background, being the 13th of 16 children, and when she was a teenager both parents died in quick succession, as the result of serious illnesses. She left school at 15 to look after her younger siblings but between the ages of 13 and 20 she was sexually abused by two of her brothers, though full intercourse did not take place.

At the time, as is surprisingly common in incest victims, she believed this activity to be normal and she currently denies that it caused her problems in later life. At 21 she met her future husband, and married two years later. Prior to having her two children she worked in a shop, and later as a cleaner. She was described as being jolly and outgoing before she became unwell, although perhaps

22

predisposed to bodily preoccupations, which might be of significance given what later transpired.

Depressed for three months after the birth of her second child, who was now aged six, she was weepy, unable to leave the house and suffered anxiety symptoms such as palpitations when alone, but she did not seek help, and her anxiety spontaneously improved. Six days before her admission to hospital, she had developed chicken-pox, with a typical rash. She did not become acutely ill, and the rash dried up and began to resolve. But at 1 a.m. on the day of her eventual admission she awoke saying she was unable to sleep and that she was seeing things on the walls. As the night wore on she became more distressed, saying that she thought she was going to die. Her husband took her to the local hospital casualty department, where she was found to be very anxious but no serious physical abnormality was noted.

She was given a small dose of a sedative and sent home. Her doc-tor telephoned to check on her and found her to be anxious but coherent and co-operative. Later she became much more disturbed, and the doctor was called to the house that evening.

She was found with her face buried in a cushion, howling for periods of several minutes at a time. In between she was more settled, then would get more distressed and start shouting. 'You're doing it again, you're making me angry . . . I've got to get angry,' before starting further howling and screaming.

She would not answer questions rationally. Over the next hour she became progressively more aggressive, hissing and clawing at the air and at those in the room. She would not allow anyone to leave the room. The GP gave her an intramuscular injection of anti-psychotic medication, after which she was a little more calm.

When seen by the psychiatrist, she was still moaning and shriek-ing into the cushion. She complained that the attention being given to her was making her more and more angry. She then stated that she was a dog and began barking for a time. This was followed by a period of being very hostile, hissing and spitting. Although she was very distressed and abusive, and therefore did not co-operate at an interview, there was no evidence that her conscious awareness of what was going on around her was impaired at this or any other stage. The fact that these symptoms were occurring in a state of clear consciousness would tend to rule out the possibility of an acute bio-logical cause, such as intoxication with alcohol or illicit drugs.

She was compulsorily admitted to a secure ward for observation.

On admission to hospital she was restless, muttering with her eyes closed. She said she was seeing the Devil, and mentioned his horns and tail. She would claw at the air, grimace and become irritable when attempts were made by the staff to question her in order to assess her condition.

She remained disturbed and uncooperative for the next two to three days, during which time she refused food, and often fluids too. She was treated with antipsychotic medication, and gradually improved sufficiently for transfer to an open ward.

At this stage it became possible to obtain an account of her experiences. She had been feeling low in mood for about three months, had initial insomnia and lost some weight. Her concentration was poor but she had no suicidal thoughts.

Her recollection of the day of admission was clear and she remembered feeling progressively more anxious, fearful and irritable. Early that morning she saw snakes coming out of the walls, but there were no lycanthropic experiences until the evening.

Later, as she was howling, she began to believe that she was a dog. So far as could be ascertained, the howling preceded the belief, not vice versa: the delusion appeared to arise secondary to the exhibited behaviour. She continued as a dog for between 30 minutes and an hour. She then became calmer for a similar length of time, during which she experienced hallucinatory voices of absent members of her family talking to her. The voices made encouraging comments to her; at times they sounded like her brothers and sisters during their childhood.

During this relative lull, she again began to become more worked up and angry. Eventually she felt herself turning into a cat, and hissed and spat at those in the room. At this point the psychiatrist was present and it appeared to him then that she was behaving like a snake, though this was not in fact the case, as she later recounted.

The period of being a cat lasted a few minutes and was again followed by relative calm, during which she had further auditory hallucinations. Again she gradually became more agitated, and started to stamp her feet and kick out at people. This behaviour was accompanied by the conviction that she was a horse. A short while later she calmed down for 30 minutes or so, but once more became disturbed. She now found herself snarling and curling her lips back as if she had fangs. She believed that her hands had changed into wolf's claws, and that she had become a wolf. When she looked at her hands, they appeared to her like real claws. It is not clear how long this stage lasted but there do not appear to have been any lycanthropic experiences after her removal to hospital.

During the evening it also appeared to her that her husband was the Devil, but when this occurred in relation to the sequence of events was unclear. After transfer to an open ward, recovery was rapid. One week later she was normal, apart from possibly some suspicious ideas about other patients. Ten days after admission she was her normal self: there were no features to suggest psychosis, and she did not appear depressed either. She was eventually discharged to outpatient follow-up on a small dose of antipsychotic medication.

A feature of this case, and some others in the literature, is an associated visual perceptual disorder, where subjects see part of themselves or their reflections as having turned into the animal. Why this is reported in some cases but not others is unclear, but it is more readily understandable if the lycanthropic delusion is regarded as a disorder of self-identity. Some psychiatrists point out that it could even be referred to as a kind of 'species identity disorder'.

It is known that the virus which causes chickenpox, which this woman had shortly before, can also infect the brain tissue, producing an inflammation that could possibly produce delusions and hallucinations. As we are evolved from animals, perhaps the brain dysfunction produced by something like a virus rekindles sensations more appropriate to our evolutionary past.

But the diagnosis in this case was not entirely clear. The acute onset and rapid resolution of symptoms, in an individual who had evidence of physical illness, still suggest a transient organic, physical or biological condition. Against this is the fact that she was fully conscious throughout and her recall of events was clear. Like many who have experienced a psychotic episode, with time this woman became reluctant to discuss her experiences. She appears to have had a psychosis (possibly linked to a physical illness, e.g. the chickenpox virus) which was probably precipitated by the three-month history of depression preceding it. This suggests that this lycanthropic episode was part of some kind of mood disorder, a conclusion supported by her previous history of depression and the possible family history of depressive illnesses. But why should this patient have developed these particular delusions at this particular time? It seems that depressive illnesses later in life are more likely to be associated with delusions: this might partly explain why lycanthropy (or other psychotic features) did not feature in the patient's previous episodes.

Previously reported cases exhibiting lycanthropic delusions have had the experience of turning into only one species of animal. This appears to be the first case officially reported where several species are clearly implicated. This might suggest that lycanthropic psychotic experiences are basically about a regression to a primitive animalistic level of functioning and that the animal chosen has more to do with cultural influences than with any strict biological correspondence. So the fact that werewolves are a well-known part of culture means that in an undifferentiated psychotic state the mind might fasten on to this myth to explain what is happening to it.

This leads to a curious circular argument. Perhaps psychosis in ancient times was first described as appearing like a transformation into animals, myths like the werewolf developed and as these became a widespread part of culture they in themselves influenced the content of delusions, so becoming a self-reinforcing phenomenon.

Beliefs about transformation into animals are widespread in pre-industrial cultures and it is interesting to note that many reported cases of lycanthropy involve individuals from isolated rural backgrounds. In this respect this patient was typical, as she was unsophisticated and led a lonely life in a tied cottage on a country estate.[18]

In contrast to this background characterized by lack of sophistication and education is the following remarkable case reported by Dr Aaron Kulick and colleagues of the Department of Psychiatry at Harvard Medical School in Boston where someone undoubtedly of high IQ believed that they were not human.[19]

The man who believed he was a crazy tiger

The patient was a 26-year-old single man gainfully employed as a research scientist, who was admitted for outpatient treatment because of a recurrence of major depression. He recalled his first episode of depression occurring in his freshman year at college. However, in the initial interview he reported that as a child he had always suspected that he was a cat, and that this was confirmed by the family cat, Tiffany, after she taught him to 'speak cat' at age 11.

Later he recalled an even earlier period, as a toddler, when he was frequently tied to a tree alongside the family dog and pretended to be a dog himself. He was harnessed in this fashion until he was of school age, but denied other physical abuse. He recalled these events with rage and sadness, but excused his mother as she was often bedridden, due to menopausal problems. While denigrating his parents he idealized Tiffany, whom he perceived as a surrogate parent. When he was alone he regularly began to hunt with cats, to eat small prey and raw meat, to take part in sexual activity with cats in serial monogamous relationships and to converse with them by mewing and making feline gestures.

He says that the activities have been continuous and are not confined to episodes of depression. He frequently visits tigers at zoos, talks with them in tiger language, pets them through the bars and collects their loose fur. While previously unsure what kind of cat he was, by the age of 17 he had concluded that he was a tiger due to his large size and affinity with tigers. For the past seven years his greatest but unrequited love has been a zoo tigress named Dolly, whom he had hoped eventually to release. When she was recently sold to a zoo in Asia he was inconsolable and attempted to hang himself. His infatuation with Dolly followed the painful break-up of his closest sexual relationship with a woman who left him at the age of 18 when she attended college some distance away.

Publicly the patient dresses in characteristic tiger-striped clothes and states he feels more comfortable in them. He is carefully groomed but sports bushy sideburns, hair, moustache and beard; these, together with his long nails, make him look distinctly cat-like. He regards himself as a tiger with a very deformed body. He hypothesizes that his true parents were tigers, but that he was adopted, or had a tiger ancestor. For fear of ridicule or incarceration, he kept his cat identity secret until he was 17, when he began to confide in close friends and psychiatrists. Tiffany also encouraged him to engage in human as well as cat activities, and this is how he rationalizes his human behaviour.

He ascribes many human abilities to cats, including language and higher intelligence, and idealizes cats as more beautiful, sensuous, honourable, nurturant and playful (albeit in a sadistic way) than humans. Notably, he believes that cats never lie and are excellent parents, unlike humans.

Due to profound depression and attempted suicide, he has required four psychiatric hospitalizations since the age of 19. During his first and third he hallucinated a visual, tactile and auditory tiger companion which gradually dissipated as his depressive symptoms cleared. Before this, during the third hospitalization, he growled and crouched in feline positions for several days. He then began to communicate in English from a crouching position and finally resumed a human posture. Subsequently he believed that Dolly had escaped from the zoo, was living in the hospital grounds and was slipping into his psychiatric unit to have sex with him in the shower early in the morning. He believed that he impregnated her, but that the cubs were born dead and she left. Eventually he concluded that he had been psychotic and worried that he was a crazy tiger. Between these more psychotic presentations he exhibits a preoccupation with cats and tigers, yearns for a tigress mate, laments his lack of fur, stripes and a tail and expresses dismay that he has outlived many cat friends.

Except for the isolated delusion of being a tiger-like cat, his thought processes and perception are usually logical.

For the past eight years he has received almost continuous psychotherapy and medication, including courses of numerous antidepressants and mood stabilizers as well as electroconvulsive therapy (ECT). In the past, depressive symptoms responded partially to some medication alone and transiently to ECT. His delusion of being a cat, however, has remained completely resistant to treatment.

It is notable that in his family a paternal grandfather and first cousin committed suicide and two paternal aunts died in psychiatric institutions with unknown diagnoses.

During his hospitalizations he received frequent visits from a small circle of friends and colleagues and appeared socially appropriate. Between ages 15 and 21, he had been involved in several satisfactory sexual relationships with women lasting one to three years. However, he found them far less attractive than cats.

Currently he remains in treatment with weekly psychotherapy and medication. He has returned to his job where he is functioning well and he has returned to an apartment he shares with two friends . . . and a cat.

Dr Kulick, who reported the case, speculates that this particular pathology could have arisen because this patient may have failed to identify with either parent, due to both parents' own disturbances, and subsequently targeted his favourite cat as an object to idealize during childhood, so the cat replaced the role of parents. This process was perhaps superimposed on a pre-existing neurological vulnerability, and this may have produced his remarkably persistent lycanthropic delusion.

Perhaps if an individual has had an unusually close relationship with an animal when young, alongside distant relationships with humans, this leads to a particular affinity with animals and in this context animal delusions might develop. Similarly, widespread culturally shared beliefs in lycanthropy appear to be more common in traditional societies where people live in closer relationship with animals.

For primitive societies witnessing frightening behaviour where a person was obviously no longer himself, it would perhaps have been most convenient to assume that what they were seeing was a transformation into a more bestial or animal-like state. For the patient, an accessible explanation for their own conduct might be that they had been taken over by an animal spirit. Historians have traced the origins of lycanthropy to Greek mythology, in which Zeus transformed the devious Lycaon into a wolf in retribution for his cannibalism and for attempting to trick Zeus into eating human flesh. The Greeks may have adopted the myth from the even more ancient Phoenician cults so the belief is probably extremely old. Several mythological monsters, including centaurs and the Minotaur, had mixed animal and human characteristics. This syndrome gave rise to the folk belief in werewolves or sanguinary man-animals, who were said to change into their animal state under the influence of the full moon. In Irish folklore St Patrick is reported to have transformed Venetius, King of Gallia, into a wolf for his transgressions. In the Middle Ages, reflecting the spirit of the Inquisition, lycanthropy was ascribed to the influence of Satan.[20]

During the sixteenth and seventeenth centuries doctors could not agree as to whether human beings could really be transformed into werewolves by the forces of evil and demonic possession – a prevalent religious view which clashed with the fledgling attempts at a scientific and non-religious explanation. More 'scientific' doctors wondered whether people through warped beliefs came to convince themselves they had been so transformed, and so behaved like a werewolf without actually being one. In fact this 'disease' with its non-supernatural theory was not at all new: the ancient Greek physician Paulus Aegineta had classified lycanthropy as a form of depression and suggested bloodletting as an effective treatment.

The problem was how to interpret the spectacular cases which would be reported at least every few decades. In the sixteenth century came the cases of Garnier, Burgot and Verdun, three men in France who confessed to having turned themselves into wolves and eaten parts of nine children.[21] At the same time lycanthropes were also mentioned from Constantinople, Germany, Greece, Asia and

Egypt. In the suburbs of Cairo, for example, men reportedly transformed themselves into asses.[22]

The case of Garnier raises the question of whether the werewolf delusion was present more in the audience than in the victim, providing a convenient way of disposing of undesirable or feared eccentric members of the community. The similarities with the epidemics of witchcraft so characteristic of the time, and subsequent burnings as a way of eliminating the odd and purifying communities of undesirables, are striking.[23]

In a gruesome case in sixteenth-century France, the remains of two boys' and two girls' bodies were found scattered around the outskirts of a small village. The nude remains had been partly eaten, with large chunks having been torn from their arms and thighs. One boy's chewed leg had been ripped from the torso and carried off. Suspicion fell on an elderly hermit, Giles Garnier, perhaps because he was a loner, and feared for being different, or he may have been isolated because he was what we would regard today as eccentric or disturbed. When he was arrested more than 50 villagers testified that they had seen him, in the shape of a wolf, eating meat that they later found out was human flesh. Garnier 'freely confessed' under torture that he had killed and eaten the children while transformed into a wolf. He was quickly condemned and burned to death.[24]

Because the religious and demonic possession view held sway, lycanthropes were often tried, convicted and burned alive. Outbreaks of mass hysteria or 'collective psychoses' occurred, resulting in one instance in the execution of 600 people suffering lycanthropic syndromes in France during the Middle Ages. In another case of apparent hysterical lycanthropy in 1700, a large gathering of nuns residing in a French convent apparently mewed and behaved as if changed into cats. Even in a culture as far removed from these stories as Japan, very similar cases were described.

These widespread panics ultimately led to the death of hundreds of innocent people, perhaps blamed for the activities of local animals. Yet those suspected of being werewolves were often ripped to pieces in the search for the wolf fur that supposedly grew on the inside of the skin. Authorities estimate that between AD 1520 and 1630 more than 30,000 werewolf cases were reported in Europe.[25]

The werewolf legend basically refers to a hybrid combination of man and wolf. A psychological attempt to explain it is to see the syndrome as the product of a split-off of unacceptable sexual and aggressive urges within an individual. One way the unconscious or perhaps even conscious mind could reconcile violent or other un-acceptable urges within the self is to see these as part of an animal the person becomes transiently from time to time: It is not I who am violent or sexual but this animal I have been transformed into. It is interesting to acknowledge that many if not all forms of unaccept-able human behaviour are commonly viewed as 'bestial', or as belonging to our more 'primitive' or 'animal-like' evolutionary past.

So perhaps the werewolf legend is a convenient way to understand depraved behaviour: but it is the same individual who is the source of all this behaviour. It is simply easier for observers, and indeed even for the participant, to classify rages or phases of unacceptable comportment as belonging to another being that the person becomes for a while. In many ways the werewolf legend can be seen as an ancient anticipation of multiple personality disorder.

There are also possible medical rather than psychological ex-planations for the werewolf myth. For example, doctors have suggested that the rare medical disorder of congenital porphyria might be the origin of the wolf legend – and porphyrias have also been invoked to explain away vampirism. Affected individuals would only come out at night because of sun sensitivity, and the disease is associated with progressive scarring of the skin and increased hairiness. Due to a metabolic deficiency a group of chemicals called porphyrins accumulate in bones, fingernails and teeth, resulting in red-brown discoloration. There is also an associ-ated psychosis that due to the accompanying iron deficiency anaemia victims may have tried to cure themselves by drinking an iron-rich food source, such as blood.[26]

Other syndromes associated with excessive hairiness may also have been the basis for the werewolf legend. For example, in-dividuals with congenital generalized hypertrichosis, a rare X-linked dominant disorder, have been described as 'human werewolves'.[27] However, these explanations do not help us to understand the modern lycanthrope, who is usually normal in appearance, and there is no evidence of any other metabolic diseases like porphyria in any of the reported cases, including the case reports which follow.

Another explanation relies on the transformative effect on the psyche, not the body, of mind-altering drugs. Delusions of animal transformation associated with ritualistic drug ingestion have been described by shamans from traditional societies around the world, particularly in Latin America. Animal metamorphosis or transformation is linked to spirit possession leading to trance states and convulsions but the key point is that by transforming temporarily into an indigenous animal a healer or shaman enhanced his personal power and aided others. As shamans chose their special vocations, it is possible that they may have experienced self-induced dissociative and hypnotic states using psychotropic agents, or suffered seizure disorders. Hallucinogenic plants are widely used by Peruvian and Brazilian Indian tribes with frequently reported lycanthropy.

In the past it was observed that dogs and wolves tended to skulk around cemeteries at night, especially during times of hurried mass burials such as wars, plagues and famines. Driven by starvation, they would undoubtedly have been attracted by the odours of decomposition. There is no great mystery as to why they should be found so frequently sniffing and digging at grave sites. This provides a naturalistic explanation for the superstitious belief that the dead in the guise of beasts could rise from the grave. The sight of disturbed earth and signs of digging, and animal paw prints around the grave, would surely be interpreted as evidence that some hideous thing had risen from the dead. The wolf in the graveyard could easily be seen as having emerged from the disturbed grave rather than having tried to dig its way in for dinner.

But if the werewolf becomes part of mythology for these mundane reasons it would seem there could even be a drive at some level, for those suffering from psychological problems that leave them feeling weak and powerless, to identify with a feared and powerful entity, like a wolf. Along with two colleagues, Dr Kiran Rao, a psychiatrist at the National Institute of Mental Health and Neurosciences in Bangalore, India, recently reported not one but two cases of lycanthropy presenting as part of a depressive disorder.[28] In both cases, a positive history of dog bite influenced the presentation of symptoms.

Dr Rao and his colleagues propose the fascinating speculation that the psychological defence mechanism of identification with the aggressor is operative in this kind of case. 'Identification with the aggressor' is the mechanism invoked to explain why for example those who were sexually abused as children by adults appear to go on to abuse other children. The theory is that when you find yourself in the presence of a superior force which has the power to crush you there is a powerful incentive to learn to become like that power in order to protect yourself from future destruction. This also explains why politically some minority groups who have historically been bullied by others turn into bullies themselves later.

The man who became a werewolf after being bitten

Mr L. was a 17-year-old single male from a lower socioeconomic, rural background with 10 years of formal schooling. He complained of feeling fearful that he might turn into a dog, and had decreased sleep and appetite of four months' duration. Three weeks prior to consultation, the patient failed an examination, following which there was an increase in the intensity of his symptoms. He had had a dog bite one year prior to the onset of symptoms and was preparing for his school examination when family members noticed that he was not talking, was remaining withdrawn and eating less than usual. He also expressed the idea that he might become a dog. Suspecting black magic, the family took him to a local faith healer. He was made to vomit to remove the effects of the 'evil eye'. However, he did not obtain significant relief.

The youngest of three siblings, the patient was described as being shy, anxious, sensitive to criticism and having few friends. He was a hard-working and responsible well-groomed individual of frail build. The volume, tone and tempo of his speech were decreased. The patient reported feeling fearful and sad. He expressed the idea that he was half-man and half-dog and felt worthless and hopeless. He was diagnosed as having a moderate depressive episode, was hospitalized for four weeks and treated with Prozac.

Psychological testing revealed that he had an average level of intellectual function with a very high level of aspiration. Tests also suggested marked dependency needs and negative thoughts about the future, such as becoming poverty-stricken or having some serious illness.

In an exploratory interview, he was initially shy and inhibited. On being reassured that adolescence was a difficult period for most individuals, he responded by expressing several doubts and concerns. He reported that he was teased by peers and called a sissy because while most of his classmates sported a moustache, he did not have any hair growth on his face and body.

In the next session, the topic of sex and heterosexual relations, culturally a taboo topic, was raised in a matter-of-fact manner. The patient reported guilt feelings regarding masturbation. He subscribed to a commonly held belief that one drop of semen was equal to a hundred drops of blood and that he might have exhausted all his semen, resulting in physical weakness.

In the third and last session before discharge, the patient reported a sense of relief at having been able to talk things over. He said he had wanted to become a doctor, but, in the light of his poor academic performance and the financial constraints, realized the need to make alternative career plans. He was discharged on anti-depressant medication and advised to come a fortnight later. However, the patient did not report for follow-up.

Lycanthropy could be seen as a severe form of depersonalization – a state well known in psychiatry when the experience is that you are no longer real and have lost your identity. Depersonalization is found in a variety of conditions, most commonly in severe anxiety states.[29]

Lycanthropy however is not specific to any disorder and in the above case did not seem to have any bearing on the outcome or prognosis. The 'fear of becoming a dog' was part of the depressive syndrome. A significant difference from earlier reports is that the patient had been bitten by a dog. Moreover, he was a shy, anxious introvert with marked feelings of inadequacy and strong dependency needs. It is possible, therefore, that here the defence mechanism of identification with the aggressor may have been operative; or that he had so effectively repressed his aggressive sides that the werewolf delusion was the only way of dealing with this aspect of personality.

In psychiatric terminology, the difference between a delusion and an overvalued idea is that a delusion is an unshakeable conviction in the face of clear opposing evidence that your belief is erroneous. An overvalued idea is an unlikely belief to which you have attached more weight than would be usually expected, but you can be dissuaded from your position if others work hard enough at it. The case reported by Dr Rao appears to be more an example of an overvalued idea than a delusion. That you hang on to your idea or delusion, despite evidence to the contrary, indicates that the way your mind processes and organizes evidence has altered in some substantial way compared to those around you. This point goes to the heart of a common error made by the lay public and indeed many psychiatrists in their understanding of delusions. Delusions are not elicited or confirmed by questioning sufferers about what they believe. This merely elicits the content of a belief system and – although strange, unfamiliar or bizarre – the content of a belief system is not sufficient to categorize thinking as delusional. The key issue is how you arrived at your belief. So it is not so much the fact you believe you are turning into a wolf that marks you out as deluded: why you subscribe to this belief is much more important in determining your mental state.

Others have viewed lycanthropy as an expression of primitive instincts being expressed literally on an animalistic level through a splitting mechanism. In other words the unacceptable hostile, aggressive, animalistic part of us is split away from our usual sense of personal identity, and separated into an animal-like transformation – the werewolf. Freud postulated what is referred to as a topographic view of the mind where repressed unacceptable impulses are stored 'down below' in the id, while the higher conscience where lofty ideals and morals are found is the superego. The ego is conscious everyday awareness – a kind of resolution of the id and superego.

It is easier for us to reconcile our aggressive and even homicidal impulses with ourselves if we see ourselves as temporarily transformed into an animal that is not like us at all. In fact the werewolf and the host person are not two completely different entities: the werewolf is a side of the other that the host usually rejects or does not allow to reach conscious awareness.

In English-speaking countries, particularly the USA and the UK, delusions are defined mainly in intellectual terms, with the disturbed nature of the belief being stressed. It is the derangement in logical thought and rational reasoning that is thought to be the primary problem. In contrast, the European concept of delusion is based on a broader notion that involves disturbance in the sense or perception of self: 'a transformation in total awareness of reality'. Thus, lycanthropy has been referred to as a 'delirium of metamorphosis'. This European tradition suggests that delusional utterances should not be interpreted as false statements about reality, but as true statements about the personal experience, i.e. as disorders of the self.

There have been intriguing case reports of lycanthropy where brain scanning has revealed alterations in the part of the brain where body shape is represented.[30] Besides the experience of altered body shape or self-identity another strange sensation that could lead to the delusion of lycanthropy is the experience of being able to communicate with animals, or animals speaking to you. Psychiatrists Dr T. R. Dening and Dr A. West of St Crispin Hospital, Northampton in the UK recently reported several individuals with severe psychotic illnesses who experience hallucinatory voices from animals. They propose the term 'Dolittle phenomenon' to describe this.[31]

This series of case reports is important because there is no previous mention in psychiatric texts or recent medical literature of individuals who experience hallucinatory voices from animals. Yet this interesting phenomenon could provide yet another pathway to the werewolf or similar delusion.

The man who believed animals knew about his illicit affair

A 46-year-old married bricklayer was admitted informally to a psychiatric ward with delusions and hallucinations, feelings of being persecuted, depressed mood and suicidal thinking. The onset of episodes was hard to date precisely as he had been a heavy drinker for years but relatives thought he had displayed paranoid ideas for five years.

There was no known psychiatric illness in his family but six months before his admission, he had an affair with a neighbour. At this time he reduced his drinking and his symptoms first appeared. He believed that people in the street, on television or in passing cars knew about his personal affairs and were discussing him, either openly or by CB radio. He knew this because people would go red or fall silent when he approached. He experienced auditory hallucinations, hearing voices swearing at him and commentating on his actions; he also believed that he was able to kill.

An isolated man, his main recreation was walking his dogs. He noticed that one young dog had some grey hairs, indicating that it knew about plots against him and that it was worried about the danger. The dog sometimes moved its ears in a way that meant that it was sensing the danger and communicating it to him. He perceived it as being on his side in a hostile environment, and mentioned on several occasions that the dog (and possibly other dogs too) talked to him, although later he denied this. He also heard blackbirds speaking to him. His wife, a rather simple woman, noticed nothing untoward until she came home one day to find him teaching the dogs to read. He explained that he was encouraging them to read a hunting book, so that they might become better hunters.

The provisional diagnosis was paranoid psychosis and he was treated with various antipsychotic medications, eventually responding satisfactorily. After a few days, he wished to discharge himself. In view of the severity of the symptoms, lack of insight, suicidal thinking, thoughts about killing, and the presence of a shotgun at home, he was compulsorily detained. On recovery he became reticent about dog-related symptoms, whilst continuing to have

36

other auditory hallucinations and telepathic experiences. While he no longer felt people were discussing him, he maintained that they had been at the time of admission. He also remained convinced that the dog had been aware of the conspiracy, because of its grey hairs.

After six weeks he was relatively well and was discharged to out-patient care. Application for the return of his shotgun was refused.

The man who didn't like the way birds looked at him

A 74-year-old retired businessman was assessed at home for severe depression. He normally lived outside the area, but for two weeks had stayed with his daughter, as he was on bail after attempting to strangle his wife.

He had no previous psychiatric history, but probably a family history of depression (his half-sister possibly committed suicide). He was a kindly but anxious and hypochondriacal man and had had marital problems for years; his wife, he said, was a difficult person. At 17, he contracted venereal disease from her. She had left him briefly on one occasion and was now refusing to live with him again.

Over two years, he became increasingly withdrawn, with feelings of depression for several months. He also suffered from sleep disturbance and poor concentration.

His disorders of perception and thinking included frightening dreams about deceased friends. While awake, he saw horrible faces condemning him for unspecified crimes. Once he felt the room was full of gas. A misunderstanding over a hospital bill led him to a belief that he had breached the Masonic oath and he developed a morbid fear of venereal disease. During this period, his sister suffered a heart attack, fell into her fire and burned to death. This led to worsening of symptoms and the patient had suicidal thoughts, twice going to sea with the intention of drowning himself. He also made a rope noose, but thought a knife would be better. Concerned at how upset his wife would be to find his body, he decided to kill her first. He attempted to strangle her in the night, rendering her unconscious, but then changed his mind and rang the police.

Animal-related symptoms began one morning when he noticed pieces of fibreglass on the lawn. He believed that birds were taking away the roof insulation and heard three thrushes condemning him, although he did not know why. Later, a blackbird came and looked at him as if he had been condemned. His wife reported that he

37

thought the birds were pecking him and trying to tear him to pieces.

Initially, he was charged with attempted murder, altered later to actual bodily harm, in view of the circumstances. Diagnosed as having depressive psychosis, he was treated as an outpatient with antidepressants. There was much improvement, though occasionally he voiced further thoughts of suicide. However, there was no recurrence of animal-related symptoms. Eventually he was placed on probation for 12 months, was reconciled with his wife, and returned home.

The woman who spoke to an owl

A 29-year-old woman had schizophrenia. Her family had moved to England from Italy when she was two years old, and she had to bear much responsibility for her six younger siblings. There was no known family psychiatric history.

At 20, she developed a belief that the house was haunted. It was thought at first that she was probably suffering anxiety symptoms due to a stressful family situation. However, three months later she was admitted to hospital with bizarre behaviour, panic symptoms and suspected auditory hallucinations. Since then she has had multiple admissions to hospital, and is often either mute or very hostile. Recent admissions have been to an intensive-treatment unit, in view of her aggressive and dangerous behaviour, and she is currently an inpatient.

Much of the time she appears to be a charming and humorous girl who dresses fashionably and flirts with staff. However, she consistently believes that she is controlled by outside forces, that her husband was killed by Jack the Ripper, and that God has spoken to her. She has talked about past lives and of being put on the throne at the Battle of Hastings. She believes herself to be an angel, but also to have risen to life having been cremated at birth. Several ferocious assaults have been made upon nursing staff. One male nurse was nearly strangled with his tie, and another felt himself closer to being killed by her than by anyone else.

She has heard animals talking to her, saying 'You have got to come back.' An owl has spoken to her, and at other times she has received messages from a special pigeon, but is unable to recall the content of the messages.

There are of course several biblical examples of animals talking to humans with the serpent talking to Eve in the Garden of Eden

(Genesis 3: 1–5) probably the most famous. St Francis of Assisi preached on occasion to the birds, exhorting them to praise and love their Creator. During one sermon, the swallows made so much noise that he could not be heard. He charged them 'to be quiet until he had finished, whereupon they meekly subsided'. However, despite ample evidence of the saint talking to creatures, he did not seem to have special understanding of their speech.

In fairy tales, transformations into animals occur frequently, and usually take the form of humans who are the victims of witchcraft. In classical mythology, animals often converse with people and it is normal in mythical settings for creatures to be understood by any human to whom they speak. Some talking animals are transformed humans, whilst others seem to be fairly ordinary animals, such as the wolf in 'Red Riding Hood' or the cat in 'Puss-in-Boots'; nevertheless, they are readily understood by ordinary people.

Wagner's hero Siegfried became able to understand the song of birds in the wood after he slew the dragon Fafner. He bathed in the dragon's blood, and when he licked the blood off his hands, he heard the birds giving him advice. Examples in myth and fable in which creatures can be comprehended are numerous. Perhaps in the past the idea of understanding animal speech was acceptable, and only in the modern, realist age has it lost its cultural sanction.

The most striking literary example of understanding animal speech is provided by Hugh Lofting's Dr Dolittle, who could understand and speak with many species because he had been taught animal languages by his talking parrot. This differs from the cases reported above where the creatures spoke in English, but the net effect of private understanding is similar; hence our eponym. (Although this is not a literary pathography, it is interesting to speculate upon the mental state of John Dolittle, MD. He began in medical practice, which progressively failed as he accumulated animals and neglected his human patients. As poverty and ruin approached, he had the sudden experience of conversing with the parrot and later with other animals. This may have represented a swing from depression into mania, although other interpretations are possible.)

The above cases were accumulated over a few years and demonstrate that identification of animal voice hallucinations does not have specific diagnostic value. Hallucinations were associated with severe episodes of psychosis, and the subjects indulged in dangerous acts in accordance with either the animal voices or other elements of the psychopathology. Several deaths could easily have occurred. Thus, identification of the Dolittle phenomenon is a legitimate cause for concern. In many cases the voices come from birds, but the significance of this is unclear. Birds are traditionally associated with communication, e.g. carrier pigeons: possibly the 'threshold' for experiencing voices from birds is lower than for hearing talking beasts. Often the hallucinations are not the only element of animal-related psychopathology; various delusions are also present.

Patients were often reluctant to recount details of the experience, especially when recovering, even though other phenomena were more readily recalled, such as persecutory delusions. A further patient, who believed that the pet terrapins on the ward were going to eat him, probably had auditory hallucinations from the terrapins, but would become violent when questioned about such experiences. This may be a recognition of how bizarre the experience of hearing talking animals is considered to be: other types of hallucinations or delusions or persecution may be more culturally 'acceptable'.

Cases of the Dolittle syndrome or phenomenon tend to emphasize the tendency of humans to project human characteristics on to animals, so-called anthropomorphism; hence the belief that animals can speak.

This view neglects another issue: it is notable that in many cases of the werewolf delusion, sex plays a prominent part. Furthermore, the basis for lycanthropy is that the animalistic delusion allows previously repressed and unacceptable sexual impulses to be acted out. Animals have sex in an uninhibited way compared to humans so the delusion of becoming an animal ensures that sexual feelings can be expressed more freely.

Psychiatrist Dr Harry Rosenstock of University of Texas Medical Branch in Houston, and Dr Kenneth Vincent, a psychologist at Houston Community College in the USA, recently reported a case that illustrates bizarre and chaotic sexuality expressed in a primitive way through lycanthropic symptoms.[32]

The woman who offered herself

A 49-year-old married woman was admitted for urgent psychiatric evaluation because of delusions of being a wolf and 'feeling like an animal with claws'. She suffered from extreme apprehension and felt that she was no longer in control of her own fate. 'A voice was coming out of me,' she said. Throughout her 20-year marriage she experienced compulsive urges towards bestiality, lesbianism and adultery.

The patient chronically ruminated and dreamed about wolves. One week before her admission, she acted on these ruminations for the first time. At a family gathering she disrobed, assumed the female sexual posture of a wolf, and offered herself to her mother. This episode lasted for approximately 20 minutes. The following night, after sex with her husband, the patient suffered a two-hour episode, during which time she growled, scratched, and gnawed at the bed. She stated that the Devil came into her body and she became an animal. Simultaneously, she experienced auditory hallucinations. There was no drug involvement or alcoholic intoxication.

The patient was treated in a structured inpatient programme. She was seen daily for individual psychotherapy and was placed on antipsychotic medication. During the first three weeks, she suffered relapses when she said such things as 'I am a wolf of the night; I am a wolf woman of the day . . . I have claws, teeth, fangs, hair . . . and anguish is my prey at night . . . the gnashing and snarling of teeth . . . Powerless is my cause, I am what I am and will always roam the earth long after death . . . I will continue to search for perfection and salvation.'

She would peer into a mirror and become frightened because her eyes looked different: 'One is frightened and the other is like the wolf – it was dark, deep, and full of evil, and full of revenge of the other eye. This creature of the dark wanted to kill.' During these periods, she felt sexually aroused and tormented. She experienced strong homosexual urges, almost irresistible zoophilic drives, and masturbatory compulsion, culminating in the delusion of a wolf-like metamorphosis. She would gaze into the mirror and see 'the head of a wolf in place of a face on my own body – just a long-nosed wolf with teeth, groaning, snarling, growling . . . with fangs and claws, calling out "I am the devil." ' Others around her noticed the un-intelligible, animal-like noises she made.

By the fourth week she had stabilized considerably, reporting, 'I went and looked into a mirror and the wolf eye was gone.' There was only one other short-lived relapse, which responded to re-assurance by experienced personnel. With the termination of that episode, which occurred on the night of a full moon, she wrote of her experience: 'I don't intend to give up my search for [what] I lack . . . in my present marriage . . . my search for such a hairy creature.

I will haunt the graveyards . . . for a tall, dark man that I intend to find.' She was discharged during the ninth week of hospitalization on antipsychotic medication.

On psychological testing the patient's performance showed normal intellect and no evidence of organic brain damage. On other tests the performance was indicative of an acutely psychotic schizophrenic with distorted body image and gross sexual preoccupation, obsessional thinking, marked feelings of inferiority, and an excessive need for attention and affection.

What is of particular interest is that the delusional material was organized about a lycanthropic core with the following classic symptoms:

- delusions of werewolf transformation under extreme stress;
- preoccupation with religious phenomenology, including feeling victimized by the evil eye;
- reference to obsessive need to frequent graveyards and woods;
- primitive expression of aggressive and sexual urges in the form of bestiality;
- physiological concomitants of acute anxiety.

Significantly these symptoms occurred in the absence of exposure to toxic substances. Furthermore, the patient responded to the treatment used for acute schizophrenic psychosis. Her doctors believed that the metamorphosis she underwent provided temporary relief from an otherwise consuming sexual conflict that might have resulted in suicide.

Nowhere is the strong link between sex and unacceptable 'wicked' or 'immoral' feelings, producing guilt, and therefore perhaps delusions that accommodate sex and guilt, more clearly expressed than in delusions of having sex with the Devil. These are usually combined with delusions of possession by evil spirits and there are clear similarities with the notion of being transformed into another creature – perhaps being possessed by one after being bitten by an animal.

A central problem with the psychiatric understanding of the werewolf delusion, and many others, is that it is a belief that is already prevalent in a society or culture before the patient arrives at the so-called pathological belief. The delusion appears 'borrowed' or shaped by the culture in which the patient was already living. So many non-medical lay members of the public might well agree with the patient that they are possessed by a demon, have turned into a werewolf or some other non-psychiatric interpretation. This means that the delusion is no longer idiosyncratic but shared with others. Classically a delusion shared by one other person besides the sufferer is referred to as a *folie à deux* and is perhaps most frequently witnessed in the context of delusions with a strong religious flavour. For here religious leaders or priests might agree with the patient, and disagree with the psychiatrist, that this is not a delusion but a justified true belief. Religious delusion surrounding demon possession or demon worship is particularly prone to this problem.

THE DEVIL DELUSION

Historically, and even today, the experience of having had intercourse with the Devil has been regarded as evidence that the individual is a witch. Those investigating cases of witchcraft were advised to seek the judgement of doctors, and the verdict of physicians became a test for the presence or absence of witchcraft.

The woman described in the following case study presented by psychiatrists Dr Paula H. Salmons and Dr David J. Clarke of the University of Birmingham suffers from cacodemonomania and might well have suffered the death penalty in former times.[33] Cacodemonomania is the delusion of being possessed by a demon. She is unusual because of her belief that she had had intercourse with the Devil, and because the belief was shared by her religious minister.

The woman who believed she had made love to the Devil

A 38-year-old married woman teacher, Mrs A., was admitted from the outpatient department with a history of feelings of unreality, alterations in mood and expressions of the belief that she was possessed by an evil god that made her carry out actions against her will. Two years previously, while she was reading the New Testament, a 'force' inside her suggested that she could have more pleasurable sensations than those to be obtained while reading the Bible. She lay down on the bed and had sexual intercourse with the force, 'as with a man', and with the physical sensation of

43

penetration, resulting in orgasm. Since then there had been about 12 similar instances, some pleasurable but most not. She said it had not been pleasurable recently and described it as 'filthy'. Her sexual relationship with her husband had declined, and she now felt that intercourse was repulsive.

Five years previously, Mrs A. had felt depressed, lethargic and detached from events occurring around her. A diagnosis of depersonalization syndrome with atypical depression was made. Treatment with mood-elevating medication succeeded, but was accompanied by overconfidence and aggression.

Over the next two years the feelings of unreality and depression persisted, and treatment with another form of antidepressant was started. Shortly afterwards, while lying in bed, the patient became convinced that her husband had physically altered. He felt scaly to the touch, and when she looked at him she saw several extra eyes and limbs. The episode passed after some minutes but was followed by marked mood swings lasting a few days at a time, with periods of elation and hyperactivity alternating with lowered mood and lack of energy.

One day while sitting in the bath, Mrs A. became convinced that she was shedding large pieces of skin, which she could see and which were blocking the plug-hole. Shortly afterward all drugs were stopped because she had become pregnant with her third child. There were no complications during the pregnancy and labour, and a normal female infant was delivered.

Mrs A.'s psychiatric condition remained unchanged until the child was four months old. While sitting at home, she suddenly smelt an overpowering odour, 'just like a newborn baby', although her daughter was in a different room. Later she had the conviction that her daughter's skin was peeling off and that some of it was wrapped around the refrigerator in the kitchen.

Until this time, Mrs A.'s religious beliefs, which were of an orthodox Christian nature, had not changed. However, a few months later, while attending a Bible class, she began to feel that her god was different in some way from the God that other people experienced. She said, 'The word Jesus is now anathema to me.' She had been forced by her god to tear up the New Testament section of her Bible, which she put in a brown paper bag and posted through her religious minister's door.

Mrs A. had a miscarriage in the following year (her fourth pregnancy), and a few months later she suddenly knew that the baby would be presented to her by her god if she searched for it in some nearby woods. She rushed from the house in night attire and bare feet, ripping her clothes and cutting herself in her struggle through the woods.

Mrs A. often had 'funny turns', in which she would feel unwell and have a sense of unreality. In three of these she was made to turn the gas taps of her cooker on 'by the god in possession of me', and in another, the sleeve of her pullover caught fire while she was cooking and burned her skin.

When later admitted to hospital Mrs A. said that over the previous six months the god that possessed her had had intercourse with her several times. She described how one evening she became convinced that her own face had changed, the left side below her eye becoming horny and detached from the rest of her face.

The patient had married at 23. Her husband, who was four years older, was a teacher, a quiet man who had little contact with people outside the family. The marriage appeared stable. At the time of hospital admission, the couple's three girls were aged 10, 7 and 3 years. Mr A. appeared unconcerned about all the peculiar happenings and continued to go to work regularly.

Mrs A. was neat and well dressed. Her appearance and behaviour were appropriate, and superficially she established reasonable rapport. Her speech and language were normal, although she was evasive when asked to describe her abnormal experiences; it was difficult to clarify her emotions and experiences. Her mood was emotionally 'cool'. Physical examination and routine investigations were entirely normal. Electroencephalogram (EEG) investigations indicated there were mild brainwave abnormalities present but these were not typical of epilepsy.

The patient declined treatment after her admission examinations, saying that her problems were spiritual, not medical. Her young religious minister agreed that Mrs A. was possessed by a malevolent force, which was responsible for all the events. On several occasions, he claimed, his treatment with prayers had stopped her peculiar feelings – especially her hatred of Jesus. He felt that medical treatment was inappropriate, and he clearly reinforced her beliefs.

There is evidence that a belief in witchcraft is still prevalent in modern Western society and several recent cases have been reported in the press in which tragedies occurred as the result of attempts at exorcism. The popularity of the occult as a subject for plays, films and books is evidence of widespread lay interest, yet there is a lack of recent discussion of these phenomena in medical and psychiatric journals.

Earlier this century, three types of possession were distinguished: hysteria, anxiety nightmares and those due to a dissociative process. Dissociation refers to the tendency to split off consciousness so that you are unaware of some of the things happening to you or even of actions you are performing. Its cause is generally a traumatic event such as sexual or physical abuse in childhood. The popular theory is that during sexual abuse the severity of the trauma is better dealt with if the victim's psyche splits their consciousness so that another personality develops within the same mind. The abuse occurs to this and not to the main personality. Taken to the extreme, this ultimately produces multiple personality disorder.

Several French authors have described different types of cases of possession, and some viewed possession states from the position of orthodox Catholic psychiatrists and accepted the co-operation of exorcists. They distinguish 'true' possession from 'false' possession, identifying the former as instances where a psychiatric explanation was not adequate or plausible. These views appear to be shared by more recent clerical writers who feel that a major difficulty in cases of possession presenting to the clergy is diagnosis. The standard clerical practice is that except in cases of emergency, causes other than true possession by an evil force should be excluded by con-sultation with the patient's doctors. Yet, they argue, there seems to be a small and increasing percentage of cases in which the presence of objective evil is the only reasonable conclusion to draw. Most advocate the intelligent use of exorcism in co-operation with the medical profession.[34]

More recently, cacodemonomania has been described in five children. In at least three of the cases, the belief in demon possession was initiated by someone other than the child. The authors describe the clinical situation as a *folie à deux* syndrome: one or more members of the family shared the child's delusion. All five children had suffered the loss of a natural parent; in three of these instances the remaining parent had remarried. Other psychiatrists have also drawn attention to the link between parental deprivation and delusional sexual experiences. This link was first interpreted by Freud, in his paper 'A Seventeenth-Century Demonological Neurosis'. He described the possession of a young man with melan-cholia who had made a pact with the Devil. Freud interpreted the Devil in this case to be a substitute for the father, whose death had originally precipitated the melancholia. This idea is extended from the individual to the cultural when psychoanalysts suggest that

Christianity attempts to resolve Oedipal conflicts with the concepts of a good God-father and an evil or sexual Devil-father.[35]

But there are also similarities between possession states and multiple personality. In both conditions, the individual experiences a period of time in which traits sharply contrasting with the 'normal' are exhibited, and normally unacceptable impulses or wishes can be expressed.[36]

Delusions of possession can indicate a psychotic illness, in which the notion of being possessed may be symptomatic of the disturbance of ego functioning that occurs in schizophrenia – a passivity experience. In the schizophrenic passivity experience the patient moves a limb but believes the limb has been moved by an outside force operating on their body. This is a classic psychotic symptom of schizophrenia and could be the basis of possession delusions or thinking. Severely neurotic patients may also exhibit hysterical and other symptoms resembling those occurring in a possession state.[37]

Possession states are more prevalent in some cultures than others. A belief in demonology and the occurrence of these syndromes has been thought to be coincident with an oppressive social structure and an inability to cope with its evils. Reports from other cultures show that such states may provide a socially sanctioned behavioural outlet for repressed impulses and needs and do not necessarily represent psychiatric illness. What is interesting, though, is that even in a Western culture in which demoniacal belief is not an active part of orthodox religious practice, such syndromes still arise, so similarities occur between patients from widely differing cultures.[38]

In the case of Mrs A., discussion with her minister illustrates a problem occasionally encountered in psychiatric practice. The psychiatrist's belief system had no common ground with the patient's belief system or her minister's. Her minister asserted that he had read the world theological literature on possession states and that he had no doubt that Mrs A. had a spiritual and not a psychiatric disorder.

Several psychiatrists investigating these disorders have felt that the efforts of a single discipline are inadequate to deal with such complex spiritual problems. They have developed a working group comprising members of the clergy, psychiatrists with religious convictions, and agnostic psychiatrists, so that a better understanding of patients' problems could be achieved. Although patients like Mrs A. present infrequently, psychiatrists should realize that a broader

47

perspective is required, which takes account of the patient's inter-personal difficulties, subculture and spiritual life.[39]

Studies of the occult go back to antiquity. By advocating a more enlightened approach to the insane than pyrotherapy (burning at the stake), Johannes Wiero's sixteenth-century treatise *De praestiglis daemonum et incantationibus ac veneficiis* stands as a landmark in the history of Western medicine. Much later Freud provided a psychoanalytic foundation for understanding the occult when he observed that the 'states of possession correspond to our neuroses . . . the demons are bad or reprehensible wishes, deriv-atives of instinctual impulses that have been repudiated and repressed.'

Others have pointed out that since the belief in witchcraft is cul-tural it should perhaps be considered pathological only when maladaptive. Belief in witchcraft and demons can be viewed as a defence mechanism that permits the projection of unacceptable feelings and wishes on to a scapegoat. Belief in possession could represent an attempt to deny responsibility for 'internal devilishness' through externalization; the ritual of exorcism then becomes appealing because it confirms the victim's innocence.[40]

In the early 1970s the film *The Exorcist* heightened public interest in the occult and four cases of traumatic neuroses which developed after viewing the film were presented in the medical literature. One case is that of a 15-year-old boy who believed he was possessed by 'demons of Satan'. The suggestion by his doctors is that this delusion was a hysterical defence against his incestuous attraction to an older sister and his resentment of his family's religious beliefs.[41]

This point is reinforced in a study on cacodemonomania and exorcism in children by psychiatrists Dr Eric Schendel and Dr Ronald-Frederic C. Kourany of Vanderbilt University in Nashville, Tennessee.[42] They argue that despite its popularity in the lay media, alleged possession of children has received scant attention in the scientific literature.

The boy exorcized with violence

A seven-year-old boy was admitted to the child psychiatry inpatient unit because of fighting, poor peer relations and aggressiveness towards his mother. His parents divorced when he was less than a year old but the mother remarried and was having multiple marital and psychiatric problems. She reported that her son's behavioural problems had become bad: she had tried 'everything' to correct him, but to no avail. Among unsuccessful attempts she listed arguing, spanking, and other punishments. (Child abuse was suspected, as the child had been brought to the emergency room with a broken clavicle and multiple bruises.) About one month prior to admission she was told by her fellow Church of God members, and quickly believed, that 'demons have taken possession' of the boy and that they needed to be driven out.

At a church service the members of the congregation prayed together and 'drove the demons out of him'. The boy was reported to have been 'flung across the room by some force', which left a 'mark' on his face. The boy said he 'was glad that the demons were gone' and that he 'saw angels after they left'. His behavioural problems worsened and ultimately led to his psychiatric hospitalization.

The boy was found to be alert, verbal and co-operative but found it difficult to talk about his relationship with his mother, and was confused about his chaotic home environment. A diagnosis of severe anxiety reaction was considered and some improvement during hospitalization was noted. He was discharged against medical advice on his mother's insistence and the State Department of Human Services was notified of suspected abuse.

The badly behaved girl

An 11-year-old girl from a small rural community in Mississippi was admitted to the child psychiatry inpatient unit because of headaches, violent outbursts and poor peer relations. On one occasion she swung her small nephew by his feet and banged his head on the ground. On another occasion she stuck a thorn in her mother's leg. The patient stated that she was aware of what she was doing during these 'spells' but could not control her body and that 'someone else' was responsible. Her grandparents and mother decided she was possessed by the Devil. She agreed.

Her parents had divorced when she was less than two years old and her mother later remarried. Contact with the natural father was sporadic, then lost. The family's religious background was fundamentalist, Church of Christ and Pentecostal. When the family doctor could not find anything wrong with her and after it was agreed that she was possessed by the Devil, she was taken to the Pentecostal church where she was prayed over for three consecutive nights so that she could be 'healed' and 'regain her faith'. Afterwards she reported she felt better for a few days. When she started to have her spells again, she was brought to the emergency room and subsequently admitted to the hospital.

Examination revealed a well-developed girl, appropriately dressed and groomed, who appeared older than her stated age and behaved in a seductive manner. She was soft spoken and articulate, and talked about having 'spots before her eyes'. Her mood was bland and indifferent but she was alert, oriented and appeared to be of above average intelligence. Medical and neurological evaluations were negative and a tentative diagnosis of conversion reaction was made. (A conversion reaction is a term used to describe the psychological process whereby an emotional experience like stress could be dealt with by 'converting' it to a physical symptom – like the paralysis of a limb for no biological reason.) In this case, the girl improved rapidly but was discharged against medical advice upon her mother's insistence.

Freud felt one of his patients used the Devil as a replacement for his dead father. Commenting on this and the fact that the book and film *The Exorcist* involves possession of a girl who has lost her father, psychoanalytic thinkers have suggested that the belief that one is possessed represents the retention of a past object as a defence against loss.

In some cases, belief in demon possession was initiated by someone other than the child, either a family member or a religious figure. The other families were heavily invested in the occult. The defence of cacodemonomania may thus be primarily a manifestation of parental pathology. It appears to be a shared delusion, a form of *folie à deux*. One suggestion is that in a *folie à deux* the primary dependent partner feels increasingly taken advantage of and becomes angrier at the other. Because of his dependency he cannot express hostility directly but instead projects it on to an outsider. When the secondary partner initially refuses to accept the paranoid delusion, the primary partner's accusations 'begin to shift toward the secondary partner, who finds this more direct hostility extremely anxiety provoking ... A point is reached where the tension becomes intolerable, and the secondary partner accepts the delusions.'[43]

In the case of children who, their parents believe, are possessed by demons, the second portion of this dynamic process occurs. The child reacts to the loss of one parent and the ambivalence of the other with growing hostility. This mobilizes anxiety and guilt in the parent. To reduce the anxiety and guilt, the parent accepts the proposition, usually suggested by a third party, that the child is possessed. It is easier to believe that the anger comes from a demon than from one's own child. The child in turn finds that the delusion offers him a chance to reduce his anxiety by resolving the conflict between his hostility and his dependency needs.

A recent Japanese study found that 21 per cent of 1,029 inpatients had a 'delusion of possession'.[44] Most of the subjects were under 30 years of age and diagnosed with schizophrenia. In a US study of 61 chronically psychotic outpatients the authors found a 'delusion of possession' in 25 subjects.[45] The comparison of these 25 'possessed patients' with 36 patients without a history of delusional possession revealed significantly more reports of childhood sexual abuse, higher dissociation scores, more cannabis abuse, more experience of thought control, and more voices heard inside their heads.

The use of terms such as 'possessed patients' or 'delusions of possession' suggests that such beliefs are primarily pathological phenomena. However, does the term 'delusion' really help to make sense of 'possession states' in psychiatric patients? Obviously, delusions are difficult to define. They could reflect 'wrong beliefs': being convinced of ideas which are not shared by one's subcultural system.

Moreover, many so-called normal people hold delusion-like ideas. The more a delusion is investigated, the more understandable and less bizarre it becomes; often it is interwoven with very individual patterns of experiencing relationships, adversities and suffering. Finally, for every delusion, as bizarre and remote as it may appear, there may be a cultural niche in which the same delusion is considered legitimate and reasonable.

According to Dr Samuel Pfeifer of Basle, who conducted a survey of the prevalence of demonic possession, it is surprising to see the high frequency of demonic attributions not only in delusional disorders, but across *all* diagnostic categories of psychological difficulty. The more intense the feeling of an outside influence alien to the patient's own personality, the more frequent are ideas about an 'occult' influence.[46]

The results of recent studies support the observation that belief in possession or demonic influence is not confined to delusional disorders. The difficulty of defining spirit possession as a delusion is perhaps best exemplified by the problem of classifying belief in God. Is this the ultimate delusion?

HAVE NEUROLOGISTS FINALLY FOUND GOD?

In Dostoevsky's *The Idiot* a character describes what it feels like to experience a particular kind of epileptic attack – 'I have really touched God. He came into me, myself; yes, God exists, I cried . . . You all, healthy people . . . can't imagine the happiness which we epileptics feel during the second before our attack.'

Dostoevsky himself suffered from epilepsy, a brain disorder characterized by random rapid electrical discharges in one area which may spread to engulf the whole brain, sometimes producing hallucinations and widespread muscular convulsions. So his descriptions of epilepsy in *The Idiot* are probably autobiographical. Dostoevsky appears to have anticipated recent discoveries from modern neurology, which is establishing a link between religion and particular brain areas. Some neurologists are even claiming to have finally found the location of God.

Epilepsy was known in ancient times as the 'sacred' disease, perhaps because modern research has found that around 25 per cent of those whose epilepsy involves the brain's temporal lobes (the parts of the brain nearest the ears) develop a distinctive religious fervour. Drs Jeffrey Saver and John Rabin from the UCLA Neurological Research Center argue that substantial numbers of founders of major religions, prophets and leading religious figures display symptoms suggesting they suffered from epilepsy.[47] Saver and Rabin's list includes St Paul, one of the first Christian missionaries, Mohammad and Joan of Arc among 12 other major religious figures of the last 2,000 years.

Dr Vilayanur Ramachandran, Professor and Director of the Center for Brain and Cognition at the University of California, agrees there is a link between neurology and religious experience, and points out that many of his patients have deeply moving spiritual experiences as part of their epileptic attacks. These include a feeling of divine presence and the sense that they are in direct communion with God. Everything around them is imbued with cosmic significance. They may say, 'I finally understand what it is all about. This is the moment I've been waiting for all my life. Suddenly it all makes sense,' or, 'Finally I have insight into the true nature of the cosmos.'[48]

Does this syndrome, linking a form of epilepsy that originates in the temporal lobes of the brain and religion, imply that our brains contain some sort of circuitry that is actually specialized for religious experience? Is there a God programme in our heads?

In an attempt to answer these questions Dr Ramachandran has recently attempted the first scientific experiments directly related to religion. He compared the emotional responses, measured by skin sweating, of temporal lobe epileptics and normal controls to various pictures and words. The temporal lobe epileptics had a heightened emotional response mainly to religious words and icons. Their responses to the other categories, including sexual words and images, which ordinarily evoke a powerful response, was strangely diminished.

Ramachandran believes his and other experiments suggest human beings may have evolved specialized neural circuitry for the sole purpose of mediating religious experience, and temporal lobe epileptics lie at an extreme end of the spectrum of activity in this brain area. After all, human belief in the supernatural is so widespread throughout the world that it is tempting to ask whether the propensity for such beliefs might have a biological basis.

In national surveys in the US, Britain and Australia, between 20 and 40 per cent of individuals report having had mystical experiences, and this figure rises to more than 60 per cent when in-depth interviews of randomly selected individuals are conducted.[49] Studies in identical and fraternal twin pairs, raised apart, suggest that 50 per cent of our religious interests and attitudes are determined by genes.[50]

Dr Michael Persinger, a Canadian psychologist, has recently found that one of the main differences between the 19 per cent of high school students who had religious experiences before their teens, and the rest, was the presence of a head injury or a blackout at least once during childhood.[51] When Dr Persinger stimulated his own brain's temporal lobes using a transcranial magnetic stimulator (a helmet which shoots rapidly fluctuating and extremely powerful magnetic fields onto a small patch of brain in order to activate it) he experienced God for the first time in his life.[52]

Feeling that one is in the presence of God usually involves the strong emotional experience of awe, which is the kind of mood likely to be mediated by the temporal lobes. But what about the other emotions involved in mystical sensations, like the sense of connectedness with the rest of the universe?[53]

Drs Andrew Newberg and Eugene d'Aquili of the Nuclear Medicine division at the University of Pennsylvania have been conducting brain imaging experiments on highly proficient meditators in order to identify those other brain areas where activity is linked to religious experience. One of their most interesting findings was decreased activity in the area of the brain that controls our sense of distinction between self and world.[54]

The mystical literature of all the world's great religions describes a state of ultimate unity. When a person is in this state he or she loses all sense of discrete being: even the difference between self and other is obliterated. Such experiences are often described as perfect union with God, and appear to be mediated by the posterior superior temporal lobule, which is what helps us differentiate between self and non-self. Altered activity in this area might be linked with a sense of unity with the world.[55]

A decreased awareness of the boundaries between the self and external world could also lead to a sense of oneness, generating a sense of community and cohesiveness. This accounts for why a religious sentiment could have positive evolutionary benefit for primitive tribes' survival and could explain why natural selection favoured the evolution of a religious centre in the brain.[56]

But Drs Newberg and d'Aquili have an even more parsimonious neurological explanation for God. They point out that one natural function of our brains is constantly to infer the causes of events we witness. We can then act upon the world or anticipate future events. As our fate is at the mercy of an often capricious universe, we are driven to try to understand the laws upon which our environment turns, so that we can calculate how to ward off future disaster.[57]

But when we find ourselves at the mercy of a world governed by no clear rules we can use to our advantage, we construct myths to help orientate ourselves. We construct demons, spirits, gods or other personalized power sources with whom we can deal contractually, via prayer and penance, in order to gain apparent control over a capricious environment.[58]

But even if the final location of God is in the temporal and parietal lobes of the brain, it may not be a final victory for atheists. Discovering a neural structure which sustains religious experience could simply be evidence that a higher power constructed humans with the capacity to experience the divine. Given that we are now almost certain such a structure exists and that probably it is inadvertently removed as part of the brain surgery frequently done to cure intractable epileptics, what happens, asks Dr Ramachandran, to patients' spiritual leanings when we remove these parts of their temporal lobes? The research to answer this question has yet to be done, but have we basically performed a Godectomy?

DO VAMPIRES EXIST?

In 1975 a case study was published of cacodemonomania presenting as *folie à deux*. The primary partner was an 18-year-old dependent schizophrenic girl who used the delusion as a paranoid defence against the hostility she felt towards her hysterical mother, who in her turn accepted the delusion in order to maintain their relationship. More on this case in the next chapter, but psychoanalysts have drawn on popular literature, utilizing the novel *Dracula* as the framework for elaborating on the theory which explains this kind of dynamic.

Count Dracula constantly changes from a charismatic desirable figure to a killer, and in so doing psychologically represents the internal conflict between the need to destroy and the desire to love. Certainly a psychological explanation might be sought to explain the perennial popularity of this genre, for like a bat out of hell, vampire mania hits town whenever 'Dracula' films are released every few years.

In the modern age, vampires have become media stars. Published in 1897, *Dracula* by Bram Stoker made the word 'vampire' a household term. More recently, a vampire trilogy by Anne Rice became a bestseller. On the silver screen, W. Murnau's *Nosferatu* (Berlin, 1921) remains a classic and then there is the hit TV series called *Buffy the Vampire Slayer*. Our enduring fascination with vampires evolved from beliefs and superstitions dating back to medieval Europe and to humankind's most archaic myths. Curiously, while providing inspiration for the arts, their legacy is also found in the rare clinical condition of vampirism, which combines some of the most shocking pathologic behaviours observed in humanity. What these films don't tell you is that vampirism is actually a rare disease treated by doctors.[59]

The word 'vampire' owes its etymology to Slavic languages; periodic vampire scares agitated these regions and the superstitious inhabitants of Central and Eastern Europe as late as the nineteenth century. A prevalent belief was that a person who had died would leave his tomb at night to attack his victims, often friends and relatives, in order to suck their blood to retain his own immortality. The vampire returned to his coffin before sunrise or risked paralysis and total helplessness.[60]

Some superstitions give the vampire the power of metamorphosis, the ability to transform into animal form (most frequently a butterfly or a bat) or into vapour and mist. In addition, because the vampire is 'dead' and soulless, it has no reflection. Those whom the vampire attacks are generally in a trance and are almost sensually embraced while their blood is sucked. The victim eventually dies and, unless proper measures are taken, will in turn become a vampire. Other ways to join the 'undead', depending on local tradition, are to commit suicide, practise black magic, be cursed by parents or the church, be a werewolf, or even be an unlucky corpse in Greece on the way to the cemetery and have a bird or cat cross in front of the procession.[61]

To counter vampires, schemes ranging from the crude to the elaborate were designed. Garlic and the crucifix were considered effective apotropaics (protective measures against evil). Identifying vampires in many ways paralleled witch-hunting techniques. Telltale signs indicating a possible vampire were unusual birthmarks, infants born with teeth, red-haired and sometimes blue-eyed children, tall and gaunt people, and epilepsy. Tombs were often opened to see if the cadaver had moved, if it had fresh cheeks or open eyes, and if the hair and nails were still growing. Such rituals were performed in Connecticut in the eighteenth and nineteenth centuries.

Suspected vampires or suspicious corpses faced a variety of measures, from symbolic exorcism to brutal mutilation. If already buried, the cadaver was unearthed and the head severed and placed between the feet. If necessary, the heart was also boiled in oil and dissolved in vinegar. The most popular response was to impale the vampire on a wooden stake with a single blow through the heart. Sometimes a priest was called on to shoot the vampire with silver bullets.[62]

In Bram Stoker's original story Dracula's antagonists are two psychiatrists, and even today psychiatrists see clients who fervently believe they are pursued by vampires, while others have symptoms which are professionally diagnosed as 'clinical cases of vampirism' or 'haemosexuality'. A survey of doctors in the 1970s uncovered two cases of clinical vampirism, and a handful of similar instances are reported every decade. The syndrome consists of compulsive blood-taking, uncertain identity and an abnormal interest in death – often manifested in necrophilia or necrophagia (pleasure derived from the eating of parts of dead bodies). Although the full-blown syndrome is rare, elements of the vampire myth are frequently encountered in psychiatric clinics. For example, many lovers in a sexual frenzy bite each other during intercourse until blood flows, and on occasions this is sucked during sex. In fact some can only achieve orgasm following the taste of blood. This very real phenomenon contributed an essential element to Bram Stoker's creation.[63]

'Auto-haemofetishism' occurs in intravenous drug users who are sexually aroused by watching their blood sucked into a syringe. 'Auto-vampirism' is self-mutilation followed by consuming blood and is not uncommon. One report tells of a patient who enjoyed puncturing his neck veins and watching in a mirror the sight of blood gush. He later moved on to piercing an artery and then lying on his back, so he could catch the spray of blood in his mouth and drink it. One woman stored her own blood so that she could look at it in times of stress, as this seemed to have a calming effect. Between the wars an arrested murderer confessed to regularly visiting slaughterhouses to drink a glass of warm blood, believing this would keep him in good health.[64]

Another element of vampirism – necrophilia, or sexual relations with the dead – is also rare, but every few years psychiatrists record such cases. In the 1920s Leger mutilated the genitalia of a young girl and drank her blood after necrophilia; Sergeant Bertrand in 1845 dug up corpses to aid his masturbation; Henry Blot in 1886 desecrated the grave of an 18-year-old girl and sexually abused her; Peter Kurten between the wars stabbed sheep whilst sexually molesting them, and indulged in necrophilic and vampiristic activities with numerous humans. Even in modern times prostitutes report that some clients ask them to play the part of a corpse.[65]

Perhaps the only comfort one can derive from this terrible litany of behavioural oddity is that these symptoms of vampirism are extremely rare, but this itself presents a puzzle: if vampirism is so exceptional, why should almost all cultures throughout history possess a version of the legend?

Some features of vampirism may have been more common in past times. For example in ancient Egypt, to discourage sexual intercourse with corpses of deceased beautiful women their bodies were not given to embalmers until several days after their deaths. King Herod was said to have slept with the corpse of his wife Marianne for seven years after her death, and similar stories are told of Charlemagne.[66]

Records of vampire-like figures exist in several ancient religions. The first pictorial evidence of the vampire appears on an Assyrian bowl showing a man copulating with a female vampire whose head has been severed. There are ancient Babylonian, Semite and Egyptian beliefs involving a dead person that continues to live in its original body and feeds off the living. Similar beliefs can be found in ancient European, Chinese, Polynesian and African cultures: most refer to demonic female figures and fused relationships between the living and the dead, expressed through blood rituals as well as sexualized and aggressive exchanges. Current manifestations of these ancient beliefs exist in voodooism and associated practices in the Caribbean and in Latin America. In Catholicism, wine continues to symbolize Christ's blood and is consumed by priests and congregations during mass.[67]

The psychoanalysts argue that necrophilia is an extreme manifestation of a frantic attempt to deny the death and separation for ever from a loved one.

But even the prevalence of this idea does not explain the mysterious epidemics of vampirism which broke out periodically in Europe before the nineteenth century. For example from 1720 to 1730 the numerous sightings of the walking dead in Hungary and Slavic regions have never been satisfactorily explained.[68]

One possibility is that the many plagues which swept the land in those days led to hasty disposal of bodies in makeshift graves, which were shallow and easily exposed. Premature burial before death was probably quite common and the victims would have awakened, struggled to the surface and wandered back to their homes clad in mud-smeared and bloodstained burial shrouds, triggering the vampire legend. A nineteenth-century surgeon demonstrated that one person in every 200, even in places like New York, could expect to be buried alive. Doctors then had no sure proof of death short of putrefaction, as was reaffirmed by the British Medical Council as late as 1885, not long before Bram Stoker commenced work on *Dracula*. Many of the normal effects of biochemical change and decomposition of a corpse may have led the ancient mind to diagnose vampirism: hair and nails continue to grow, the body can become warm and blood liquefy again, cheeks redden and eyes open where before they had been closed.[69]

Another explanation, which we have already seen invoked for lycanthropy, is that the rare genetic disease known as *erythropoietic protoporphyria* was confused with vampirism. This fatal disorder induces the body to produce too much porphyria (pigment) which results not only in redness of the eyes, skin and teeth, but also a receding upper lip and cracking skin which bleeds when exposed to light. It has been suggested that physicians in the past could treat such patients only by secluding them from light of day and persuading them to drink blood to replace that lost by their bleeding; these features, plus the episodes of insanity the victims were prone to, could easily have been the basis for the vampire story.

However, the problem with this theory is that clinicians have described cases that involve acts that are strongly reminiscent of some aspect of the mythical vampire's behaviour but where no medical or biological explanation such as porphyria disorder can be found.[70]

Clinicians have defined vampirisms as all sexual or aggressive acts – whether or not there is blood suction – committed on a deceased or a dying person. This view tends to cover a variety of behaviour – necrophilia, necrosadism, necrophagia and vampirism. In the 1820s, the case of Antoine Leger, who drank his victim's blood but also raped, murdered, mutilated, and partially devoured a young girl, supposedly illustrates an instance of polyvampirism.

A more recent case fitting this broad definition of vampirism is described in detail in the psychiatric literature. In 1978, during a two-day rampage in the Mayenne region of France, a 39-year-old man attempted to rape a pre-adolescent girl, also biting her deeply in the neck, murdered an elderly man whose blood he drank and whose leg he partially devoured, killed a cow by bleeding it to death, murdered a married couple and almost succeeded in doing the same with their farmhand. Arrested on the third day, he also admitted to strangling his wife almost a year before and disguising her death as a drowning.[71]

Others propose a definition that excludes overt necrophilic activity and emphasizes a libidinal component. They see clinical vampirism 'as the act of drawing blood from an object (usually a love object) and receiving resultant sexual excitement and pleasure'. In this view, the sucking or drinking of blood from the wound is often an important part of the act but not an essential one. They report a case of a young man serving a prison sentence who came to the attention of prison authorities after several inmates were caught stealing iron tablets and expressed a fear of developing anaemia. The investigation showed that the young man had been trading sexual favours with these inmates in return for the opportunity to suck their blood.

Others have attempted to identify vampirism much more closely with the Dracula myth, defining it as a recognizable, although rare, clinical entity characterized by periodic compulsive blood-drinking and an affinity with the dead. Relying on the modern vampire myth, they reject associated features such as desecrating graves, violating corpses, eating human flesh or having sexual intercourse with the living. One clinical sample expressed no interest in sex; for them, blood ingestion was a compulsive behaviour that brought mental relief, though they had no ability to psychologically comprehend the experience or ascribe it any meaning.

A fourth definition involves autovampiristic behaviour. This condition is distinguished from self-mutilating behaviours, intentional suicide attempts, dramatic gestures in the context of treatment of borderline patients, and manipulative self-harm that may take place for secondary gain in prisons.

One young woman was hospitalized during her fourth pregnancy, following repeated vomiting of considerable amounts of blood. She apparently enjoyed these haemorrhages and the sight of her blood. She also voluntarily disconnected transfusion equipment, let her blood drip, and stated she would prefer to drink it. At first no investigation was able to determine the source of the bleeding. Finally a mouth examination by a specialist revealed several bleeding wounds at the base of the tongue. Staff inferred that she sucked these wounds, swallowed the blood, and then vomited. Apparently sometimes she just kept the blood in her mouth before rejecting it. Eventually she developed severe anaemia and when she died two years later, an autopsy revealed that her stomach was bloated with blood. A psychological feature of critical diagnostic importance was the patient's mythomania. It is likely that this patient suffered from the rare syndrome of *L'asthénie de Ferjol*, found exclusively in female patients, often paramedical staff, who bleed themselves surreptitiously and wrap themselves in a web of non-truths. In addition to hiding the condition, they also make up stories regarding important aspects of their lives.[72]

Regardless of which definition is adopted, overt vampiristic and autovampiristic behaviour are rare phenomena. One survey uncovered 53 cases, all but one man having acted out almost exclusively on deceased women various blends of necrophilic vampirism. An informal inquiry into the incidence of vampirism in Great Britain, mainly based on forensic mental health specialists, found seven cases, one of which was a third-hand account. Another study found four cases of vampirism, which was viewed as an all-male phenomenon as opposed to autovampirism, which is a gender-blind but predominantly female behaviour.

Dr Philip D. Jaffé, a psychologist at the University of Geneva, and Dr Frank DiCataldo of Bridgewater State Hospital, Massachusetts, report a case of clinical vampirism. They describe someone they feel warrants the full description of a 'modern vampire'. Both authors were directly involved with him at a maximum-security forensic hospital in the US.[73]

The man who was a vampire

Jeremy, currently 35 years old, was raised in a seemingly ordinary middle-class family. His father worked as an electrical engineer, and his mother was a mathematics teacher. He harbours an intense hatred of his mother and believes that her testimony sealed his conviction for the murder of his paternal grandmother. He has often alleged that his mother was physically abusive during his childhood. Descriptions of the abuse vary over time and are coloured by delusional thinking. For instance, he alleged that she belonged to a witchcraft club, when in fact she also taught astrology. During the club's occult seances, Jeremy claims that blood was drawn from him. He has openly expressed his wish to kill his mother and fantasizes about her death. He has written her letters seething with hatred from prison and from the maximum-security hospital where he now serves his sentence.

Jeremy first demonstrated his fascination with blood at the age of five when he was hospitalized with pneumonia. While convalescing, he drew pictures of hypodermic needles dripping blood and buttocks with open wounds oozing blood. In school, he drew goblins, bats, witches, and scenes of violent deaths from gunshot wounds. To this day, he paints vampires ravaging helpless females. He also became an avid reader of witchcraft literature and horror novels, including most of the classics.

His mother testified that when he was 13 he started killing

small animals, such as cats, squirrels, fish and birds, and ate them. He also became nocturnal and wandered the streets of his home town.

By the time he reached adolescence he was using illicit drugs on a daily basis and was arrested for shoplifting and vandalism. At 15 years of age, he was caught stealing a case of tear gas from the local police station. This led to the first of several court-ordered hospitalizations. After his discharge, he began showing signs of psychosis. He developed the delusion that a transmitter in his head was controlled by someone in outer space. He felt something was wrong with his head, and built and wore a cardboard pyramid in the hope that it would somehow protect and heal him. He was in and out of treatment until he was 17, when he disclosed to a therapist that he was thinking of killing his father.

After a two-week hospitalization, he returned home. However, his family was alarmed when he began keeping an axe at his bedside. They installed locks for their bedrooms and even slept in shifts so that one family member would be awake at all times. Eventually Jeremy's mother obtained a court order to remove him from the home. He moved into his own apartment and then travelled to Florida.

From Florida he called his parents, telling them that vampires were trying to kill him. A year later, at the age of 19, he returned home and lived with his family again. His mental condition deteriorated rapidly. He was unable to sleep, became withdrawn and neglected his hygiene. He reported hearing voices for the first time. These voices warned him to beware of his family and friends, because they were vampires. His interest in consuming animal and human flesh was rekindled. He killed several cats and removed their brains to see if he could learn how to correct his own brain, which he believed was dysfunctional. He also reportedly drank horse blood.

His obsession with the ingestion of blood, especially human blood, seemed to come from his belief that he could become a vampire and so escape the torment of voices in his head and be granted eternal life. Initially he obtained human blood through accidental circumstances. Later, in psychiatric hospitals, he cut elderly and infirm patients with small staples and traded sex for blood. He also bought a handgun with the intention of shooting someone to draw blood.

After another court-ordered hospitalization for killing, dissecting and eating a cat, he was released into the custody of his now-divorced father. Auditory hallucinations kept warning him that some people were vampires: they ridiculed him because he had never killed anyone and told him that to become a vampire he must kill and drink someone's blood. Furthermore, he believed that his grandmother used an ice pick to steal his blood while he slept. That she was an invalid and in a wheelchair did not shake this belief. He also believed that she was trying to poison him. A few days later, he murdered her.

Jeremy's verbatim account of the murder, in the court-ordered forensic mental health evaluation, reveals his psychotic state of mind:

> I took out a gun and painted the bullets gold. I asked my grand-mother if she wanted anything done and she said she wanted me to do the laundry. I did the laundry and asked her if she wanted any-thing else done. She said 'no.' So I put on my suit and shot her. I thought she wanted to die. When I pulled the gun on her I was sur-prised. She said 'no, no, don't do that.' But it was too late. Once I pulled the gun on her, I had to do it. I shot her in the heart, and she was wiggling and screaming at me. Then I shot her three more times real fast. Then I started saying a bunch of weird things to her real fast. I whispered in her ear something about the devil, something I had read in a witchcraft book once. I gave her the last rites and said a short prayer

The coroner's report indicates that his grandmother was also stabbed, but Jeremy has always denied this. Currently he denies drinking her blood, but at one point he admitted trying to suck her wounds but gave up because she was 'too old'.

He dragged the corpse off the sofa and into a bedroom where he poured dry gas on it. He ignited the corpse, which eventually led to the whole house catching fire. He then disposed of the gun in a nearby river, picked up his father, and drove him to his house. He was with his father when the police called to report the tragedy. Jeremy and his father drove to what remained of the torched house. Jeremy tried to enter it to retrieve a box, telling the police it contained tax returns. The box had already been confiscated by the police and contained among other things gold-painted bullets. The next day Jeremy went to the police station and forcibly tried to recover the box. A struggle ensued, and he was arrested and charged with assault and battery on a police officer. He confessed to the murder the following day.

His trial showcased a battle of mental health experts. Jeremy pleaded not guilty by reason of insanity and his lawyer introduced four expert witnesses who testified that he suffered from paranoid schizophrenia. The prosecution, in an attempt to get a murder conviction, introduced their own expert who testified that Jeremy suffered from a borderline personality disorder and was criminally responsible. The jury convicted Jeremy and he received a life sentence, with a concurrent lengthy sentence for arson.

He was sent to a maximum-security prison and managed rather well for three years on antipsychotic medication. After stopping medication, he developed the bizarre delusion that a prison officer was stealing his spinal fluid. He also believed that the left side of his body was dying, and that by consuming human flesh or spinal fluid he could reverse the process. He armed himself for protection but shortly after almost killed the prison officer he feared. Jeremy was charged with attempted murder but this time was found not guilty by reason of insanity. He was committed to a maximum-security forensic hospital. Considerable therapeutic effort has brought behavioural stability. However, he still believes he is a vampire and needs to consume human blood and flesh. There are no plans to discharge him from this hospital in the near future.

The problem for psychiatry in diagnosing this kind of behaviour is that the relationship of vampirism to psychopathology is complicated by the low incidence of this phenomenon. Psychoanalytic explanations draw attention to the early biting oral stage during which the infant uses his teeth with a vengeance.

Despite the speculative nature of this theoretic approach and regardless of whether early psychological and/or physical abuse actually takes place, it is interesting to note that psychotics often manifest persecutory delusions of incorporation, devouring and destruction. Lacking the capacity for more abstract or symbolic thought, the ingestion of blood and/or body parts may be a way for the schizophrenic psychotic to literally replenish himself. This feature may also be a more regressed manifestation of the peculiar dietary habits exhibited by some schizophrenics. Another consideration is the lack of a stable sense of self. Some schizophrenics succumb to extremely concrete forms of testing their very existence, such as cutting through the skin to determine that blood flows and merging with and living off dead or dying victims.

Other aspects often observed in schizophrenic patients and related more directly to the vampire myth are a preoccupation with mirrors (another sign of profound identity disturbance) and reversal of the day–night cycle.

The psychodynamics of vampirism are quite different for the cases featuring psychopathic and perverse personality traits. Psychopathy is a personality disorder characterized by grandiosity, egocentricity, manipulativeness, dominance, superficial emotions, poor inter-personal bonding, lack of empathy, anxiety and guilt. Psychopathic and perverse personalities carry out more integrated and organized behaviour than schizophrenics, and contact with reality appears mostly intact.

Emphasizing the strong libidinal component in vampiristic be-haviour, some psychiatrists label it a perversion. The perverse aspects can be observed in a few cases, specifically when the subject apparently draws sexual satisfaction from drinking a live victim's blood. Here, the subject's history may be the key to understanding the fixation on blood and its idiosyncratic meaning.

Depending on the actual circumstances, a strong desire to control the victim may be the most important feature. This may account for the popularity of sadomasochistic scenarios involving aspects of vampirism. In mainstream sexuality, love bites between amorous partners may be highly symbolic remnants of vampire sensuality. However, in the case of necrophilic and necrosadistic vampirism, even when cadavers are sexually violated, the link between vampirism and perversion is not clearly established.

Yet as far as vampirism is concerned, sexual behaviour appears almost completely subordinated to a destructive and sadistic drive. The cases of Jeffrey Dahmer, the Wisconsin multiple murderer of the early 1990s, and Sergeant Bertrand in the mid-1850s in France illus-trate this predominance.

When vampirism is embedded in a psychopathic personality dis-order, the potential for extremely dangerous behaviour seems to be compounded. In cases of vampirism, subjects frequently have the common childhood impulse control difficulties, are under-socialized and demonstrate an early tendency to violate limits and rules. More often than not, there is a history of animal abuse including mutilations. These features tend to persist into adulthood: lack of empathy with others becomes very noticeable, and criminalization can occur. The use of physical force and the propensity to act out on innocent victims without the capacity to foresee and without concern for unpleasant consequences create the conditions for lethal behaviour.

While there may exist medical, psychiatric or psychological explanations for real vampires, their rarity means that they cannot account for the grip on our imagination of the vampires. Not only have massively popular films and novels been created, but the theme has been exploited in serious literature by the Marquis de Sade, Goethe, Southey, Byron, Baudelaire, Keats and Coleridge. Perhaps the force of the story lies in the combination of necrophilia, necrophagia, serial killing, blood, sex, death and cannibalism. Every possible taboo is violated: the vampire is the freest of all characters to do just what he or she pleases.

But how to reconcile the combination in one character of our two most intense emotions – lust and cruelty? Well, perhaps Bram Stoker simply anticipated the modern hero who must be capable of great violent and sexual feats. He mixed this seductive cocktail with modern disillusion with religious answers to the problem of the afterlife. Vampires live on after death, but do not go to heaven or hell, an ambiguous position which is closest to how most come to terms with death in a post-religious age. The powerful paradox symbolizes the wish for life and renewal, accompanied by the hideously self-centred desire for survival, through the destruction of a living human being if necessary.

The vampire and the werewolf are among the strongest images of our times, as they are both portraits of the struggle for life at the expense of others.

2

IT TAKES TWO TO TANGO:
WHEN DELUSIONS ARE CONTAGIOUS

When you live in the shadow of insanity, the appearance of another mind that thinks and talks as yours does is something close to a blessed event.

Robert M. Pirsig, *Zen and the Art of Motorcycle Maintenance*, 1974

We have seen that beliefs about being possessed by the Devil or a demon may be delusional, but they can also be shared by others, not just in wider culture, but by many who have a close relationship with the patient. This naturally raises the thorny issue: how can a belief be a delusion if it is also widely shared by others? Delusions are meant to be the idiosyncratic production of a 'fevered mind', or in more modern parlance the confused output of disordered biochemistry found in a disturbed brain. That others could 'catch' a delusion, or share it, calls into question these biological theories, and raises the troubling issue of whether delusions can be contagious.[1]

But if you can pass on a delusion to another is it also possible to drive someone crazy 'on purpose'? This is referred to as the Gaslight Syndrome after a play in which a husband coldly and calculatedly tries to drive his wife insane – an intriguing syndrome we shall explore later in this chapter. But before that we need to address the more general issue of whether two people share a delusion they both really believe in.

Folie à deux, in which two people report the same false beliefs, was first formally reported in 1860 and then named in 1877 by French psychiatrists Laseque and Falret in a paper entitled 'La Folie à Deux ou folie communiquée' published in the *Annals of Medical Psychology*.[2] The paper described seven cases in each of which a dominant deluded person recruited a submissive 'normal' person who entered willingly into and fully participated in a deluded world.[3]

Since this paper the typical presentation has remained remarkably constant. This is usually of a dominant person (the inducer) suffering from a psychotic illness whose delusions become incorporated into the thinking of 'healthy' members of their family, and so become shared by others with varying degrees of intensity.

Commonly the recipients are not regarded as psychiatrically ill in the way the 'inducer' is, as the recipients' symptoms subside on separation from the inducer, although there are reports of the recipients also suffering from a psychotic illness needing treatment. Psychological interpretations have focused on the idea that recipients identify so closely with, or are so dependent on, the 'inducer' that they are willing to take on their ideas, no matter how bizarre.[4]

No condition illustrates more dramatically our deep need for relationships, as it seems we will even sacrifice our understanding of truth on the altar of maintaining a connection with someone who has lost their grip on reality. In order to preserve the relationship we take on their delusions, so minimizing conflict and disagreement with them.[5]

Psychiatrist Dr D. H. Ropschitz in the 1950s reported a case of *folie à deux* in which three other people came to accept delusional ideas, though two of them were already psychiatric patients.[6] In this case it was a manic-depressive doctor who affected both colleagues and patients with his grandiose thinking – a symptom itself characteristic of manic depression.

The doctor who knew best

Dr A. was a young physician with a special interest in psychiatry because of his own manic-depressive disorder. Unfortunately, his symptoms began recurring while he was visiting Ms B., an old friend and a chief nurse at a large psychiatric hospital. His former therapist was ill at home and unable to see him, and the hospital director Dr J. was vacationing in Italy. As Dr A. entered his manic phase he became loud, talkative and full of energy. He bragged that no case was too difficult for him – he possessed magical curative powers. Soon he took complete charge of the psychiatric unit and began treating patients.

Nurse B. was enchanted and followed him around in a state bordering on ecstasy, observing what she believed to be his miraculous healing gifts. She brooked no criticism from any of the staff, attributing it to petty professional jealousy. Dr A.'s first case was an ex-airline pilot who had developed a fear of flying. Over a 24-hour period the pilot was implored, threatened, lectured to and browbeaten into believing his phobia was cured. The next recipient was a man with sexual problems in his marriage who was similarly convinced that he was cured. Now Dr A., the two cured patients and Nurse B. became a mutual admiration society, the forerunners of a new era in psychiatry. They flew off to Italy to share their new discoveries with the vacationing Dr J., who, aware of Dr A.'s medical history, immediately arranged with the British Consulate to ship the quartet home. Nurse B. and Dr A. by now were uncontrollably hyperactive, euphoric and delusional.

Back at the hospital, when Dr A.'s former therapist was unable to persuade him to sign himself into the hospital voluntarily, the therapist reluctantly signed involuntary commitment papers. Now Dr A. was interviewed by a panel of psychiatrists. He talked for a solid hour without a pause, denying that he was mentally ill, accusing the panel of professional jealousy and claiming that he had royal blood which gave him special powers. He also said that he was working undercover for the British Foreign Office, which protected him from being judged by normal standards.

When Nurse B. was asked her professional opinion, she did not agree that Dr A. was ill and demanded that the panel contact the Foreign Office. When she was asked whether he would be less mentally ill if he really did work for the Foreign Office, she was silent. Finally Dr A. was sent to another psychiatric hospital, whereupon Nurse B., well into denial, claimed that she had known all along that he was psychotic. No longer under the spell of the charismatic doctor, Nurse B. and the patients soon returned to their previous selves.

Despite this extraordinary case and the close proximity of many who are in a deluded frame of mind in psychiatric hospitals, the illness of *folie à deux* has always been thought to be extremely rare. Yet it generated much interest, as in the twentieth century approximately 200 papers were written on the subject.[7] Most were concerned with the method by which delusions were transferred from one person to another. Obviously it was also possible that subclinical forms were more prevalent and might be found in isolated groups under charismatic leaderships, such as cults.

Using the nineteenth-century definition this illness had to meet the following criteria:

• the presence of a high degree of similarity in the general motif and delusional content of the partners' psychosis;
• the presence of positive evidence that the partners have been intimately associated.

Few people in close association with deluded individuals acquire their delusions. Other terms for *folie à deux*, now often known as Induced Psychotic Disorder (IPD), are (and were) infectious insanity, psychic infection, contagious insanity, collective insanity, double insanity, influenced psychoses, mystic paranoia, induced psychosis, associational psychosis, epacti psychosis and dyadic psychosis. One investigator reported 29 individuals with *folie à deux* in 1,700 consecutive admissions to a psychiatric hospital (1.7 per cent).[8] But many cases may go unnoticed because they are classified individually or because only one member of a pair is admitted. The more a hospital is oriented towards family evaluations and diagnoses, the more likely a partner in a shared psychotic disorder will be found.

Perhaps the first literary description of *folie à deux* can be found in the relationship between Don Quixote and Sancho Panza in *Don Quixote* by Miguel Cervantes, published in the early seventeenth century.[9] The nobleman, Don Quixote, represents loss of reason; his squire, Sancho Panza, is the personification of common sense. Sancho comes to be the companion of the craziest man in the world. When Don Quixote, on his deathbed, seems to regain lucidity and tries to persuade Sancho that all his previous delusions, like walking knights, do not exist, Sancho, now raving mad, answers by encouraging his master to live long in the world of his dreams. Sancho has accepted and completely shares Don Quixote's delusional ideas of greatness.[10]

Cervantes was born in Madrid in 1547 and may have become knowledgeable about psychiatry because his own life was filled with incredible situations reminiscent of those of his literary creations. In *Don Quixote*, his second novel, he provides a deep and thorough description of the delusional ideas of greatness and persecution, auditory and visual hallucinations, along with melancholia and cognitive impairment, which suggest several neuropsychiatric diseases (paranoid schizophrenia, dementia).

The influence of Cervantes on the work of writers (Borges, Dostoevsky, Joyce, Twain), musicians (Purcell, R. Strauss) and painters (Picasso) is important and well known. However, there has been little appreciation of his influence on some key figures in psychiatry, such as Freud. Certainly Freudian ideas are often used to try to explain the dynamics between two people that allows them to share a belief that is palpably untrue.[11]

Psychiatrist Dr S. J. Kiraly of the Clarke Institute of Psychiatry in Toronto reported a case of a delusion shared by a mother and daughter in the form of demonic possession, which could be explained using Freudian ideas.[12] The case could be described as arising out of the relative isolation of the daughter and mother, who came to live in a relatively closed world of their own making. Psychoanalysts maintain that because of social and psychological isolation, partners in *folie à deux* develop an excessive dependence upon each other, due to the lack of outside sources of gratification and the stabilizing influence of external reality checks.

Inevitably in a close suffocating relationship one partner becomes convinced that the other partner is taking advantage or exploiting them. The first partner's hostility remains unexpressed for fear of driving the other partner away, which would be terrifying for a dependent person. So the hostility is denied and instead is projected outwards on to others in the form of paranoid delusions. The deluded person comes to believe that others are out to get her because she is projecting her own hostility instead of recognizing it for what it is – anger at her own dependency.[13]

Because of the closeness of the relationship, if one person develops delusions the other comes under abnormal pressure to take on and believe these delusions as well. Failure to do this threatens the relationship. The problem is that once the other person accepts the delusion this is seen as triumphant proof of its reality by the first patient.

The mother and daughter who shared a delusion of possession

An 18-year-old female high school student presented at the drop-in service of the Clarke Institute of Psychiatry, accompanied by her mother. Their chief complaint was that they were hearing voices and they were controlled by an evil spirit. The patient felt herself to be under great pressure from two sources: financial difficulties at home and school exams. A week prior to admission she and her mother had started to perform experiments taken from a book of exercises related to occult phenomena. These involved a cross and a ring tied to a string dangling from the patient's finger. Both the patient and her mother felt they were gradually being 'taken over' by an archangel who later became a fallen angel or demon.

Four days before admission they heard voices and the daughter experienced involuntary movements of the hand. The spirit started to give instructions to the daughter: he wanted her to take over all the money in the world and bring it under his control. The daughter followed some of the instructions. For unknown reasons she dug a hole in their yard and beat her head against the side. She did not experience fear at the time but over the next few days both her and her mother's anxiety mounted. On the day of admission they went to the family lawyer to obtain help in contacting the publisher of the book in order to gain more information on the subject of demonology. He referred them to a radio journalist who had given lectures on the subject, and he in turn sent them to the Clarke Institute, a famous Toronto psychiatric clinic. The daughter was admitted on the same day and the mother was sent home accompanied by a nurse. As her anxiety settled with reassurance, she was treated as an outpatient by another psychiatrist.

The daughter looked younger than her age and appeared exhausted. She seemed to be vigilant, anxious and fidgety, and talked rapidly. Her intelligence, judging from her vocabulary, was judged to be average. She interrupted the interview, waved her arm and exclaimed 'There he is, doing it again . . . I do the opposite of what he wants . . . Can't you hear him?' She could not explain what the 'demon' wanted her to do but said she was influenced by an alien force and was being controlled: the demon not only moved her arm but guided her in other actions. Other delusions included fear that the demon would kill her, or harm her mother or brother, if she did not comply.

When interviewed separately, the mother and daughter gave identical descriptions of the delusions. Together, they collaborated each other's stories and interrupted one another. There was some evidence of role reversal.

The mother looked older than her stated age of 53. She was exhausted, anxious, fearful and preoccupied. She was fully oriented and alert, with no memory disturbance. Like her daughter, she claimed that the demon constantly relayed messages to her. She gave a history of auditory hallucinations which were identical to those of her daughter. She was also afraid that she would harm someone or that some harm would come to her. She was very reluctant to be separated, even temporarily, from her daughter.

Following admission the daughter's personal history was obtained with difficulty. She was born in Toronto and moved to a small town at the age of two. The family lived opposite a graveyard. Her early development was uneventful as recorded by her mother, but the patient vividly recalled some disturbing childhood memories: getting lost in a lane, almost being run over by a car and being threatened by her brother. Her brother, 18 months older, was a close playmate throughout her pre-school years. She was very close to her mother, who was overprotective; she considered her father to be distant and wrapped up in his own problems. She began school at the age of six at a girls' school. Although there were schools in their community the mother chose to send the patient to one in Toronto which necessitated 400 miles of driving per week. The mother explained that their neighbourhood was full of drug addicts and bullies.

As a teenager the patient lacked peer relationships. Her mother was overly concerned about her daughter's social life and had many sexual fears. Socially isolated, the patient attended one dance throughout her high school years. When she was about eighteen years old, she saw an advertisement in a newspaper for a book on the occult, which she purchased, hoping to solve her problems. It was not until two months later, one week prior to admission, that the mother, at the patient's invitation, also started to experiment with the occult.

The diagnosis was *folie à deux* presenting as a paranoid psychosis. In the case of the mother there was a hysterical overlay. In the daughter, the diagnosis of schizophrenia was made.

Psychiatrists feel that in *folie à deux* it is important to separate the partners and this was effectively done by hospitalizing the daughter. The mother was followed up by another psychiatrist, and made a rapid recovery. Following admission, the daughter's anxiety and thought disorder were brought under control with antipsychotic medication. The patient's delusions were accepted without argument but she was encouraged to concentrate on here and now reality and to keep active.

The family was assessed by a social worker, who confirmed that the mother was dependent, easily swayed but verbally dominant over other members of the family. The father was extremely passive. Family therapy was offered and carried on past discharge, to encourage the mother's acceptance of her daughter's activities outside the home; to help the parents overcome their own social isolation; to assist the parents in setting realistic limits to their expectations of their daughter's performance at school; to encourage them to let their daughter make her own decisions. The patient began attending school from hospital. She continued to do well on medication and there was no recurrence of delusions or thought disorder. She was discharged from hospital six weeks after admission.

In this mother–daughter relationship they were both overly involved in each other's lives. The daughter in particular seemed to have no outside interests and the mother was very dependent on the daughter. Eventually the daughter began to feel stifled and put upon so this stress probably contributed to her nervous breakdown. Given the hostile feelings towards her mother, these emotions were projected outwards on the world in general, so explaining her paranoid delusions involving the view that the world contained danger to her. But the illness also served a useful function in that it helped to bind the mother to her because she was now ill and needed looking after. It also helped shift the balance of the relationship a little so that the daughter could rely on her mother a bit more for help rather than the other way around. It is this kind of dynamic which is thought to underpin many *folie à deux*-type delusions.

A recent viewpoint supports the idea that there is no difference in the quality and content of *folie à deux* if the partners are not blood related. As early as 1880 the syndrome was noted in non-genetically-related groups such as husband and wife, and this surprised early clinicians, who until then had explained almost all mental illness on the basis of hereditary taint. *Folie à deux* came to be called 'morbid interpsychology', a disorder previously unknown.[14]

In the 1950s terms such as 'mental contagion' were introduced, and within a decade the illness was divided into four categories: the *forme imposée* – cases in which delusions were transferred from a mentally ill person to a previously healthy person; *forme simulantée* – cases in which partners became deluded together without either one initiating the process: *forme communiquée* – in which the recipient of the delusion went on to elaborate on the delusions after separation from the inducer; *forme induite* – cases occurring within insane asylums.[15]

Psychiatrists Dr Landrum S. Tucker and Dr Thomas P. Cornwall of the University of North Carolina School of Medicine, Chapel Hill, North Carolina, recently reported the case of a mother and son plotting to murder the father.[16]

A homicide pact between a mother and son

Bobby A. is a 10-year-old boy who was admitted to a juvenile psychiatric unit after he had been detained for allegedly burning down his father's house. Two years before this admission Bobby's parents had been divorced after a stormy marriage of 18 years. His mother's own mother had been diagnosed as paranoid schizophrenic and her older brother was felt to be 'somewhat strange'. Mrs A. had always felt 'very close' to her mother. Her father was a hard-working man who was away from home often, including an absence of several years during Mrs A.'s adolescence when he was out of the country. During that time he became extremely ill and almost died.

When Bobby was born, Mrs A. felt 'abandoned' by her husband because he was away on business just as her father had been. She was depressed for some time. Bobby was a healthy child, met all developmental milestones and did well during his early school years. When he was eight his parents separated and divorced, and he and his mother moved to a town nearby.

Six months prior to admission, Bobby and his mother moved to the west coast, where they lived in various cities for short periods and kept to themselves. She began to tell Bobby that his father wanted to kill them. She started staying up all night with Bobby, telling him that Mr A. had put razor blades in their beds, cut her hair and poisoned their pets. Bobby did not believe his mother at first since he knew his father was living across the country, but he was afraid to disagree for fear that his mother might hurt him.

Slowly Bobby began to feel his mother was right and they began to plot to murder Mr A. They decided to burn down his home while he slept. After several months of planning Bobby flew alone across

75

the country to his father's home town and set his father's house ablaze that night. Mr A. barely escaped in his nightclothes and Bobby was found by the police walking away from the flames. Mrs A. returned to the state and was placed in a mental institution.

When Bobby was seen initially he was very anxious, with poor eye contact. In therapy he drew a spaceship heading towards a large sun. From the ship came a cord that attached to a small ship. Bobby said the smaller ship went ahead of the big ship to check things out. He was concerned that the big ship's outer shell was melting away. The mission of the ships was to destroy the sun, but they were being destroyed. Bobby wished the ship could get back to earth safely. In addition to individual therapy Bobby was treated by therapeutic milieux, including school and recreation. One especially important factor in his treatment, a point that has been stressed before, was separation from his mother. On the ward Bobby was at first over-controlled, polite and bright (his IQ was above average). In the first few weeks he was inadvertently allowed to receive two letters from his mother, and at those times he again manifested severe anxiety.

After two months the themes in Bobby's play began to change. He staged recurrent battles using a giant soldier from outer space who came with a flamethrower to destroy a 'special' house full of smaller soldiers. He talked directly of his fear of his mother and his disbelief that he could have had the 'crazy' thoughts about his father being so bad. At this time his thoughts were organized and he was relaxed and more open with his feelings.

At the end of three months, Bobby had shown no overt psychosis for several weeks and so, after careful consideration, he was sent home to his father. His father had worked closely with the hospital, including participation in weekly individual therapy. In the nine months of Bobby's outpatient therapy since discharge he has moved from battles to playing checkers and talking about school and activities. Bobby also has begun writing songs. His first one said, 'I'm lonely since I left you – but I've got my feet back on the ground.' Bobby is doing above-average work in school, participates in sports, has made friends and gets along well with his father. His mother remains hospitalized.

Past efforts at explaining criminal activities involving a *folie à deux* situation have focused on the projection of delusions by a psychotic, more intelligent, dominant partner on a less intelligent, passive partner who identifies with the dominant one. Certainly, some of this is evident here. Another factor in this case is a 'fit' in the dominant and passive partners' unconscious motivations: the wish to kill the father figure in order to possess the mother. Bobby wished to destroy his father to win an Oedipal victory while Ms A., so strongly attached to her own mother psychologically, wished to destroy her father symbolically to gain a negative Oedipal victory. In the regression to psychosis both acted on their unconscious wish to destroy the father figure, while the conscious delusion was that he wanted to destroy them.

These Freudian ideas are based on the notion that the pre-existing intensity of the relationship is a vital factor and this could explain why induced psychosis is surprisingly rare among non-related patients in psychiatric hospitals. After all, one would have thought that those most vulnerable to delusional thinking would transmit delusions to each other readily, but this does not appear to happen at all frequently. More than 90 per cent of the reported cases in the literature are of related individuals. The most common relationships are, in descending order, two sisters, husband and wife, mother and child, two brothers, brother and sister, pairs of friends and whole families.

Dr Adriana Neagoe, a psychiatrist at the Boston University Medical Center, reported the following intriguing case of a *folie à deux* – which was pieced together after the death of one of the couple, though they appeared also to have had a suicide pact arranged.[17]

The man who believed that he and his wife had been abducted by aliens

The 'inducer' in this case, Mr J., is a 46-year-old Catholic widower who referred himself to the Emergency Department in the middle of the night, and was voluntarily hospitalized because he was suicidally depressed. A junior salesman, he was living in a public shelter. Following admission, he said his wretchedness was caused by the first anniversary of the death of his second wife, Cathy. He had been depressed for periods of time at the age of 17 and in his twenties, and was hospitalized for severe depression and attempted suicide following an overdose when aged 37 on the first anniversary of the death of his first wife, Linda.

He had never seen a psychiatrist before. He had no known previous family history of psychiatric problems and he was proud that he was the only one in the family to obtain a college education in the form of a degree in mathematics. He grew up in a rural area and described long-standing conflicts with his family due to their 'low level of education' compared to himself. However, Mr J. seemed only to have held down jobs that were of a much lower level than would be expected from someone of his educational background, like being a taxi driver and a flower delivery man. Yet he had always harboured the desire to discuss existential issues and had wanted to be a priest when he was younger. He had never pursued this ambition because he was too depressed about being away from home. Indeed in the last few years he had lost his faith and now described himself as an atheist.

He met his first wife, Linda, in high school and married her when in college. After 15 years of marriage, Linda died from a post-surgery embolism. His father-in-law had always blamed Mr J. for the death of his only child because Mr J. had not advised Linda to go to see the surgeon sooner. Mr J.'s guilt roused by this accusation led to his suicide attempt and to his first psychiatric admission. Soon after this he met Cathy and they were married two years later. For the next six years until her death she was bedridden with a severe form of juvenile onset arthritis. During this time he provided 24-hour care.

It was during this enforced isolation from the outside world that a shared delusion developed. Mr J. and information from 19 audiotape recordings he made of his wife's recollections document an elaborate delusion involving UFOs and aliens on the part of Cathy and Mr J., whose interest in UFOs dated back to his high school years.

He claimed to have seen a UFO with his first wife, although she did not share this belief or his idea of a possible 'reunion through UFOs' after death. He reported that he had lost interest in UFOs after Linda's death and resumed the study of them four years into his marriage with Cathy. Following Cathy's death he moved to another state where he found a job as a grocery store salesman. He planned to save money for psychotherapy sessions with a local expert who wrote popular and controversial books about 'alien abductions'.

When examined by psychiatrists Mr J. was depressed and unable to talk about his second wife without tears. He had a suicidal plan on the night of his admission, believing there would be a '50 per cent possibility of joining his second wife on another planet or a UFO' if he jumped off a high building.

During his hospital stay, when he and his psychiatrist listened to the tapes of Cathy, he spoke about the terminal period of his wife's life with considerable detachment. During ward rounds, he appeared more like a scientist, repeatedly returning to his haunting by UFOs. He felt an obligation to share with professionals his and his wife's extraordinary experience: it gave a purpose to the rest of his life. He appeared enthusiastic when visited by one of his six friends, all alien believers. He was started on mood-stabilizing and antipsychotic medication and his depression and suicidal planning rapidly improved. However, his fixed belief in aliens remained.

Data from her husband and the tapes enabled a 'psychological autopsy' of Cathy. She grew up the only child of a middle-class family and graduated from college with a degree, majoring in psychology. She was a social worker in her home city for many years and was 39 years old, single and living alone when she met Mr J., who was two years younger. Cathy was diagnosed with juvenile rheumatoid arthritis when she was still a teenager. After two years of friendship, they decided to marry despite the grave prognosis of her illness. Mr J. described their marriage as perfect, as they never argued and Cathy never opposed him. He said they shared the same enjoyment of reading. Neither had ever used alcohol or drugs.

Two years before Cathy's death, Mr J. began to show her pictures of aliens who resembled owls and discovered that she was very afraid of owls. She began to experience a nightmare in which she screamed out her 'memories' of alien abduction. Mr J. asked her interview-like questions to elicit more information and recorded the 19 tapes while she was 'sleeping' and speaking loudly with wide-open eyes. She remembered nothing in the morning, but when confronted with the tapes, Cathy and Mr J. elaborated the conviction that she was an alien, born 3,000 years ago. Furthermore, Mr J. had met and married her because aliens induced him to do so, as he was the right person to help her 'remember'. The couple then came to believe they were in contemporary contact with aliens. During an average day, nothing happened by chance; for example, if they could not find an object in the house, it was a sign 'They' exist.

They both saw objects disappearing and reappearing in their house. Mr J. said that when one day an aide asked Cathy to prove she was in contact with aliens two objects spontaneously and simultaneously dropped off her bed in front of everyone, which shocked them. Later, Mr J. came to believe that he might also have been abducted thousands of years ago and might currently be an alien himself. Cathy asked her husband to help her die if she were ever in extreme pain and signed a will to attest to this. Mr J. had a plan to press a pillow against her face when the moment of extreme suffering came and then to kill himself by jumping off the building. This did not happen because Cathy died peacefully in hospital.

Six months after his discharge from hospital when he was seen by psychiatrists again for a follow-up appointment his mood seemed to have remained stable since his discharge. When his psychiatrist told him that his chart and notes were missing he suggested that some day the chart would reappear, making reference to the aliens' manner of becoming noticed on earth. He was somehow right: his chart 'miraculously' reappeared in the next few days, returned from the outpatient clinic where he had had a follow-up visit for his diabetes.

Although these partners largely shared the same content of their delusion, it had bizarre, persecutory qualities in Cathy's case, as indicated by her unpleasant 'nightmares'. For Mr J. the delusion seemed linked to a sense of grandiosity. The belief that Cathy was a child abducted 3,000 years ago who later came to Earth as an alien with human appearance has a superficial similarity to the Capgras delusion (see Chapter 14) in that there is the same delusional denial of the authenticity of the identity of a clearly recognized person. The cosmic content of the delusion seems to be shaped by a theme from popular culture of alien abduction and 'spirit possession' found in other so-called more primitive cultures.

Shared religious delusions pose a high fatal risk in suicide pacts between family members. Here the similarity with the religious types of delusion is worrying: the aliens replace God and a UFO or a mysterious planet replaces heaven (a place of rest when one dies).

In *folie à deux* one theory is that the recipient learns abnormal behaviour from the inducing dominant partner and subsequently begins to behave and think psychotically. From this learning theory perspective Cathy could not ignore certain habitual behaviour of her husband, such as his interest in literature about aliens and his fascination with strange pictures of aliens whose faces resembled owls. From wondering about her owl phobia to constructing a false belief about aliens was probably only a step. When no corrections to these fantasies were forthcoming because of her seclusion, for Cathy the borders between reality and imagination could have become increasingly blurred.

Picturing Cathy in her submissive bedridden position accepting and building upon the delusion of her husband to preserve their gratifying relationship is not difficult. Her childish screams on the tapes provide evidence of the regression she may have experienced as a result of her physical disability, her psychological isolation and her possible depression. We can observe how in fantasy Cathy achieves her wish for attachment; however, the result is a pathological one in that she follows Mr J.'s delusion and contributes to its elaboration from her own repertory of childhood events.

The circular character of *folie à deux* described in the literature applies in this case too, so 'shared psychotic disorder' is more accurate than 'induced psychotic disorder'. The circular causality of the phenomenon makes the terms inducer and inductee somewhat blurred and the delusion itself is elaborated by both partners until it is owned by them as a believable symbiotic reaction. Mr J., who on his own had never before thought he might be an alien, came to believe it through the couple's mutual delusion.

Mr J. shared his delusion with six peers, which saved him from total withdrawal. We don't know the degree to which the six friends shared and accepted his beliefs but the bond was strong enough for one of them to visit him in a locked psychiatric unit. The current endeavour of Mr J. to make public the extraordinary experience he shared with his wife seems to be the sole meaning of his life. The narrow focus of his preoccupation prevents him from forming connections with people other than those who fit into this unique purpose. His parents and sibling are almost non-existent for him and his belief in God now has no meaning for the former good Catholic who wanted to become a priest. This progressive limitation in so many areas leads to a reduction of personality and to an investment in a single belief system, which if overturned can pave the way to suicide or a suicide pact.

Suicide pacts are not found only between husbands and wives. For example, cases of *folie à deux* among identical twins were first reported in 1947, and in these the dominant and submissive dynamic interpretation applied and might still apply today, as witnessed in the recent sad example of a suicide pact between twin brothers in Britain. Paul Dane helped his depressed twin brother commit suicide as part of a tragic pact but was spared jail by a Judge John Phillips at Carlisle Crown Court in September 2001. Dane, 20, agreed to help his brother Kevin take his own life by providing the tools to enable him to hang himself from the ceiling of his bedroom at their family home after their worried mother insisted they sign on for unemployment benefits.

The attempt to strangle himself with his own belt failed and Paul Dane was found by his father 'trembling' in front of his dead brother's body. Dane was sentenced to a three-year community rehabilitation order, with the judge commenting: 'The circumstances surrounding this case are tragic, difficult and to some extent unexplainable.' At an earlier hearing Dane, now 21, had admitted aiding and abetting the suicide of his brother. He was comforted by his sister in the dock as he listened to the judge explain how Dane had helped drill holes in a beam in Kevin's bedroom for the noose before feeding the rope through. Police interviews suggested that, independently, both Dane and his brother had attempted to take their own lives before this but had not succeeded.

Encouraging them to pursue a more normal life, their parents set a deadline by which they were to sign on to look for work. The twins regarded this as an invasion of their voluntary social isolation and on 3 October, the deadline set by the parents, their father found Kevin's body. In the years leading up to the tragedy the pair had led an 'unremarkable' life. Kevin decided to go to college but after a year he left and went to work in a biscuit factory in Carlisle. When the contract ended the twins gradually became more reclusive, venturing out of their locked rooms only at night, when they would 'converse, eat and watch television'. The reasoning behind their social exclusion appeared to be rooted in a mental disorder.

Certain distinguishing characteristics of suicide pacts have been described. A study of 58 completed suicide pacts in England and Wales between 1955 and 1958 found the majority, 72 per cent, were of spouses with an average age of 58. Only two cases were between friends. Previous attempted suicide was found in 10 per cent of cases. In another study only one out of 12 cases involved adults of the same sex. The interdependence of pact victims and their isolation from family and community have also been noted. Normally the presence of another person protects the subject from yielding to the suicidal urge but in suicide pacts each partner acts on the other, intensifying the urge so that it is the unit that kills itself and not the partner acting individually. They act as one.[18]

Although *folie à deux* is the most frequently encountered example of an induced psychosis, extended conditions involving more individuals or even whole families (*folie à trois*, *quatre*, *cinque*, etc. and *folie à famille*) may occur, though these are extremely rare.[19]

Robert Bryant, a lecturer in psychology at the University of New South Wales, Australia, recently reported the following case of *folie à famille* in which seven members of a family shared varying delusional beliefs.[20]

The family who 'caught' paranoia

The father was a 62-year-old Serbian-born man who lived with his wife, mother-in-law and four children. He reported that 15 years earlier he and his family had developed an array of physical symptoms following spraying of weed-killing chemicals in a property adjacent to their home by a government department. He reportedly developed headaches, skin rash, vomiting, diarrhoea and chest pains. The father reported that soon after the onset of these symptoms he attempted to seek medical assistance for his family. But, he said, doctors refused to treat his family. Independent evidence indicates that the spraying did occur and that the father did initially develop the reported symptoms. Although medical examination indicated that these symptoms abated after a short period, the father maintained that they persisted.

He received considerable medical attention but did not believe it was adequate. In the following months the doctors advised that he was not suffering a physical disorder so he began to wonder if the government intended to prevent him from receiving treatment. He became more convinced that the perceived inadequacy of the doctors to treat him was evidence of a government conspiracy against his family. He believed that the government was intentionally spraying Agent Orange as part of an experiment to evaluate the lethal effects of chemical poisoning.

The father also believed that three doctors who had agreed to assist the family had been killed. He contended that a hospital existed to treat victims of the chemical poisoning but that this was reserved for government employees involved in the experiments. He also maintained that the government was engineering a nationwide conspiracy of secrecy. He reported a greater sense of control after realizing that his poor health was a result of this conspiracy because he felt that his symptoms and the doctors' reluctance to treat him were now attributable to a salient cause.

Subsequently he felt more mastery over his situation because he believed that he could now take steps to protect himself and seek help elsewhere. In the ensuing years, the father reportedly developed a range of physical symptoms, including headaches, pain across the centre of the chest, pain behind the eyes, pain in all joints, urinary incontinence, diarrhoea, flatulence, dizziness, difficulty breathing and dry throat. Medical evidence did not substantiate any of this. Repeated medical tests indicated no organic basis for these reported symptoms. The father interpreted these reports as further evidence of the conspiracy between doctors against his family. In the ensuing 15 years he consulted medical specialists from many countries because he believed that local doctors would be prevented from helping the family.

Although the overwhelming medical opinion was that the father did not suffer a physical disorder, he did obtain some reports that were consistent with his beliefs, but only from obscure medical authorities in less developed countries. He had been referred to several psychiatrists, and a diagnosis of paranoid schizophrenia had been established. It was noted that whereas he had initially suffered transient physical symptoms following exposure to the spraying, these symptoms were short-lived and were supplanted by hypochondriacal delusional beliefs that involved a wide array of physical symptoms that were inconsistent with medical assessments following toxic exposure.

The father was the second of three children and although his family grew up under a totalitarian communist regime in Serbia, they were not allied with the Communist Party. As a result, they were constantly persecuted by government authorities. His family was denied vocational opportunities, material benefits and had little independence. He explained that he grew up with a strong suspicion of government agencies. His family had emigrated from Serbia when he was 30 years old to escape the government oppression. Approximately a year before the spraying, he had suffered a back injury that impeded his ability to work. He reported that he experienced marked guilt at the time because of his inability to provide for his family.

At the time of spraying, the children were aged 6 to 12 years, and the mother and grandmother were 37 and 60 years old, respectively. The two women developed similar beliefs: they reported that the family was suffering severe illness because of intentional government poisoning as part of a widespread conspiracy against the family. The children were reared in social isolation in which the family's physical symptoms were the focus of all activities.

Consistent with a *folie à deux*, each member of the family reported an identical constellation of physical symptoms. The family was repeatedly informed by the father that they were experiencing major health risks as a result of the poisons. He had convinced them that the eldest son had a malignant tumour and that his life was at risk. Each of the family members claimed that their poor health precluded occupational, social, sexual or leisure activities.

A key issue is that this family was from abroad and so was relatively isolated from social life by language barriers and cultural differences. This might make reality testing more difficult and as paranoid people tend to keep moving to get away from persecutors the delusion can become self-sustaining. This theme recurs in the Gaslight Syndrome, where a person who is deeply dependent on another fails to see that the other is in fact trying to drive them mad.

In 1939 Patrick Hamilton, an English playwright, wrote *Gas Light* in which he described a husband's attempt to force his wife into a 'lunatic asylum' by convincing not only her friends and those around her but even herself that she was insane. This behaviour pattern has not received attention in the psychiatric literature until recently.

Gas Light's plot is simple. It is set in Victorian London and the title symbolizes the terrifying darkness of the late afternoon in winter. Mr Manningham, the husband, is a dictatorial rogue with a mysterious past. Mrs Manningham, dependent and excessively childlike, is afraid that her husband might be correct and that she is mad. Nancy, the female servant, is sexually involved with the husband so would like the wife to be committed and out of the way. Rough, a retired police inspector, achieves resolution by rescuing Mrs Manningham and ensuring that Mr Manningham gets his just deserts.

Mr Manningham is condescending, treats his wife as a child, flirts with others in her presence, teases her sexually and intellectually and then denies the behaviour which his wife witnesses. Mrs Manningham has feelings of inferiority, is naively over-trusting, yet is suspicious of her husband's possible sexual indiscretions but without really facing their reality. She wants to retain her husband at all costs even if it means being mad. He exploits her publicly, frustrates her strivings for independence, denies her view of reality and interprets her environment to her in such a way that she is totally confused.

He creates situations which show up her madness: for example, he hides a picture and accuses her of losing it. He communicates with her in a domineering confusing way. In one breath he orders her to her room, then when she mildly protests he denies that he has done so. The pattern of a domineering sadistic partner and a dependent masochistic one is clearly drawn. Nancy the maid's sexual reason for wishing to end the marital relationship is unmistakable and the nature of the distorted communication is spelled out. They share the essential features of Gaslight Syndrome, the outcome of which is the labelling of the dependent partner as mentally ill and her removal to a mental institution.

Dr Cawthra and psychiatrist colleagues at the Department of Psychiatry at the Royal Victoria Infirmary, Newcastle, reported the following case of Gaslight Syndrome, or what they refer to as imposed psychosis.[21]

Mrs A. is a 52-year-old widow who first presented in the hospital's Accident and Emergency Department, when she expressed distress about the sudden disappearance, three months previously, of her 22-year-old daughter.

On further enquiry she stated that over a period of 6 years her late husband's spirit had returned to her house, brought her flowers and often rearranged the contents of cupboards. At times the spirit would criticize Mrs A. for her unsatisfactory housework and had even struck her on the head and pushed her by the shoulder. He also took her daughter's clothes out of her wardrobe and laid them on the bed for her. Each day he would engage the two of them in conversation and sometimes create a great deal of noise in the house by banging on doors and cupboards. Mrs A. claimed that her daughter witnessed these events, but since her disappearance her husband's spirit had not visited again.

Mrs A. also claimed that her daughter worked for famous private doctors and, through this work, had spoken to Prince Charles and Princess Diana. Indeed, her daughter claimed that she was Princess Diana's friend and that she had met Prince William when he was six weeks old.

Mrs A. was asked to attend a psychiatric case conference, following which it was agreed that her symptoms were suggestive of a psychotic illness, possibly a kind of late onset schizophrenia otherwise known as paraphrenia.

On the day of her admission into hospital Mrs A. was given antipsychotic medication and, in view of her concern about her daughter, an attempt was made to contact the young woman. Two weeks later, Mrs A.'s daughter, Miss B., telephoned the hospital to enquire about her mother's health. She insisted, however, that her mother was not told of her whereabouts as she was attempting to build a life of her own away from home. Miss B. claimed that her mother had prevented her from leaving home and had stopped her from claiming unemployment benefit. However, in the year before she left, Miss B. had begun to claim her unemployment pay and told her mother that this money was earned from her work with famous private doctors. To direct questioning about her late father, Miss B. stated that his spirit had returned and had spoken to both her mother and herself. She also confirmed her mother's contention that the spirit had rearranged various articles in the house.

During a further conversation with Miss B. she was asked about her mother's reference to Princess Diana and Prince William. Miss B. admitted that she had never met them but had told her mother that the doctor she worked for knew them. Miss B. agreed that she may have given the impression that she also knew them personally. She eventually admitted too that she had never worked for private doctors.

In order that this mother/daughter relationship might be more accurately assessed, Miss B. was invited to meet with doctors so that they could obtain a detailed psychiatric history and gather information about her mother.

Towards the end of this meeting, Miss B. was asked specifically about her father's spirit. Initially, she reiterated that her father's spirit had returned and added that he sometimes left notes of instruction for her mother. However, after she had been asked to confide in the doctors, and after being assured that what she told them would be held in the strictest confidence, Miss B. suddenly became distressed and tearful. She then admitted that she had been speaking in her father's voice to make it appear as if her father was talking to her mother and herself. She also confessed to rearranging things in the house and to leaving notes for her mother that were ostensibly written by her father.

Miss B. gave a number of reasons for doing these things. She was afraid of her mother and felt she could not cope with her by herself; she needed more freedom for herself, and in the notes supposedly written by her father explanations were given for her absence from home during the day.

Formal assessment of Miss B. revealed no mental illness. Indeed, she was of average intelligence and co-operative. Her history, however, showed that her earliest childhood memories were of feuding parents; they shouted at each other and these disagreements frequently culminated in violence. This was the situation until her parents separated when Miss B. was 8 or 9 years old. Her father died two years later of a brain tumour and, although Miss B. stated that she cried after he died, before his death she had experienced feelings of anger towards him for the way he had treated her mother. However, she admitted that her father had never mistreated her and after his death she held fond memories of him.

With regard to her mother, Miss B. stated that when she was 12 years old her mother began threatening to put her into a children's home because she would then be free to get a job, sell her house and move away if necessary. This led Miss B. to feel vulnerable and insecure.

With regard to Mrs A.'s own history, she recalled that starting school and separating from her own mother had been extremely difficult. As a child, Mrs A. was only able to remain at school when she was secure in the reassuring knowledge that her mother would be at the school gates to see her at both break- and lunch-time. Mrs A. also recalled that her father would do some of the housework at weekends because her mother was extremely tired. Her mother's fatigue was seen as further evidence of unswerving dedication to attending and caring for her. At the age of eleven, Mrs A. refused to sit the 11-plus examination, which both her elder siblings had passed. She recalled being terrified of failing, but was unable to connect this with her mother's high hopes and, indeed, expectation that her children should do well in life.

When Mrs A.'s daughter was born, she was nursed in an incubator for the first two weeks of life. During this time Mrs A. was constantly afraid that her daughter would die. She never really understood what was wrong with her baby, and held a grudging resentment towards the medical profession for the way she was treated at the time. Mrs A. also stated that when her daughter wished to leave home in her late teens, she was totally unable to understand why she would want to do so, other than to marry or to find employment.

It is of particular significance that Mrs A.'s mother was a spiritualist and during her late teens she attended seances. She would go with her mother to spiritualist meetings where attempts were made to contact the dead.

Within a few days of her admission into hospital, Mrs A. began to have doubts about whether what she was told by her daughter was true, and she also started to have doubts about the return of her husband's spirit. She was puzzled by the disappearance of her husband's spirit the moment her daughter left home. Mrs A.'s subsequent history showed her to be free of all psychotic phenomena, but she remained angry and deeply embittered to the point of tears about her daughter's reluctance to remain in contact with her. This was despite the fact that she had been informed that Miss B. had telephoned the hospital on a number of occasions to ask the staff to reassure her mother that she was well.

Mrs A.'s life history also showed that she had severe difficulties in the process of individuation and separation. She experienced marked difficulty in starting school and in separating from her mother (whom she idealized as a totally devoted mother) and her teachers were seen as frightening authority figures. Indeed, Mrs A. idealized the mother/daughter relationship as one in which there is little or no room for separateness.

Mrs A.'s belief that her husband was visiting her from the grave seemed to serve the function of attempting to provide a solution to a complex dilemma for both mother and daughter. The 'voices' appeared to provide both with comfort and acted as a defence against depressive anxieties to do with loss and separateness.

Two further factors seem to contribute towards an understanding of why Miss B. invoked the idea of the return of her father's spirit: first, when Miss B. was 14 years old, her mother mentioned that she thought a spirit was in their house and that this was either the spirit of Mrs A.'s mother, who had died the year before, or of her husband; second, Miss B. had heard from a girlfriend who experienced her own late mother's spirit rearranging things in her house, and how this presence had been comforting to her.

This case study demonstrates that it is possible that the spreading of mental illness, or the induction of it, can serve a psychological function within a relationship. But how can this apply to situations where the abnormal mental state spreads like wildfire through a whole community? This phenomenon occurs with the extremely strange and intriguing syndrome of epidemic hysteria.

Epidemic hysteria is most commonly reported in small, cohesive social units within enclosed settings, such as schools and factories. There are two types of hysterical reaction in groups: anxiety and motor hysteria. Anxiety hysteria has a rapid onset and recovery period, usually 24 hours, and is precipitated by the sudden perception of a threatening agent, typically a strange odour or the rumour of contaminated food. Common symptoms include headache, dizziness, nausea, hyperventilation and general fatigue.

Essentially, these are physiological reactions to sudden anxiety.

Mass motor hysteria incubates more slowly than anxiety hysteria, and it develops in an atmosphere of accumulating long-term group stress. It is prevalent in intolerable social settings, most commonly in schools enforcing extreme disciplinary measures. Symptoms include altered states of consciousness, melodramatic acts of rebellion (histrionics), and psychomotor agitation whereby anxiety that builds up over long periods results in disruptions to the nerves or neurons, triggering temporary bouts of muscle twitching, spasms and shaking. Symptoms appear gradually and usually take weeks or months to subside. There were numerous reports of school and factory episodes of this type in Western countries before the mid-twentieth century, associated with strict educational policies or dehumanizing factory conditions before the rise of unions. Modern reports are rare except in non-Western schools and factories, where episodes remain prevalent under strict capitalist discipline or academic regulation coupled with limited or non-existent channels for the expression of grievances.

In theory, both motor and anxiety hysteria can be alleviated by removing the stressful agent. This may be easier said than done, due to the emotionally charged nature of many outbreaks and the difficulty often encountered in convincing sceptical group members. In anxiety hysteria, the key is to persuade those affected that the 'toxic' agent has either been eliminated or never existed. Episodes of motor hysteria are frequently interpreted by the affected group as confirming the presence of demonic forces, making it vital to convince group members that the offending 'spirits' have been eliminated or appeased.

Collective frenetic emotional displays labelled as mass hysterical outbreaks have been recorded in Japan in particular, in 1705, 1771, 1830 and 1867. These coincided with oppressive feudal regimes and accompanying social crises. These events were identified as a combination of hysteria and ritual through which collective catharsis was achieved under the guise of *okage-mairi*, a custom involving a pilgrimage to give thanks to the Sun Goddess. Outbreaks were characterized by collective frenetic dancing, crying, singing, obscene and bizarre behaviour, amnesia, trance states and transient ailments.[22]

Stress frequently plays an important role in cases of mass hysteria. Japanese youth are under tremendous academic and social pressures to achieve; students with low or mediocre grades have been known to kill themselves. However, reports of mass hysteria among

Japanese students are relatively rare and the incidents reported are linked to sudden anxiety from strange odours.

Stress as a cause is also problematic. Groups of people are under great stress all the time, including platoons of soldiers and communities experiencing floods or famine, yet there are few if any reports of mass hysteria affecting these people. Why? Because extraordinary stress *per se* does not and cannot trigger epidemic hysteria. Psychosocial stress occurs in combination with a specific context in which there is a perceived harmful agent.

Benjamin Radford of the Center for Inquiry in Amherst, New York, and Dr Robert Bartholomew, a psychologist at the University of North Queensland in Australia, recently reported on a mass psychogenic illness outbreak on 16 December 1997, involving more than 12,000 Japanese children. They had various signs and symptoms of illness after watching an episode of a popular animated cartoon, *Pokémon*. While photosensitive epilepsy was diagnosed in a minuscule fraction of those affected, this explanation cannot account for the breadth and pattern of the events. The features of the episode are consistent with the diagnosis of epidemic hysteria, triggered by sudden anxiety after dramatic mass media reports describing a relatively small number of genuine photosensitive-epilepsy seizures. The case indicates the importance of the mass media in precipitating such outbreaks.[23]

The word Pokémon is a shortening of the term 'pocket monsters', from the original Japanese name *poketto monsuta*. It was created in 1996 as a video game for the hand-held Nintendo Game Boy system and within a few months became a bestseller. A television cartoon version of the game débuted in Japan on 1 April 1997. Sales of Pokémon products generate more than $1 billion annually for Nintendo. Pokémon has become a global icon that is so popular in the United States that *Time* magazine featured it on the cover of a 1999 edition. The TV cartoon centres on young boys and girls who wander the world of Pokémon looking for small creatures (Pokémon) to capture, befriend, and train for battle against other trainers (and their Pokémon). The ultimate goal is for the children to collect one of every 'species' and become Pokémon Masters. There are at least 151 Pokémon characters, each with unique powers and individual personalities. The most popular character, Pikachu, resembles a yellow rat and has the ability to shock opponents with electricity.

EPISODE 38

At 6.30 p.m. on 16 December 1997, *Pokémon* episode 38, 'Dennou Senshi Porigon' (Computer Warrior Polygon), aired in Japan on TV Tokyo. The programme gained the highest ratings for its time slot, with an average market share of about 15 per cent. In the episode, Pikachu and its human friends Satoshi, Kasumi and Takeshi have an adventure that leads them inside a computer. About 20 minutes into the programme, the group encounters a fighter named Polygon. A battle ensues, during which Pikachu uses electric powers to stop a 'virus bomb'. The animators depict Pikachu's electric attack with a quick series of flashing lights.

Millions watched the programme. In one city, Toyohashi, more than 70 per cent of the 24,000 elementary school students and 35 per cent of the 13,000 junior high school students watched the programme. In Tokyo, the Kawasaki education board investigated all public kindergartens and primary and middle schools in the area and found that 50,174 students, or 55 per cent of the children, watched the episode.

At 6.51 p.m. the flashing lights of Pikachu's 'attack' appeared on television screens. By 7.30 p.m., according to Japan's Fire Defence Agency, 618 children had been taken to hospitals complaining of various symptoms. News of the illnesses spread rapidly throughout Japan and became the subject of media reports later that evening. During the coverage, several stations replayed the flashing sequence, whereupon even more children fell ill and sought medical attention. The number affected by this 'second wave' is unknown. Reported symptoms included convulsions, altered levels of consciousness, headaches, breathlessness, nausea, vomiting, blurred vision and general malaise.

The following day TV Tokyo issued an apology, suspended the programme and said it would investigate the cause of the seizures. The programme's producers were questioned by police about the cartoon's contents and production process. The Japanese Health and Welfare Ministry held an emergency meeting, discussing the case with experts and gathering information from hospitals. Video retailers across Japan removed the series from their shelves.[24]

Outraged mothers accused TV Tokyo of ignoring their children's health in the quest for ratings; other parents called for the implementation of an electronic screening device to block intense animation. Japanese Prime Minister Ryutaro Hashimoto expressed concern, stating, 'Rays and lasers have been considered for use as weapons. Their effects have not been fully determined.' Although a Nintendo representative quickly explained that the only link between its game and the cartoon was the characters, the company's shares immediately dropped nearly 5 per cent on the Tokyo stock market. TV Tokyo also placed warning labels on all future and past *Pokémon* episodes.[25]

Bright, flashing lights have been known to trigger seizures in epileptics. In 1994, British commercial television advertisements and programmes were limited to a rate of three flashes per second following an incident in which a noodle advertisement featuring fast-moving graphics and bright flashes triggered three seizures. After several teenagers had seizures while playing Nintendo video games, the company began including warning labels on much of its software. The notice stated that the games' graphics and animation could cause a *shigeki*, a strong stimulation resulting in unconsciousness or seizures.[26]

The *Pokémon* case was of concern. But although bright flashes seemed to be the likely culprit, these had been used hundreds of times before without incident. The use of different coloured lights flashing alternately to create tension is common in the distinctive Japanese animation technique used in *Pokémon* (and many other cartoons). 'During editing, that particular portion didn't call my attention or bother me,' producer Takemoto Mori said. All *Pokémon* episodes were screened before airing, and no problems were reported.

A clear genesis of the panic remains elusive. After four months, Nintendo announced that it could find no obvious cause for the outbreak, and *Pokémon* returned to the airwaves. Further research was left to the scientific community. The researchers concluded that some of the children had latent photosensitive conditions which had predisposed them to have seizures when exposed to the flashing lights. One local estimate of the incidence of seizures triggered by *Pokémon* was 1.5 per 10,000, 10 times the incidence found by British researchers.

'The jerks' was a term used to describe an hysterical epidemic in which many who attended emotionally charged nocturnal religious revival meetings during the seventeenth and eighteenth centuries in parts of the southern United States had psychomotor agitation of the arms or limbs and often collapsed afterwards. Researchers suggest that among the throngs of participants there were perhaps some who had epilepsy. Some meetings were held during the evening with only light from torches flickering in the night. Did this trigger any seizures? Did those few with epilepsy trigger mass hysterical response in others?[27]

The outbreak of illness symptoms coinciding with the broadcast of *Pokémon* fits the profile of mass anxiety hysteria triggered either by observing someone having a genuine seizure or by learning of the illness from mass media reports or word of mouth. While such epidemics are often triggered by the sudden stress and uncertainty surrounding a single case of real illness, a few have a viral, bacterial or toxicologic component. For example, in 1998 three fourth-graders at a California school inadvertently ingested lysergic acid diethylamide (LSD) and were hospitalized. Eleven other students who had sampled a white powder from a vial believed that they too had ingested LSD and were also hospitalized. Despite symptoms ranging from violence to hallucinations, test results were negative and the students were released within a few hours. In other instances, actual events such as a chemical leak have served as a trigger.[28]

While the mass media are rarely implicated in triggering epidemic hysteria outbreaks, their reports often exacerbate the situation. Publicity fuels hysteria as news of the affliction spreads, planting concern in the community through public meetings and the reporting of misinformation. In the *Pokémon* episode, the jump in the number of reported cases is strong evidence for the role the mass media played. According to the news accounts of the time, the number of children said to be affected remained around 700 on the evening of the *Pokémon* episode and the next day. The next morning, the episode dominated the Japanese news and the seizures 'were the talk of the schoolyards'. When the children heard panicky accounts through the mass media, their friends and their schools, the number of children reported the next day to have been initially affected increased by 12,000.[29]

One common component of mass hysteria is an exaggerated over-estimation of risk. For hysteria to spread, those affected must not only perceive the risk as real and present, but also believe they are vulnerable to it. Researchers surveying epileptic patients have found that 'more than a quarter of those surveyed indicated that they thought that a substantially greater proportion of people with epilepsy were at risk from [video games] than the estimated real risk suggests. One in 13 perceived that every individual with epilepsy is at risk of a seizure as a result from playing video games . . . [T]he proportion . . . who saw themselves to be at risk from video games is two to three times the estimated real risk.' This risk over-estimation may have been associated with the cartoon version of *Pokémon*.[30]

The late Canadian cultural theorist Marshall McLuhan observed that the technological revolution has made the world into a 'global village'. The continuing reliance on mass communications, especially television and the Internet, gives the novel nature of the *Pokémon* illness outbreak added significance. Technological inno-vations have the potential to influence far more people than traditional mass hysteria episodes. Rapid and perpetual innovations are changing how and where we work, how we interact with others, how we play and many other facets of everyday life. Although a small number of persons affected by the *Pokémon* animation were confirmed as having photosensitive epilepsy, most clearly were not. So what were the vast majority of children experiencing? Inexplicably, no outbreaks of mass illness symptoms associated with viewing television were reported before and none have been reported since the episode.[31]

Given the chameleon-like nature of hysteria, it is not surprising that, as we enter the new millennium, it should manifest in a television-related setting. Epidemic hysteria has been known to take many forms: these include shaking, crying and glossolalia accompanying Melanesian cargo cults and Holy Spirit movements, running and laughing fits in central and southern Africa, demon possession in Malaysia, fainting in response to imaginary bug bites in the southern United States, clay eating among Australian Aborigines, and strange odours in modern Western schools and factories. The *Pokémon* illness symptoms are unusual because of the large numbers affected, and may be a harbinger of future techno-logical hysterias that have the capacity to affect massive numbers of people at a phenomenal speed.[32]

3

The Phantom Lover Syndrome

O, I see that nose of yours, but not that dog I shall throw it to.
Othello to Desdemona's alleged lover, Cassio, in *Othello*, IV i, 141–2

> *I will set My jealousy against you . . .*
> *They shall remove your nose and your ears,*
> *And your remnant shall fall by the sword . . .*
>
> Ezekiel 23:25

> *I will chop her into messes! Cuckold me!*
> *Othello*, IV i, 197

Classically, the strongest emotions – the deepest passions – are what were thought of as causing madness. As a result love – perhaps the greatest passion of all – was held responsible for much insanity. For doctors since Hippocratic times, lovesickness was a real diagnosis, and all about fixation. Its victims would find themselves unable to rid themselves of obsessive thoughts about some unattainable object. Sleep and appetite would depart, eventually rendering the body seriously diseased. The consequences could even be fatal, as in the case of Thomas, Archbishop of York, who supposedly died of the malady in 1114.[1]

Historically the cure for lovesickness was sex: the humoral excesses could be cured by discharge of the reproductive fluids. Pagan Greek and Roman doctors felt no compunction about prescribing intercourse for their lovesick patients. As Galen insisted, health-conscious men make love even when the act gives them no particular pleasure. King Louis VII of France, distanced from his queen by military duties, was thought to have fallen ill due to this lovesickness, so his doctors suggested that a substitute woman might cure him. He preferred to die faithful to his wife.[2]

In Arabic countries in the Middle Ages lovesickness was diagnosed not just by loss of weight, appetite and interest in life. A sufferer would also have their pulse taken by the physician, who would recount at the same time all the names of eligible members of the opposite sex in the local community – the name at which the pulse quickened would establish the diagnosis. The cure for this form of lovesickness was marriage.[3]

Lovesickness has not made it into the modern lexicon, so was it real, or did it simply evolve into what we now call erotomania or stalking?

Certain forms of love appear to be the most vulnerable to delusion. We all can recall times when we acted irrationally while in the grip of passion. Some even argue that love itself is a delusion. In fact several different forms of love delusion are so well known to psychiatrists that they have attracted their own terms. These include Phantom Lover syndrome, erotomania or De Clérambault's syndrome, incubus syndrome and Othello syndrome. Delusions regarding interpersonal relationships and disordered sexuality are not uncommon in schizophrenia illnesses. Sexual delusions (mainly delusion of imposed intercourse) have been found in 44 per cent of hospitalized patients suffering from schizophrenia or a paranoid state.[4]

In contrast to the common delusion that there is love between two people when the real relationship is much less passionate, having a phantom lover means feeling loved by someone who does not exist at all. Less extreme perhaps is loving someone who once existed but who has died or moved away and whose death or departure is delusionally denied. A variation on this is loving a stranger: although the stranger exists, he or she remains someone unknown or never spoken to.[5]

Perhaps the most common of all is loving someone and being convinced that one is loved in return. The object of love may be a former suitor whose change of heart is not believed, or someone who is an interested professional, like a doctor, lawyer or teacher whose attentions are not intentionally amorous but are interpreted as such. I have been consulted by numerous female lawyers who were stalked by male clients who mistook the professional interest of the woman as a more intimate personal engrossment. At least in that case there is some possible understanding of why a man might make such a mistake, no matter how clumsy. However, there are syndromes in psychiatry where the error appears totally inexplicable.[6]

Erotomania is the erroneous conviction that someone is madly in love with one but the delusion has no basis in reality whatsoever. It can apply to someone the sufferer has never even met, like a newscaster on television. De Clérambault's syndrome is another name for this disorder, and historically it was often reserved for those cases in which the deluded woman considers herself the victim of the active erotic pursuit of a man of much higher professional status. The following case, originally reported by De Clérambault in the 1920s, illustrates the major themes characterizing the disorder.[7]

The woman who believed a king was in love with her

A 53-year-old fashionable dressmaker with a paranoid disorder of ten years' duration was convinced that King George V of England was madly in love with her. She believed that the soldiers and sailors and tourists she ran into on the streets were really his emissaries, sent by the King to proclaim his love for her. Prior to this royal romance, she had been convinced that King Edward VII was in love with her, and his predecessor had been an American general. She pursued the unfortunate King George from 1918 onwards, paying several visits to England hoping to meet him. Frequently she waited for him outside Buckingham Palace. Once she saw a curtain move in one of the palace windows and interpreted it as a signal from the King. She claimed that all Londoners knew of their royal affair. She vividly summarized her passion for him as follows: 'The king might hate me but he can never forget. I could never be indifferent to him, nor he to me . . . It is in vain that he hurts me. He is the most distinguished of men . . . I was attracted to him from the depths of my heart. I wished to live under the same heaven as he and in the midst of his subjects. If I have offended him I have suffered in my heart.'

This particular disorder will be discussed in greater detail in Chapter 5 but a key issue is that it must be differentiated from simple infatuation. In infatuation you fancy someone but are aware of the possibility that your fondness may not be returned – though you hope fervently it will be. In erotomania you believe the other person loves you, and only after you become aware of this do you consider returning the affection. Obviously the psychological mechanism involved has something to do with projecting your own wishes on to an unsuspecting target.[8]

The essential point about all delusional love syndromes is how our imagination becomes so exercised about mythical relationships – it seems our mind readily fills in the gaps in what we desire so that we believe our non-existent lovers or their love exist. Although the delusional syndromes of love are obviously extreme manifestations of disturbed behaviour they raise questions about how many of our normal relationships are imaginary. In other words it may be that for our relationships or even society at large to work, mechanisms in our minds 'fill in the gaps' and permit us to believe positivity towards us exists from others much more than it really does.[9]

All relationships involve some inference about what is going on in the other person's mind when they think of you. We only become aware of this when the activity becomes grossly disordered, as it does in the psychiatric love delusions. Perhaps the most extremely delusional is phantom lover syndrome because in this disorder the other lover doesn't even exist at all, while in other emotional disturbances the other person exists but their attitude to love or a relationship with the sufferer is misunderstood. The phantom lover syndrome is a common delusional pattern classically encountered in middle-aged single women. Dr Mary Seeman, Clinical Associate of the University of Toronto, reported the following two illustrations.[10]

The woman who believed in an overseas lover

Angelina K. is a 33-year-old single woman. First generation Canadian, she is the youngest of four children and the only one left at home with her mother. The father is deceased. Angelina has led an isolated life with few girlfriends and no boyfriends. Her mother seeks medical attention for her when Angelina barricades herself in her room with stacks of cut-up newspapers and refuses to come out. Angelina reports that several years ago she went out on a blind date. The young man was smitten with her but because of the jealousy of girlfriends had to remain hidden. He has therefore over the years resorted to communicating his love by blinking car lights, dimming

99

and brightening neighbours' house lights and visiting the house in various disguises, posing as a salesman, telephone repairman, boarder and so on. Recently he has been moved by malevolent forces to another country so they now communicate using coded words in the daily paper announcing aeroplane trajectories over Angelina's house. Either he himself or friends sent by him pilot these planes to assure Angelina of his undying love.

The woman in love with an officer

Carole M., a 35-year-old divorcee, was admitted to hospital after being found hiking to a town many miles away in pursuit of a truck about whose shifting position she was kept informed by code via the headlights of passing cars. She stated that she had met a man that summer; he was in the Marines and was to follow her west after she returned home. After many months of waiting with no answer to her letters, she thought there must be danger in exposing their love and that he could only come for her in camouflage. When she saw the truck she knew immediately that he was in it and that she must follow.

Though these cases clearly represent grossly disordered thinking, they do contain some of the illogical elements in the early stages of adult love. Belief in telepathy between lovers, reading meanings into natural events, explaining the lover's lack of ardour by face-saving rationalizations, wallowing in passionate daydreams: all are characteristic of adolescent crushes and continue to form a part of many adult love relationships.

Pop-singer fads and movie-idol crazes are related phenomena. The real personality of the loved one is immaterial – how can you know someone you have never met? This early adolescent immature state of love – after all, adolescence is when most people develop crushes on distant figures – is in fact self-centred, not other-directed as we often prefer delusionally to believe. One needs desperately to love – and whom one loves is inconsequential.

Related to phantom lover syndrome is incubus syndrome, where again not only is the love imagined, but the lover as well. The incubus syndrome is the delusion of having experienced sexual inter-course in one's sleep with an imaginary lover – but the key point is that when you awake you continue to believe that the lover really exists. Certain cases of erotomania feature this delusional thought; such cases may form a specific clinical syndrome linked to paternal deprivation.

The concept of the demon lover or incubus seems to have a universal appeal and has been known since pre-Christian times. In classical mythology the ancient Greek myth of Cupid and Psyche describes sexual activity with an unseen lover who visits under the cover of night. The description of the incubus by Caelius Aurelianus in the fifth century was based on the ancient belief in the demon who, in the guise of a man, seduces women. It was related to the spirits of the woods, the sylvans and fauns.[11]

In the Christian era the incubus was defined as an angel who had fallen from heaven because of his lust for women. Galenic humoral theory and demonology were combined by Arnauld de Villanova in the thirteenth century. He stated that if certain warm humours develop in the body the incubus is likely to seize upon the person. In the fifteenth century Pope Innocent VIII described sexual intercourse between witches and incubus devils in his papal bull *Summis Desiderontis Affectibus*.

Kramer and Sprenger, in the book that inspired the epidemic of witch burning during the Middle Ages, *Malleus Maleficarum*, tell of witches having sexual intercourse with the incubus and getting their strength from him, and also describe the efforts of the incubus to subvert other women. Thus the belief in the incubus contains elements of dangerous and uncontrollable sexuality as well as of persecution. Women accused of being witches and having intercourse with the Devil were burned at the stake since at least 1275.[12]

The following case presents features which relate to erotomania and delusions of imposed intercourse similar to the medieval belief in incubi and is reported by psychiatrist Dr L. B. Raschka of the Clarke Institute of Psychiatry in Toronto.[13]

The lover who disturbed the bed linen

A 52-year-old seamstress was admitted to hospital five months after she had begun to feel that people were trying to kill her. Her physician prescribed antipsychotic medication but she soon became convinced that he was trying to kill her and she went to another doctor. Eventually he too was considered to be among the group of her potential killers. She moved away to escape her persecutors. She complained about getting electric shocks from the refrigerator when she touched it. Once she saw a man on television laughing and telling her she would be killed.

There was no history of mental illness in the family. Her father had died when she was 15 years old, and her relationship with her mother was distant. Sexual development was normal although she was shy and socially withdrawn. She married at age 20, subsequently bore two daughters, and was divorced at 26. At 30 she remarried and had a further three daughters. She frequently accused her second husband of infidelity, and at the age of 44 obtained a separation from him. Since then she had been living alone or with her daughters, whom she also accused of trying to kill her.

On admission, the patient complained that her family physician had fallen in love with her and on occasion had come to her bed during the night for sexual intercourse. This was proven by the fact that her 'bed linen was disordered and that she felt hot in the morning'.

She was found to have impaired judgement and auditory hallucinations. She described her experiences with resentment, expressed her indignation over the selfish behaviour of her 'lover' and complained about her unfulfilled sexual needs. A diagnosis of schizophrenia was made and medication and psychotherapy started. In response to the treatment her condition improved and although most of her delusions have faded, her belief in the reality of her sexual experiences has persisted.

In the following case, showing the coexistence of erotomania and schizophrenic sexual delusions, the patient's behaviour is discussed from the point of view of social significance as well as potential dangerousness.

The Capgras syndrome is another uncommon condition: it is characterized by the delusion that a person, usually closely related to the patient, has been replaced by an exact double. Psychiatrist Dr Atul Pande of the University Hospital of the West Indies reports such a case, in which a feature of additional interest was that the patient's father was cast in the role of the incubus.[14]

The woman whose imagined lover was her father

A 20-year-old single female clerk was admitted with a history of disordered behaviour which had developed over a period of one month. Described by her mother as being a shy, sensitive person, the patient had begun to exhibit unusual aggressive outbursts towards her father, whom she perceived as rigid, over-religious and an advocate of puritanism. She complained that her father had compelled her to have sexual intercourse with him a year before. She seemed vague as to whether this had occurred on just one or several occasions, and she inferred it from the sensation of a hand moving over her body and touching her genitalia while she was asleep. She further stated that the lady accompanying her was her stepmother and was posing as her real mother. No amount of reasoning could convince her that she was mistaken.

She was the eldest of three children. Her relationship with her father was distant, largely because of religion. The family belonged to a Christian sect known as the Brethren, whose code of conduct included total renunciation of worldly possessions and avoidance of social intercourse with anyone except fellow Brethren. The father attended religious meetings daily and exhorted his family to do the same, equating their reluctance with evidence of sin.

At puberty her father began to restrict his daughter's social contacts and made repeated allusions to her (imaginary) male friends. Each day he insisted upon having a detailed account of her movements, including people she had spoken to. This aroused great resentment in her and she told her mother, who, though sympathetic, expressed her helplessness in the face of the father's overpowering ways.

Mental examination on admission showed emotional blunting, thought disorder, auditory hallucinations and a total lack of insight. The patient was given antipsychotic drug therapy and improved significantly over the next few days. Though her emotions continued to be flat, her thinking became clearer and the hallucinations disappeared. Interviewed at this stage, she reiterated that her father had had sex with her during her sleep and that her mother was not her real mother. But she also admitted that everything seemed like a dream and that she was experiencing difficulty in distinguishing between dreams and reality. Three weeks later these phenomena had disappeared and the patient denied that her father had ever had sex with her or that she doubted her mother's identity.

In her schizophrenic-like psychosis the unsatisfactory relationship with her father gave rise to the longing for a loving father and the delusion of incest, which put her in competition with her mother for her father's affections. The delusion that her mother was her stepmother, and therefore an impostor, helped acceptance of the competition. The basic defect in reality testing is illustrated by the patient's own admission that she could not tell dreams from reality.

The complete resolution of symptoms with antipsychotic treatment lends support to the conclusion that the incubus and Capgras phenomena shown by this patient were the outgrowth of an underlying psychotic process.

The word 'love' derives etymologically from words meaning desire, yearning and satisfaction and shares a common root with 'libido'. Thus, the psychological sense of love can be interpreted as referring to the satisfaction of a yearning, which for the present purpose we will formulate as the obtaining of certain sensory stimulation.

Some psychologists claim that as children we form templates of the characteristics (e.g. appearance, movements, expressions) of those individuals, most often family members, whom we love. As adults, when we encounter someone who matches a part of the template, it reminds us of the absence of that person and creates a yearning to have the template filled again. Love comprises that yearned-for component, plus another, difficult component: the acceptance of the totality of stimuli provided by another person.

In his 1956 book *The Art of Loving*, the psychoanalyst Fromm pointed out a contrast between love and anxiety. In his view, anxiety is the fear of impending isolation, e.g. that which results from separation, abandonment or ostracism. The antidote for anxiety is loving contact in physical or symbolic form. Thus, distilled to its essence, perhaps love is a desired form of sensory stimulation, real and/or symbolic.

What then is the consequence, if the forms of loving stimulation that one craves are absent, or one is thwarted from obtaining such stimulation? The individual may seek stimulation actively. However, our body evidently has another system that is designed to generate a substitute. This can take the form of conscious physical or mental stimulation. For example, as most gratification is derived from stimulation, not the lack of it, people deprived of sensory experience hallucinate it. Consistent with this, in children who show compulsive excessive masturbation (10 to 15 times per day) there was a common theme of withdrawal of affectionate parental tactile stimulation; this was reversed by reinstatement of affectionate non-sexual tactile contact by the parents. In other words, the reinstatement of the parents' loving stimulation to their child reduced the child's compulsion to provide self-stimulation.

Perhaps, however, the most common manifestation of a phantom or imagined lover occurs when you delusionally imagine your spouse has taken a lover. This time the imagined lover is not your own, but belongs to a person for whom you feel possessive love, so the notion that they have a lover causes strong upset and the often dangerous pursuit of this imagined lover.

Othello syndrome is a psychiatric condition in which the degree of jealousy and/or belief in the infidelity of one's spouse reaches delusional intensity. While delusions of infidelity and jealousy have been known since antiquity, only in modern times have they acquired a popular name. In the psychiatric literature, Othello syndrome has appeared as, among other things, delusional jealousy, sexual jealousy, erotic jealousy syndrome, morbid jealousy, psychotic jealousy, pathological jealousy, conjugal paranoia and the delusion of infidelity.[15]

Othello syndrome refers to delusional belief systems where the most prominent theme is the infidelity of a sexual partner. It is named after the central character of Shakespeare's tragedy *Othello, The Moor of Venice*, where the initially trusting Othello is consumed by suspicion and jealousy and eventually murders his guiltless wife, Desdemona, at the prompting of an evil courtier.

While this occurred in the context of a marital relationship, Othello syndrome can be applied to any general situation involving sexual, or otherwise intimate, partners. There is, however, no clear demarcation of 'normal' from morbid jealousy. In a classic study of 30 cases, the typical Othello patient was described as follows: older than 40 with no prior history of mental illness; the apparently sudden onset of delusion, though probably with a history of increasing suspicion for several months; retrospective misinterpretation of past events and minimal clues to prove the spouse's infidelity; and the spouse's imagined lover being unidentified, with the patient making no effort to secure proof of infidelity.[16]

Jealousy in marital and other interpersonal relationships is a common phenomenon. Excessive or morbid jealousy is less common and can be quite distressing. In marital therapy, jealousy sometimes presents as the focal problem, and sometimes emerges as a factor contributing to the marital disharmony. Othello syndrome implies that sufferers pose a danger to spouses or significant others. After all, Othello killed his wife as a result of her alleged infidelity. The dangerousness presented by Othello syndrome individuals ranges from serious verbal threats to homicidal acts. Moreover, the target of the Othello delusion can be someone besides a spouse or significant other.[17]

The following case was reported by psychiatrist Dr Gregory

Leong and colleagues from the University of California at Los Angeles.[18]

The man who believed his family conspired to conceal his wife's lover

Mr B., a 48-year-old man, was evaluated for exacerbation of psychotic symptoms and aggressive behaviour. He had been falsely accusing his wife of extramarital activity for the past three months. Mr B. further alleged that his three sons conspired with Mrs B. to hide her infidelities. The family reported that as a result of his wife's assumed infidelities Mr B. had threatened to hit a male stranger with the butt of a rifle as the stranger passed in front of Mr B.'s house. Fortunately, the gun was otherwise in a non-working condition and subsequently it was removed from the home by his family.

Mr B.'s thought processes were tangential and he denied hallucinations. He had no criminal history involving physical violence or the desire to hurt anyone. There was no family psychiatric history. About a year prior to the evaluation, Mr B. had experienced the sudden onset of dizziness, headache, vomiting, ataxia and left-sided weakness. On neurological examination it was found that he had a long-standing history of hypertension. His head CAT scan revealed left brain haemorrhage. The patient agreed to an outpatient psychiatric referral, but failed to keep his follow-up appointment.

There are several psychological influences associated with the genesis of the Othello syndrome. Low self-esteem and feelings of inadequacy have been suggested as significant factors involved in its development regardless of the presence of other organic factors. Associated psychological features include sexual inadequacy or dysfunction and a passive personality. The frequently observed concurrence of alcohol abuse and Othello syndrome has suggested a possible link between the conditions. Even though some cases of morbid jealousy have been known to subside upon cessation of alcohol consumption, alcohol usage has not been identified as a sole causative agent. Nonetheless, it is certainly an exacerbating factor in many cases.

Othello patients often harbour hostility towards others. Such hostility may escalate to serious physical violence, including towards the two primary Othello targets: the unfaithful spouse or significant other and the alleged paramour. Family members or others who are delusionally identified as accomplices of the putatively unfaithful spouse or significant other also become potential targets. Finally, bystanders who are not part of the delusion can inadvertently be injured when a person with Othello syndrome attacks an Othello delusion object.[19]

In the 1960s the British psychiatrist R. R. Mowat studied a large sample of morbidly jealous murderers and attempted murderers. Mowat found that of the 67 victims of the 63 male perpetrators, 50 were the wife or mistress, and five were the alleged 'rival'. Seven of the eight perpetrators killed their husbands. Eight of the male and one of the female murderers killed their own child. Mowat posited that the imaginary nature of the alleged rival was the reason for the infrequently observed victim rate. He calculated that the average time between the onset of the Othello delusion and the homicide was 4.53 years. A shorter period of elapsed time appeared to be associated with depression or alcoholism. In a majority of cases, the convicted murderer or attempted murderer retained their original Othello delusion long after the homicide.[20]

Mowat felt that the most important diagnostic finding was that one-third of his sample suffered from schizophrenia. With 12 per cent of all psychotic murderers suffering from the Othello delusion, Mowat stated that no other single delusion is associated with so many deaths. In a study of murder trials in 1968, 26 per cent of the cases involved sexual jealousy among both psychotic and non-psychotic defendants. Mowat's study reflects the significance of jealousy, ranging from mild to the delusional range, in the commission of homicides.[21]

The 'geographic' cure – that is, creating a physical separation between the person with Othello syndrome and the Othello target – was criticized three decades ago because many Othello patients were thought to be treatable. However, treatment interventions have shown only limited efficacy at best, leaving the Othello delusion to percolate for three to five years before erupting in a physical attack. In a similar dilemma, Dr Clérambault's syndrome or erotomania, the geographic cure may be the only viable solution. Substantial physical separation between the delusional person and the object of the delusion, however, could be implemented only by modifications in the legal system. Society will need to decide how to balance public and domestic safety with individual autonomy in cases of persons persistently suffering from Othello syndrome.[22]

Peter Butler, Director of Psychological Services, Royal Rehabilitation Centre in Ryde, Australia, reported a case of what he termed reverse Othello syndrome – a delusional belief in the fidelity of a romantic partner appearing in a 49-year-old man following a traumatic brain injury.[23]

The subject exhibited a variant of secondary erotomania that featured a prominent reversal of the Othello delusion. After initially acknowledging the collapse of an established intimate relationship he developed an intense delusional belief that his former romantic partner, who had in fact broken all contact and begun a new relationship soon after he sustained a severe brain injury, remained sexually faithful and continued as his lover and life partner. This belief was firmly held on inadequate grounds not affected by rational argument or contrary evidence and apparently not arrived at through normal processes of logical thinking. Total faith in the former lover's fidelity, and retrospective misinterpretation of co-incidental and insignificant events to affirm that faith, were the central elements of the delusion.[24]

The link between death and the delusions of love occurs because for many love is so central to life that without it life loses all meaning. This also explains the link between delusions of jealousy, adultery and violence.[25]

Dr Judy Okimura and Dr Scott Norton of the Bliss Health Center in Fort Huachuca in the USA recently reported a case which indicates that unusual violence as a consequence of adultery is still widespread in many parts of the world.[26]

The man with no nose

A 44-year-old schoolteacher visited a dermatologist for cosmetic restoration of his nose. The tip had been bitten off about 25 years earlier by his angry fiancée after his unfaithful liaisons. The open wound had been closed at the time, resulting in a distorted tip and a shortened bridge. Their engagement had ended.

Nose-biting as punishment for adultery or sexual rivalry in Kiribati has been described in several non-medical reports. Nancy Phelan's *Atoll Holiday* (1958), describing her travels in the Gilbert Islands (as Kiribati was formerly known), includes a photograph of a smiling woman from Tarawa who is missing the tip of her nose, with the caption, 'Unfaithful wives get their noses bitten'.[27]

Anthropologist Henry Lundsgaarde, who lived in the Islands in the early 1960s, described how in the past it was the local custom for a wronged wife to challenge her rival by attempting to bite off the rival's nose.[28] Similarly, a husband could punish his unfaithful wife by disfiguring and abandoning her. With the decline of traditional ways, it became more common for wives of philandering husbands to obtain justice through the judicial system rather than take matters into their own hands (or, shall we say, teeth). Nonetheless, Lundsgaarde reported in 1974 that 'from time to time, and much to the amusement of Gilbertese and Europeans alike, some instances of this traditional and favourite form of disfigurement . . . still occur'.

In 1990 Dr D. E. Lewis noted that vengeful nose-biting was no longer practised among the Kiribati islanders.[29] However, in 1996, anthropologist Alexandra Brewis reported that there were still about 10–15 episodes of vengeful nose-biting each year. Victims have become less conspicuous in recent years owing to regular visits by Australian plastic surgeons who reconstruct mutilated noses while on assistance visits to Kiribati.[30]

The purpose of biting off the nose of an adulterous wife is to destroy and disfigure an important aspect of her sexual attractiveness – her face. One of the driving forces behind this behaviour in Kiribati culture is a powerful sexual jealousy known as *koko*, 'a murdering thing' that is believed to make people insane. *Koko* is felt by both men and women and is blamed for much of the violence of men towards their wives when there is even the slightest hint of adultery. The display of *koko* is thought to be a sign of commitment to a partner and is said to afflict the ghost after death. This volatile emotion is accepted, forgiven and even socially sanctioned, especially if the woman's behaviour provokes her husband. A wife who repeatedly displays immodesty, whether by dressing in appropriately or by talking in public to another man, would probably be punished after each perceived offence, each punishment being more severe than the previous one. The first time she shows immodesty, her husband might beat her. The second time, she might be beaten within sight of her relatives, who, in an attempt to absolve themselves of the shame she has brought upon them, may cheer in support of the husband.

If she continues her behaviour, his *koko* is likely to culminate in rage, as he bites off the tip of her nose. In so doing, 'the husband not only destroys his wife's looks but also leaves her with a permanent and public sign of his *koko*'.[31]

Whether by cutting with a knife, slicing with a razor, or tearing off with teeth, nasal mutilation has been practised in other cultures throughout history. According to ancient Roman law and Indian custom, nose amputation was an acceptable penalty for adulterers, thieves and prisoners of war. As a result, the art of nasal reconstruction has its origins in India, where it was practised as early as 1000 BC, and in western Europe it was first reported in fifteenth-century Sicily. Modern rhinoplasty has been influenced by the Italian and Indian methods of nasal restoration. Nose-cutting and biting also existed among American Indian tribes (e.g. the Apache, Blackfeet and Mesquakie), the ancient Egyptians, rural Pakistanis, medieval Serbs, the Ashanti and the Chevsurs (Khvarshi) of the Caucasus. The purpose was to destroy the woman's sexual attractiveness, though in some societies the disfigurement of a woman for infidelity may also have been a marriage-mark, a symbol that a wife is her husband's property.[32]

What may seem to be a barbaric practice is not so far removed from Western society. In 1778 Thomas Jefferson wrote a bill mandating that those guilty of rape, polygamy or sodomy would be punished, 'if a man, by castration, if a woman, by cutting thro' the cartilage of her nose a hole of one half inch diameter at the least'. Injun Joe, in Mark Twain's *The Adventures of Tom Sawyer*, declares that 'When you want to get revenge on a woman you don't kill her – bosh! You go for her looks. You slit her nostrils – you notch her ears like a sow.'[33]

Punishment for infidelity has not been limited to mutilation of the nose. Facial bite wounds on men from jealous wives have been reported in the Gilbert Islands for more than 100 years. In the 1970s there was an epidemic of penile amputations in Thailand, where 'it became fashionable . . . for the humiliated Thai wife to wait until her [cheating] husband fell asleep so that she could quickly sever his penis with a kitchen knife'.[34]

How, then, did the nose become the object of the wrath of sexual jealousy? Freudian theory, it has been suggested, would equate the human nose to the phallus, both being non-paired, protruding, midline organs. This analogy predates modern psychoanalytical theory, for the ancient Romans believed that nasal size corresponded with penile length. In sixteenth-century England, a long nose on a woman was often associated with sexual impulsiveness.[35]

John Mackenzie, a surgeon at Johns Hopkins in Baltimore, Maryland a century ago, believed that tissues of the nasal turbinates and septum were analogous to penile erectile tissue, which became engorged under the influence of vasomotor nerves. In 1884 he proposed a reflex pathway that connected the nose to the genitals, and concluded that many nasal afflictions, such as nose bleeds, sneezing and congestion originated from genital engorgement. In 1893 Wilhelm Fliess, a Berlin nose and throat specialist and colleague of Freud, further developed this 'nasogenital reflex' theory, stating that nasal and turbinate disorders could lead to symptoms such as dysmenorrhoea and abdominal discomfort through activation of this pathway.[36]

Fleiss used nasal surgery to 'cure' the non-nasal symptoms of many patients, including those under the care of Freud, who was a strong believer in this concept. Although the notion of a nasogenital reflex has virtually disappeared from medical teaching, the theory was accepted and supported for nearly half a century.

Mackenzie suggested that it was the 'influence of an elegant and handsome nose as an incentive to illicit amours that led to the well-known custom of amputation of that organ in adulterers, "*truncas inhonesto vulnere nares*" [from Virgil's *Aeneid*, VI, 497], whilst in women detected in the act the disfigurement . . . was intended as a perpetual reminder of their shame'. Others have postulated that nose-biting is not merely an act of punishment but has a more symbolic role, that 'perhaps by biting off her nose the husband is symbolically castrating the adulterous wife, who has illicitly assumed the male role by taking control of her own sexuality. Or alternately, perhaps the husband is castrating the lover – biting off the symbolic equivalent of the lover's penis and so fending off the rival's attempts to appropriate his property without provoking open warfare'. Nose-biting continues to be an established cultural practice. By increasing our awareness of it doctors can become sensitive to the circumstances behind these injuries and perhaps be better equipped the next time they see a patient with a missing nose.[37]

Jealousy has long been seen as deeply undesirable in a relationship and a profoundly negative emotion, but now evolutionary psychologists like Dr David Buss, a professor at the University of Texas, argue that jealousy plays a vital role in keeping a relationship healthy. Buss argues that one fundamental and dramatic gender difference which has been concealed until now is that women are much more likely than men to try to invoke a bit of jealousy in their partner.[38]

Jealousy appears to offer many benefits to women, which might explain why it is such a popular tactic. Jealousy can bolster a woman's self-esteem because of the attention it attracts from other men. It can increase her partner's commitment by rudely awakening him to how desirable she really is, and it can test the strength of the bond. If he responds to her flirtatiousness with unconcern, this strongly suggests he lacks real commitment to her. David Buss quotes psychological research that has found the most common reaction in men whose jealousy has been aroused is to increase their attentiveness to their partners. After becoming jealous, men report they are more likely to keep track of what their partner is doing and do something special for her. In other words, as a tactic, jealousy often works.[39]

One recent study asked a sample of unmarried but dating men and women to complete a jealousy test. Seven years later, when they were contacted to check which couples had actually married, it was found that being more jealous of your partner while dating dramatically increased the likelihood of being married seven years later. Modern psychology at last seems to agree with St Augustine, who originally pointed out, 'He that is not jealous is not in love'. Indeed the total absence of jealousy now signals to many marital therapists a lack of real passion in a relationship. Some now prescribe a bit of jealousy as a way of stimulating a relationship that is becalmed. A husband would be encouraged by this new marriage guidance to demonstrate his love for his wife by expressing displeasure when she shows the slightest interest in another man. He should ring frequently from the office to check exactly what she is doing, keep an eye on her wardrobe and be openly suspicious when new clothes are acquired.[40]

A common peculiar observation of marriage therapists is that immediately after a crisis when a man discovers his partner has had an affair, the lack of excitement in the marriage sometimes disappears, and the predicament seems to revive the sexual passion of the original relationship. Another man's attention can reaffirm a woman's attractiveness in her previously bored partner's eyes.[41]

Eliciting jealousy intentionally in order to gauge how serious your partner is about you, or to get them to be more committed, is a common tactic. In one study 31 per cent of women and 17 per cent of men admitted they had intentionally aroused jealousy in their romantic partner. In Dr David Buss's own study of newlyweds, women more than men report flirting with others in front of a partner, showing interest in others, going out with others and talking to another man at a party, all in order to make their partner jealous. Another common female tactic is to make sure to mention to the boyfriend how much fun she had when out partying without him. But perhaps one of the most effective but subtle female strategies is simply to smile at other men while out with a partner.

Psychologists have found that most men misinterpret what a woman's smile really means, and make the mistake of assuming it is a signal of sexual interest. So when a woman smiles at another man, while at a party with her partner, she is skilfully using the inherent male bias in interpreting body language against them. The man being smiled at makes an advance, and the partner gets annoyed because he detects a rival, yet no-one can blame the woman who instigated the rivalry and confrontation, because all she was doing was being innocently friendly . . .

A lot depends on the motivation. One study found that 8 per cent of women try to elicit jealousy in order to bolster their low self-esteem, and an even smaller percentage do it in order to punish their partner – taking revenge for a previous wrong. A massive 38 per cent of women report they evoke jealousy to increase their partner's commitment; because it gets their partner to believe that if he does not display greater engagement, she might depart for greener pastures.[42]

The largest group of all, 40 per cent of women, report using jealousy to test the depth of the relationship. Whether you can pro-voke some jealousy in your partner produces valuable information about exactly how committed he is, which it seems is difficult to elicit in any other way. This could explain why psychological research has found that women who rate themselves to be more involved in the relationship than their partner is have the strongest tendency to use jealousy. The women who thought they liked their partner more than their partner liked them were almost twice as likely to use jealousy as a tactic in the relationship as women who felt the opposite.

So it seems that it is women who feel less desirable than their partners who are prone to using jealousy as a way of correcting the imbalance. But the true revolution produced by Professor Buss's work is the revelation that jealousy can be a good thing – it acts as a natural defence mechanism to shield love from rivals. If you never felt jealousy at all, then you would not be vigilant to possible threats to your relationship from competitors, or be aware of the signs of betrayal.

Jealousy is universal and has evolved over millions of years, Buss argues, precisely in order to help warn us of such threats. It tells us when a partner's sexual indifference might not merely be caused by work stress. It helps us to detect and recall the subtle signals that, when brought together, herald desertion, and so allows us to do something about it before it happens.

The problem is that if jealousy takes hold of someone whose mind is vulnerable to breakdown it can have extremely dangerous consequences.

A tragic murder at the University of California resulted in far-reaching changes in the law about therapist-patient confidentiality. After this case, therapists in the US were compelled by law to break patient confidentiality and warn a member of the public if they were in danger as a result of a patient's delusional system. Because the case has been extensively reported in the popular press the real names of the main protagonists are used in this account, as presented by University of Houston Distinguished Visiting Professor of Law William Winslade and Judith Ross, an associate at the Centre for Healthcare Ethics at St Joseph Health System in Orange County, California.[43]

The man who tape-recorded his imaginary lover

Twenty-five-year-old Prasenjit Poddar was an Indian graduate engineering student at the University of California at Berkeley. He grew up amidst grinding poverty in a tiny village in India as a member of the harijan or 'Untouchable' caste. His early environment was so poor that an Indian friend and mentor at Berkeley, Farrokhg Mistree, had to teach him how to use plates and how to eat with a knife, fork and spoon. Many considered Poddar to be a genius in overcoming such a background to win a rare Indian government fellowship for study in the United States and then excel in his graduate studies of electronics and naval architecture. After two years of unrelenting devotion to his work, however, he was ready to relax. He began attending weekly folk dances sponsored by the International Student Organization.

Here he was attracted to Tanya Tarasoff, a lively, outgoing 20-year-old American student. Although she continued to chat and dance with other young men, she included Poddar in her circle of admirers, occasionally even visiting him in his room to continue their conversations. Poddar had never before been involved with a woman, and he was baffled by her friendly interest. Mistree, his more worldly friend, correctly saw that Tanya was no more or less friendly to Poddar than to any of her other foreign student friends, and told Poddar she was only being sociable.[44]

However, a New Year's Eve party found Poddar and Tanya momentarily alone together in an elevator, and she impulsively reached out and kissed him for the New Year. For one glorious moment the untouchable was touchable. His first kiss! He was ecstatic, convinced now that she had at last revealed her true loving feelings for him.

But in subsequent months she behaved as before. Sometimes she stood him up, danced with others, and talked openly in his presence of her intimate involvement with other men. At other times she enjoyed conversations with him. Confused by her mood changes, he began tape-recording their talks in his room. Then he would spend long hours brooding over every word of their conversations. He began to skip meals and then classes and soon had to withdraw altogether from classes. Mistree persuaded Poddar that it was essential to make a clean break from the fickle Tanya and return to his studies.

This plan was successful for several months – until she called, saying she missed his friendship. Now he was drawn under her spell once more. He became more determined than ever to discover her true feelings, endlessly playing his tapes and even splicing them to make her voice express great love for him.

In desperation, one day he proposed marriage to a very startled Tanya, who turned him down. Now distraught, Poddar became convinced that everyone was laughing at him behind his back.

'Even you, Mistree, laugh at my state. But I am like an animal. I could do anything, I could kill her. If I killed her, what would you do?' In reply Mistree said, 'I would tell the truth.' To this Poddar said, 'Then I would have to kill you too.'

Relenting later, Poddar sought out his friend that evening and warned him that he was out of control. After that Mistree slept with a chair wedged against his door.

Alarmed by Poddar's escalating threats of violence, Mistree persuaded him to seek psychological counselling at the UC health service. Dr Stuart Gold, a staff psychiatrist, examined him and told him he was seriously disturbed. Dr Gold prescribed antipsychotic drugs and scheduled him for weekly appointments with Dr Lawrence Moore, a staff psychologist. Poddar did not think his secrets were safe with Dr Moore so while he continued to repeat his violent threats, he never revealed the identity of his intended victim. After 10 sessions he abruptly terminated therapy and told Mistree of plans to buy a gun. When Mistree told the doctors, they wrote to the campus police describing the danger and recommending hospitalization for Poddar. Armed with this information, the police warned Poddar to stay away from Tanya, but took no further action. Meanwhile, Poddar thoroughly frightened Tanya by following her around campus and loitering near her house. He decided to confront her with his pain and humiliation one last time. She met him in the doorway of her home and told him to leave, but he pushed his way inside. She ran; he ran after her and shot her, then stabbed the dying woman numerous times as she fell.

Poddar was convicted of second degree murder and served five years in prison in California before his sentence was reversed on appeal by the California Supreme Court. Rather than try the case again, a plea bargain was struck and Poddar was deported to India. He reportedly married a lawyer and resumed his life there.

His case illustrates an important point about when delusion boundaries end. Often with the delusion of love or in phantom lover syndrome, as in other delusions, it seems at first glance that the disordered thinking centres only on the issue of love. When it comes to the rest of the patient's life their ability seems intact. However, as in the case of Poddar, the breakdown in reasoning actually affects their whole world-view. Poddar began to imagine that everyone was laughing at him and this contributed to his final psychotic state.

According to Freud, falling in love is perhaps best thought of as a short-acting, spontaneously remitting psychosis, though the observed resemblance between love and madness predates Freud in legend and poetry by many centuries. But Freud observed that falling in love is not infrequently attended by a variety of symptoms which, clinically stated, sound like the characteristics of a disorder.[45] Changes in mood, physical restlessness, sleeplessness, loss of appetite, disturbances of work patterns, ruminative thinking and delusional beliefs about a person which do not correspond to others' perceptions of reality are all consequences of the state.

The exaggerated sense of well-being produced by states of love means all might not portend well in the long run if this state is used as the basis for making long-term decisions – like the choice of a life partner. But viewed from a Western perspective, falling in love is a wholly acceptable process. The vast majority of marriages in Western culture, it is safe to say, arise from an experience of falling in love, even though this might be a remarkably transient mental state.[46]

Indeed, the divorce statistics alone indicate that love is an unreliable basis for making choices, let alone the countless occasions when detached observers consider a match unlikely or ill advised. In the UK, a one in three chance of establishing a marriage which will end within 10 years is not a very good actuarial base. Nevertheless, certainly for the greater part of the last century and perhaps a good deal longer, romantic love has been the basis of such choice.[47]

If love is a common delusion then 'imaginary relationships', far from being dysfunctional or pathological, may in fact be a requirement for competent participation in many societies, including our own. Defining the imaginary as 'unreal' reflects a uniquely Western epistemological assumption – and shows that we have neglected the importance of the imaginary in everyday life.

The fan–celebrity relationship poses a particularly interesting case with which to initiate this investigation, for this relationship contains both real and imaginary elements. And rather than focus on celestial gods or dead ancestors, this relationship involves the famous who walk among us.

Since the beginning of media of any sort, there have been fans of individuals whose thoughts, words and images those media transmit. Fans differ from ordinary consumers of fame because they form especially strong affective attachments to the objects of their interest, and they can use those attachments as a stepping-stone both to relationships with other fans and to relationships with the famous themselves.

Scholars have emphasized how fans, regularly exposed to the intimate details of the lives of serial television characters, come to establish attachments to those characters that resemble their own social attachments. Theorists have implicated the use of close-ups in the taping of soap operas and the access that viewers have to the emotional lives of the characters in the formation of bonds. Soap opera worlds provide a sort of surrogate community life for viewers, as they become part of the neighbourhood in which their favourite characters live.

Dr Kerry Ferris, a sociologist at Bradley University in the USA, has conducted research into how fans – not necessarily stalkers – try to gain access to celebrities. One fan told of her use of the advertised whereabouts of one celebrity to track a whole group of others. This fan made a habit of attending local plays starring members of the *Star Trek* cast, hoping that other cast members would come to see their colleagues' shows. She was often rewarded.[48]

[Dianne] and some friends saw a play in which several of the *Next Generation* cast members performed. Afterward, they waited for them at the stage door. As they were talking with [their favourite actor], a second actor and the rest of the cast called out from across the parking lot the name of and directions to the restaurant where the cast was dining *après théâtre*. Dianne said she and her friends figured, 'Why not – they probably won't even notice us', so they used those directions and drove to the restaurant, a tiny Italian place in Hollywood where the Trek cast was the only party dining. Dianne says she and her friends were embarrassed but sheepishly stayed and had dinner themselves, never bothering the people at the other table but trying to quiet their excitement at being in the same place.

Dianne and her friends at first used legitimate means to find the actors at work and then used more dubious tactics to dine near them. She used knowledge of a celebrity workplace to gain access to the more private, intimate setting of a restaurant and thus engineered extended contact with them. Soap opera fans use similar tactics. Following actors from pre-staged events to create a fan-staged encounter involves capitalizing on attendance at official functions to get contact at a more personal level. In Dr Ferris's research into fans, a soap opera fan tells how she persevered in tracking a soap actor after a personal appearance. Despite the actor's reluctance to divulge his travel plans, she managed to see him off at the airport. Along with her friend, she went to great lengths to have contact with the actor outside of the strictures of the personal appearance situation. But they had to start at that point. They found him 'at work' and followed him to wish him a very personal *bon voyage*.

While fans can identify celebrity workplaces with relative ease, they must work harder to find out where a given celebrity lives. A grey-market traffic exists that provides celebrity home addresses: with money, luck, some elbow grease, or a bit of each, fans may learn addresses from personal cheques, voter and motor vehicle registration information, postal service delivery information or even purloined studio call sheets (the daily taping schedules that include actors' home addresses so studio limousines can bring them to work).

Although the behaviours of certain fans and those of stalkers share some similarities, the fans in this study take care to differentiate themselves from stalkers and the dangers they present. These fans recognize that they must make observable, to the celebrity and to others, the safety and sanity of their own interest, in contrast to the dangerous, unbalanced interest of the obsessed.

Is there a notable difference between fans and stalkers in this study? The fan activities discussed here do indeed bear a striking resemblance to the activities of stalkers. The asymmetrical awareness, the unilateral pursuit, the lack of reciprocity, and the search for and use of information are all characteristics of 'relational stalking'. Indeed, by its very nature, a stalking relationship is built on contested claims: each party views his contact with the other through a radically different lens. Where the victim sees threat, the pursuer sees devotion; in some cases examined in this study, these contested claims are clearly present. The attempt to control and impose a relationship on an unwilling – or at least unwitting – celebrity is also clear. In addition, the fans' attempts to reframe their unilateral pursuit as if it were a more reciprocal relationship also smack of stalking. Do these things make fans into stalkers?

Fans who acknowledge the possibility that their attentions may frighten the very people they hope to impress may try to account for their actions, to reframe them as unthreatening.

In a contemporary culture in which celebrity stalking is a ubiquitous part of the *Zeitgeist*, it seems unavoidable for fans to engage in accounts meant to put celebrities at ease. The problem with such accounts, of course, is that 'Don't be afraid!' is exactly what a stalker might say too.

The most famous obsessed fans are well known: Mark Chapman (who obsessed over and killed musician John Lennon), Robert Bardo (who stalked and killed actress Rebecca Shaeffer) and John Hinckley (who attempted to kill President Ronald Reagan to impress actress Jodie Foster).

What is the difference between dangerous and innocuous fan behaviour? The actions of these fans can be the subject of conflicting interpretation. Their own claims, as noted above, focus on the unthreatening nature of their actions, while others can and do claim that these actions are threatening. A fan may see her attempts to find a celebrity at home as purely innocent curiosity and challenging spadework, but those attempts may frighten the actor. Is she a stalker? She very well may be, but not by her own account. The essential pathology of the stalker is the subject of chapter 5 and is entitled 'The Delusion of Love'. In the next chapter we examine the delusions associated with sex, as love is often described as merely the biological facilitator of sex.

4

SEXUAL DELUSIONS:
WHEN DEATH AND SEX GO HAND IN HAND

In our town the other day
They hanged a man to make him pay
For having raped a little girl.
As life departed from the churl
The townsfolk saw, with great dismay
His organ rise in the boldest way
A sign to all who stood around
That pleasure even in death is found.

Old English poem

In the massively popular film *The Truman Show*, the everyday life of one man is broadcast live to millions watching: only he doesn't realize he is at the centre of a TV programme. It's the fact that Truman Burbank doesn't know he is being filmed which adds the spice to viewing his life. This is precisely the psychology of the voyeur, whose only pleasure is gained from secretly observing what is supposed to be hidden.[1]

The movie's prophetic vision that society is becoming increasingly voyeuristic might be even closer to the truth than the filmmakers ever imagined, and I don't mean the rise in reality voyeurism TV where participants are filmed 24 hours a day. Reality TV is not genuinely voyeuristic as the participants know they are being watched, albeit 'covertly'. However, the camera angles are designed to give a 'peeping tom' feel to the images, which suggests that the programmes are trying to pander to a kind of perverse pleasure. Perhaps this is more prevalent in the population than might be comfortable to admit.

More worrying is the fact that recent psychiatric research has uncovered a modern breed of 'video voyeur', who uses the latest miniaturized camcorder technology to covertly tape women undressing. The latest cameras with zoom capacities can be remotely activated and hidden behind imperceptible pinholes, as in smoke detectors, wall clocks or mirrors. Their ultra-low-light sensitivities present the modern voyeur with unparalleled opportunities to put public dressing rooms, bathrooms and private bedrooms under surveillance, without the need to be physically present to peep.

Case reports recently published by American psychiatrists[2] include a schoolboy who mounted a miniature camcorder above a small hole in the ceiling of a girls' school changing room. There was also the student who covertly filmed his sexual encounters with his girlfriend in his bedroom, using a miniature camera hidden in a smoke detector. The video was later widely distributed around the university campus.

But perhaps the most disturbing recent case was that of a neighbour entrusted with a house key whenever a married couple left home on holiday. While they were away he installed a mini TV camera with a transmitter, concealed within the ceiling light. He regularly taped their sexual activities for over a year, and although the couple usually made love under low lighting, their intimate activities were recorded clearly because of the sophistication of his video equipment. The camera was discovered by accident when the light fixture needed a repair.

These case reports may be the tip of the iceberg, with the vast majority of voyeurism probably going unreported. Surveys have found 50 per cent of the male population admit to voyeuristic fantasies, while 42 per cent of normal college students confess to engaging in some form of voyeuristic activity. Current estimates are that 20 per cent of women, often unwittingly, have been victims of voyeurs.[3]

Although in *The Truman Show* Truman Burbank is portrayed as relatively unaffected by his covert filming, psychiatrists usually find that serious psychological harm results from the discovery that you have been the victim of a video voyeur, particularly if you have been viewed in your home, where you are most used to feeling safe. Victims are often left suffering from a form of paranoia – they are forever unsure whether people they subsequently meet have seen a copy of the video.

Exactly why video voyeurs should be coming to light so often right now is unknown, especially as in the 1970s a dramatic drop in the rate of voyeurism was explained by the increasing availability of pornography. In Copenhagen, for example, after liberalization of pornography laws, the annual police reports of peeping plummeted from 76 to 2. The old-style peeping Tom was associated with 'anorak' type interests that combined social isolation with opportunity, such as astronomy and bird-watching. Higher than average rates of voyeurism were thought to occur in window cleaners and construction workers.[4]

Psychiatrists theorize that voyeurs lack the social skills or opportunities to develop properly intimate relationships, and so have to resort to merely observing, perhaps protecting an immature personality from the emotional risks of genuine intimacy. This would suggest that the current rise in video voyeurism is because our TV-soaked culture encourages so much passive viewing that we interact less with each other; this has helped to deskill us socially, so eventually all we are good at is watching.[5]

Widespread voyeurism is not apparent only in our interest in reality TV. The obsession of press and public with hidden lenses pointed at celebrities begs the question of whether this fascination is related to the darker preoccupations of the voyeur.

Voyeurism is a sexual perversion and is defined by deriving pleasure from secretly overhearing or spying on the sexual activity of others. There are also certain sub-types of voyeurism, like *troilism*, which is the sharing of a sexual partner while another person looks on. Voyeurs often offer to pay for clients to visit prostitutes, on the condition that the voyeur is allowed to watch.

Another sub-type is the person who derives sexual pleasure from watching the act of elimination. There are brothels, particularly on the continent, in which the act of elimination can be watched through glass panels. There is even some evidence that Hitler suffered from this perversion (though if he really had every syndrome attributed to him by enemy doctors then it was a wonder he managed to get out of bed, far less conquer half of Europe). This kind of behaviour sounds extremely abnormal, yet psychiatrists report that voyeuristic pleasures are not uncommon.

A key element of voyeurism is mediated by mystery and forbiddenness – the more difficult it is to see, the greater the compulsion of the voyeur to watch. Voyeurs have been known to fall from buildings and trains in their desperate attempts to peep.

This behaviour is not just in the shadows of society. To look, to hide and to reveal account for a considerable amount of interest in the fashion industry and the media. Freud thought that everyone was vulnerable to perversion and that there was no sharp division between pathological and normal sexuality. True enough, some studies find that 65 per cent of normal males admit that they have done some peeping.

One study of construction workers found that voyeuristic behaviour – termed by them 'watching the windows' – made up a large part of their working day. Most people go through a peeping stage during adolescence, a time when sexual drive is high and available outlets low. Women are also guilty and have their own voyeuristic activities, like 'crotch watching' – observing men's trousers.[6]

Then there is the compulsion of all these hidden cameras and secret recordings which have been the heavy artillery in the recent tabloid battles. Perhaps it was thinly disguised voyeurism (dressed up as intellectual curiosity) which led hundreds of thousands to buy the tabloid press for photographs of royalty, and thousands more to listen on a special telephone number to the *Sun's* recording of an alleged conversation between Princess Diana and a friend. After all – who has ever hung up on discovering they have dialled into a crossed line? Electronic surveillance, spying, personal surveillance, eavesdropping, opening mail, leaks – are all essentially voyeuristic acts and play a large role in novels, film and even modern government. Not only are we all voyeurs, but we vote for them as well. Given this pervasiveness, where does the unconscious desire to peep come from?

The Freudians argue that the urge dates back to the 'primal scene' – the infant observing or overhearing parental love-making for the first time. This inadvertent discovery is deeply traumatic, and the loss of innocence is accompanied by a preoccupation with uncovering what else might be kept hidden throughout life.[7]

Another theory is based on the fact that the voyeurs seen in clinics have a poor fantasy life. While most people rely on fantasy to achieve sexual arousal, voyeurs, having little imagination, rely on what they have actually seen. It might be that those with the strongest compulsion to read newspaper exposés are those unable to envisage for themselves what the great and the good might be getting up to behind closed doors.

The general population are guilty of another favourite trick of the voyeur: the denial of voyeurism by relying on second-hand observations. The study on construction workers showed how those who were not guilty of peeping relished hearing the reports of the peepers in great detail – being voyeurs by proxy. Similarly, those who look at the pictures of royalty can deny actually being in the bushes peeping, but are being second-hand voyeurs with the help of the photographer and the publisher. This is also true of those who would deny ever eavesdropping – but relish hearing secret tapes of conversations.[8]

The most famous example of this voyeur-by-proxy effect was the 1972 Watergate scandal, where President Richard Nixon and colleagues were responsible for a huge secret electronic surveillance programme. They often preferred to hear of any results second-hand from operatives, rather than view or listen to the material themselves. The very fact that Nixon ordered so much secret taping – even of self-incriminating conversations which he must have known would cause his downfall if they were ever made public – hints at the sort of compulsion to peep no matter what the risk, which finally destroys most voyeurs.

Perhaps, like voyeurs, we are sometimes too busy trying to peep on others to see those parts of ourselves which will be our own undoing.

But while 'voyeurism' is a word frequently bandied around to describe much common behaviour, the idea that it is a perversion treated by psychiatrists is often very far from what the public might imagine it to be. There is controversy over whether there is any continuity between the kind of widespread sexual behaviour found in the general population and the perversity treated in a clinic.[9]

Deviant sexual behaviour is defined as an obligatory dependence on an unacceptable or unusual stimulus for sexual arousal and satisfaction. 'Paraphilias' is the newer technical medical term for sexual deviations, which are intense sexual urges or fantasies involving either (a) non-human objects, or (b) the suffering or humiliation of oneself or one's partner or of children or non-consenting persons.

One of the categories of paraphilias is the fetish paraphilias and here the main feature is the recurrence of intense sexual urges and related fantasies towards non-living objects, or fetishes. Common fetish objects include women's underwear, shoes, stockings and clothes made of certain material such as leather. Parts of the human body can also become fetishes, such as the feet. It is rare, clinically, to find fetish objects that do not fall into these categories, although very unusual paraphilias are occasionally reported.

So the term 'sexual fetishism' refers to parts of the body, fabrics, articles of clothing, or other inanimate objects which become a focus of sexual attraction in themselves. Fetishistic responsiveness is common in normal populations and predominates in men. Although up to 18 per cent of men may report sexual fetishism, few seek any change and with the advent of more liberal public attitudes to sexual variation there is even less pressure on individuals to consider themselves abnormal or abandon their lifestyles. Nonetheless, fetishism and its relationship to other psychiatric syndromes remain an intriguing and troubling area of psychopathology.[10]

There are some 40 or 50 known different paraphilias or sexual deviations recorded. Treatment of paraphilias has been a controversial, if not a somewhat disreputable topic in psychiatry and in clinical psychology. There are a number of reasons for this. First there is a problem of definition. Deviant sexual behaviour is defined by social and cultural criteria. Sexual behaviour that is taboo in one culture may be acceptable in another. There is no absolute criterion by which to distinguish paraphilic behaviour from normal behaviour.

Secondly, there is the matter of the patient's consent to treatment. The paraphilic individual does not usually seek treatment or change. In most instances the paraphilic undertakes treatment at the insistence of society, for example in exchange for a reduced prison term. When he voluntarily seeks treatment, it is done to escape shame resulting from social censure.[11]

Thirdly, the methods used to treat paraphilic individuals have sometimes been so drastic as to raise doubt as to whether they are therapeutic techniques or methods of punishment. The legality or illegality of a paraphilia certainly has implications for its treatment. The paraphilic individual with a behaviour that is illegal is considered a sex offender and is in danger of being imprisoned. His paraphilia is thus a danger to himself and possibly to others, so treatment and cure is imperative. Persons with a relatively harmless paraphilia seek treatment because of guilty feelings, a diminished self-image and the resulting depression that has led to a breakdown of normal psychosocial functioning. Or they seek treatment at the insistence of relatives and friends.

Some examples of drastic treatments are surgical castration and aversive conditioning using strong electric currents. Treatment of paraphilias also remains controversial because of the relative ineffectiveness of psychological techniques.

Paraphilic sexual behaviour may have a biological component that does not respond to psychotherapy but requires anti-androgenic hormonal therapy as well. Interestingly, paraphilias are largely limited to men and a consistent finding in literature is the effectiveness of anti-androgenic medication, suggesting a link between testosterone and related hormones and sexually exploratory behaviour. However, double-blind controlled studies are rare, and ethical problems are raised by consequent forced feminization.

The origins of paraphilias remain mysterious but a classical learning or conditioning model might explain the development of such conduct. Briefly, this relates to the pairing of a stimulus with a particular response. Perhaps a child at a high level of arousal (e.g. anger, discomfort, or pleasure and warmth) encounters the material-to-be fetish (e.g. rubber mackintosh, baby pants or teddy bear) and experiences intense genital sensations. When the object appears again, the child searches for the feeling she or he experienced previously. If this feeling becomes available, the connection between arousal and object is strengthened. If the feeling is not available, the association becomes weakened and eventually disappears. In adulthood, when overtly sexual material produces the same genital sensations, the person classifies the fetishist association as a sexual one, even if the original association had nothing sexual about it.[12]

However, even though this model provides a starting point for examining fetishist behaviour, most psychologists caution against the suggestion that a single childhood experience could directly serve as a basis for classical conditioning or learning. In the general population, the presence of sexual fantasies is accepted as being central to the development and maintenance of sexual behaviour. According to Glenn Wilson, a psychologist at the Institute of Psychiatry in London who is one of the few scientists to have specialized in this area, perhaps those involved in variant sexual behaviour are like 'script-writers and actors in rather specialized plays' where the plot is 'as logical as those played out in conventional love-making' whilst appearing 'illogical to the uncommitted'.[13]

Perhaps the psychological reason that men are so prone to sexual deviations lies in the supposed sex difference in the use of masturbation and therefore fantasy during the years before social skills are developed enough to produce opposite-sex interaction. In young men there are many years when masturbation is used to relieve sexual tension in the absence of sexual or relationship opportunity, while adolescent girls are thought much less likely to resort to masturbation so frequently and have superior social skills to engage in relationships. Masturbation is generally regarded as a widespread sexual practice in most parts of the world, and most would not view it as a deviant sexual behaviour, although certain religions may forbid it.

Reports vary to some extent, but the early research of the famous sexologist Kinsey and colleagues from the 1940s is probably quite representative. This research found that 92 per cent of men had masturbated to orgasm at some time. Kinsey also reported that almost all males who masturbated used sexual fantasy during the act.[14]

So a central question in the psychology of sex is: why do certain objects turn us on? It is obvious why an attractive member of the opposite sex might – but how is it objects like shoes, leather, fast cars and so on also seem able to heighten sexual arousal? An obvious explanation is that perhaps these objects, for example underwear, are so strongly associated in the mind with the sexual stimulus of a naked body that the brain generalizes its excitement from the body to the underwear. Similarly, if you have a car accident your fear of driving might generalize from stress of being on that particular road again, to the vicinity, and then to all roads or all forms of transport.

The cases reported here involve unusual paraphilias of the fetish type and the extraordinary uniqueness of the fetish objects raises important issues with regard to the genesis of paraphilias and sexual desire in general.[15]

Learning is a fundamental activity of the brain, and learning involves forming connections between stimuli that were not previously associated. So our brains are evolutionarily wired up to learn not to approach that place where we noticed a lion lurking before. We now associate a previously innocuous vicinity with danger and so enhance our chances of survival.

The point of this argument is that if you are used to having sex with your partner after eating at a certain restaurant then just viewing the menu will turn you on. Sexual arousal is a very powerful reinforcement system: we are wired up to gain a great deal of pleasure from sex as this ensures we will pass on our genes, and this therefore becomes a strong drive. So anything linked to sex is something we become attracted to and this could explain our attraction to so many fetishistic objects other than actual people. It also explains why advertisers try to link their products with sexual imagery.

But there are problems with this theory. How is it a group of people become so attracted to the related object that they forget about the actual sexual act with another person? How come the businessman driven to work hard to afford the sexy car soon persistently comes home so late from the office that his sultry girlfriend in exasperation separates from him? Why are some people more attracted to the leather shoes than to the gorgeous model in them? These are examples where sexual drive does not appear to adaptively help us pass on our genes; indeed it appears positively to get in the way of proper intercourse.[16]

One intriguing possibility is that we may experience sexual pleasure from more than just genital stimulation and this means we could link such pleasure with a whole set of experiences other than simple sex. This theory goes a long way to account for the peculiar variety of fetishes so many appear prone to. Intriguingly as well, these new ideas return us to Freud's original thinking about the power of libido in our lives, but using the word libido in a much wider sense as the notion of sexual energy.

The experience of sexual pleasure while viewing or in the vicinity of an object may teach the brain to strongly associate pleasure with that object. If someone is aroused by the presence of stiletto heels and they then masturbate to them this reinforces a strong link in the brain between pleasure and these objects, so preserving the fetish for a lifetime. However, it remains unknown why certain unusual sexual stimuli are preferentially conditioned and reinforced.[17]

An interesting issue is the fact that most fetishes – the unusual attachment of the sexual drive to unconventional objects of desire – demand from the client often socially deviant or unacceptable behaviour, like voyeurism. Perhaps the danger and the consequent excitement in itself become part of the sexual pleasure? The next case of extremely dangerous behaviour appears to support this theory.[18]

Psychiatrist Dr Raj Shiwach of the University of Texas and Dr

John Prosser of Terrell State Hospital, also in Texas, recently reported the following unusual case.[19]

The man who liked to be crushed

A 38-year-old single man was admitted to a psychiatric hospital from a local burns unit after sustaining burns on his lower body approximating a fifth of his total body surface area. He told the doctors that for a long time now he would get sexually excited at the thought of being burned or crushed, and as a direct result he had frequently exposed himself to dangerous situations. For example, he would climb into refuse collecting trucks and ejaculate at the sensation of being crushed, only escaping at the last possible minute. He admitted masturbating almost daily to deviant sexual fantasies or to pictures of fire, people being burned or crushed, and even just the sight of chimneys. Recently he had been climbing into a large dumpster, pouring alcohol on the refuse and setting it on fire. He managed to masturbate and get out of the refuse bin with minor burns twice, but the plastic dumpster eventually melted and overturned, causing the injuries he now had.

When the physicians examined him they found no abnormalities (with the exception of healed burns). Routine laboratory medical tests were also normal. Standard testing using pencil and paper questionnaires for depression and obsessive-compulsive disorder also were unremarkable, indicating that his behaviour could not be readily accounted for by a clinical depression or a marked compulsive disorder.

He is the eldest of four siblings (two are married, and one brother is an alcoholic who lives on Skid Row). One of his paternal uncles was gay and died of AIDS. Personal history showed normal developmental milestones and homosexual sex abuse (oral and anal) by an older man in return for attention and gifts between the ages of 6 and 12. At a young age, the patient remembers a family member threatening to put him in an oven and 'roast him like a pig' for being mischievous. He often wondered about this afterwards as his first solitary sexual experience was at the age of 15, when he climbed into an oven, curled up in a foetal position, and ejaculated. He remembers entering a big unlit oven out of curiosity and liking the warmth and sense of suffocation but did not realize he had ejaculated until the third such instance.

He remained a socially isolated virgin and gave a history of sexual disinterest in males or females and of ignorance of sexuality in general. Once he masturbated after covering his face with a plastic bag and liked the partial sense of asphyxiation as 'the semen shot up 3 feet in the air'. The patient gave up this practice after two months as he considered it too dangerous. He had been arrested several times for climbing into the hazardous waste incinerator of the local hospital and had been treated once for a fractured pelvis (from deliberate exposure to a box compactor) and another time for significant burns. Twice, he came close to self-immolation after pouring gasoline on himself. He denied feeling guilt over his past experiences and denied getting any pleasure out of seeing other people suffer, but did admit to a desire to join an order of Benedictine monks.

He had a bachelor's degree in communications but worked in places where he could have easy access to large waste disposers, ovens and box compactors.

He was treated initially by a long-acting intramuscular anti-androgen injection. This treatment is administered roughly once a week and consists of medication that remains in the body at high enough levels over several days to antagonize the sexually arousing effects of testosterone. It had a remarkable effect on his libido, reducing the frequency of his sexual fantasies, erections and masturbation. He even stopped looking at environmental cues such as pictures of chimneys for sexual excitement.

However, later, at the patient's own request, the anti-androgen therapy was discontinued. Eight weeks after the injection he started having more erections. An antidepressant was introduced after three weeks of admission and was continued over a period of 18 weeks.

During the first few weeks of treatment and assessment the patient was seen on a weekly basis and aversive behaviour therapy was started. This treatment pairs the experiences the patient currently associates with pleasure, with displeasurable associations – a bad smell, for example – and so breaks the connection between the stimulus and sex.

After three months, the patient was instructed to keep a daily diary of the content and frequency of his sexual fantasy arousal and masturbation. A trained clinical psychologist introduced a combination of a form of psychoanalytic or Freudian-based psychotherapy, sexual education, and social skills training; this continued after the discontinuation of the antidepressant.

Aversive behaviour therapy using olfactory aversion was used as the sole therapy next, and the combination psychotherapy was re-introduced after the behaviour therapy. The patient was discharged after 34 weeks of therapy. When last contacted, he had resumed his paraphilic activities.

This description of an unusual case of paraphilia in a socially inadequate man goes some way to back up the theory that the cause of fetishes and sexually deviant behaviour is the inability of the poorly socially skilled to obtain conventional sexual relief with another person. This causes them to turn to more impersonal ways of obtaining sexual pleasure.

To my knowledge, the love of being burned has not been reported before, though there have been reports of people getting sexual excitement at the sight of fire. Learning theory best describes the development of the disorder in this patient, though psychoanalytic factors (like guilt and punishment) may be important. These issues and his possible anger at his parents over their failure to recognize, intervene and protect him from childhood sexual abuse were explored in relation to his masochistic behaviour during the insight-oriented psychotherapy.[20]

A biochemical hypothesis for paraphilias has been proposed, and drugs useful for obsessive–compulsive disorder and in difficulties with impulse control have also been reported to be helpful. The patient received such antidepressants for 18 weeks but the results were not impressive. However, anti-androgen treatment did have a clear impact on the patient's masturbation rate (zero rate coincided with low testosterone levels) and reduced his fantasies and environmental sexual scanning (recalled data). The patient was very clear about these effects, and in fact his reason for discontinuing the injections was based on them.[21]

These results suggest that anti-androgens and aversive techniques can be beneficial in the short term and may have to be continued for longer periods in situations where there is a clear risk to the patient. But reshaping the sexual behaviour and correction of the underlying social deficits may be equally important in the longer term.[22]

This man's masochism did not involve psychological humiliation or interaction with any other person in real life. Paraphilias can often have overlapping diagnoses and our patient's desire to be crushed and the subsequent experimentation with plastic bags suggest an overlapping element of autoerotic asphyxia where sexual pleasure is derived from suffocation.

This is an important element in the following case, where the experience of inhaling and so partly being suffocated by car exhaust fumes appeared to enhance sexual pleasure. In a paper entitled 'Pollution in Metroland: An Unusual Paraphilia in a Shy Young Man', psychologists Padmal de Silva and Amanda Pernet of the Institute of Psychiatry in London report an extremely unusual sexual deviation in a young man whose main sexual interest was in Austin Metro cars, which excited him tremendously.[23]

This had started about one year before referral when his family acquired a car of this make and model. Some generalization had occurred to Vauxhall Nova and Astra, Fiat Uno and Ford Fiesta cars, all of which, he said, were somewhat similar in appearance to the Metro.

He gained gratification by masturbating when possible in the car, or, more frequently, behind the car while the engine was running and exhaust fumes were being emitted. He made great efforts to find deserted car parks or other isolated places where he could get out and masturbate in this way. He denied that the inhaling of fumes was part of his excitement; but he always left the engine running and squatted behind the car when masturbating, whenever such an act was possible. He said the idea of being polluted added to his interest. The possible alteration of consciousness caused by inhaling some of the fumes hinted at a related asphyxiophilia or hypoxiphilia intertwined with the fetish for the car.

He was treated with a multiple package involving strategies like asking him to imagine the arousing scene interrupted by powerful aversive scenes (e.g. being caught by the police, his father appearing on the scene) at a crucial point in a sequence of fantasy. The second was attempted self-administered 'orgasmic reconditioning', where an acceptable fantasy is introduced to replace the deviant fantasy at a crucial point in masturbation.

As noted earlier, the development of fetishes has been explained as arising from the association of a previously neutral object with a sexually arousing object and/or a reinforcing event, in this case orgasm. One view is that the reported reinforcement of the fantasy of the paraphilic act or stimulus by orgasm achieved through masturbation is the key factor in these cases.[24]

Experimental studies have demonstrated how a sexual response can be conditioned by pictures of boots. This can be achieved most simply by presenting a slide of the boots along with slides of sexually arousing nude women. The learning model provides at least a partial explanation of the acquisition of fetishistic paraphilias. In this case, the regular masturbating leading to orgasm, both in the physical proximity of the Metro and while looking at photographs or having fantasies of it, clearly played a crucial role in maintaining and strengthening his paraphilia. However, this explanation needs supplementation.

This man probably also derived additional pleasure from the slightly altered state of consciousness caused by the inhalation of exhaust fumes. Although he denied that he had a particular liking for the exhaust fumes, he admitted that the idea of being polluted was exciting.

Reduction of oxygen intake and related asphyxiation as a sexually exciting experience in some paraphiliacs is well known. Perhaps this paraphilia had the added dimension of hypoxiphilia or the deprivation of oxygen to the brain, albeit in a mild form. This may well have enhanced orgasmic pleasure, leading to unusually strong reinforcement of the fetishistic attachment. The full-blown syndrome is known as autoerotic asphyxia and we shall return to this phenomenon in more detail later.

Sufferers from paraphilias and fetishes are often caught in a vicious cycle: their destroyed self-esteem as a result of their secret problem in itself inhibits them from engaging in social intercourse. This social isolation probably preserves the use of an unusual impersonal sexual outlet.

The treatment approach of emphasizing the development of social skills is illustrated by Dr Ratnin Dewaraja, a psychologist at the University of Tsukuba in Japan, who recently reported a case of what was termed 'formicophilia'. In this case the man derived sexual pleasure from the tactile sensations produced by small creatures (e.g. snails and ants) creeping and crawling on his body.[25]

The man turned on by crawling creatures

The patient referred himself to the psychiatric clinic at the University of Colombo in Sri Lanka, seeking treatment for what he described as 'my disgusting habit'. At the time of referral he was depressed, unemployed, had no friends, and most of the time was preoccupied with collecting snails, ants, cockroaches and frogs, and then masturbating while these creatures crawled on his body. He was diagnosed as not psychotic but suffering from a paraphilic condition. It was decided to treat him with a combination of behaviour therapy and counselling.

Because of the relative harmlessness of the behaviour it was decided that therapy should be aimed at improving the patient's psychosocial functioning and self-image, even if the paraphilia could not be eliminated. The patient reported that he could not talk with people, especially women, because he suffered from strong guilt feelings associated with his paraphilia. The aim of therapy was to reduce his feelings of guilt and to increase his social competence, especially in heterosexual relations.

He was encouraged to develop heterosexual imagery and to masturbate to heterosexual imagery and pictures. He was also encouraged to develop heterosexual social interactions, to facilitate transfer of any heterosexual fantasy into heterosexual behaviour. At the termination of therapy he engaged in his paraphilic behaviour once a week, compared with 3–4 times a week before treatment. The rate of masturbating to heterosexual imagery increased from zero before treatment to three times a week at the termination of therapy.

A key issue is that despite the intense treatment this man received his paraphilic compulsion remained, raising the suggestion that the paraphilias might share much with intense obsessional behaviour and in particular obsessive-compulsive disorder.[26]

Dr Richard Caplan and colleagues from the Southern General Hospital in Glasgow recently described a case which indeed provides evidence of an association between obsessive-compulsive disorder and both tattooing and bizarre sexual practices.[27]

The man who had no space left on his body

A 27-year-old man who had been unemployed for five years was referred with symptoms of complex rituals and daily checking of routine events in his flat, such as washing, cleaning, door-locking, bed-making and placing an item of furniture in a particular position at particular times. The referral followed the man's increasing distress, which had resulted in bouts of heavy drinking in an effort to suppress his symptoms and subsequent attendance at the accident and emergency department.

He was unmarried, of normal intelligence and average educational background. He showed resistance to his compulsive urges, which he felt were irrational.

Further enquiries revealed a 10-year history of obsessional tattooing. He had his first tattoo at the age of 15 with some friends on a visit to the seaside. At this age he was still functioning normally

134

and was not disabled by compulsive behaviour. Over the subsequent years he had further occasional tattoos, always at the same local parlour.

He began to attend at the same time each week to spend the same amount of money. He would ultimately spend about one-third of his weekly wage of £180 on tattoos. As parts of his body were filled, he wanted the remaining spaces between the drawings to be shaded by the tattooist. When these were filled he wanted all the line drawings to be coloured and eventually even skin in drawings of people was coloured with flesh-coloured ink. He felt driven to have most of his skin covered.

The weekly ritual of compulsive tattooing lasted almost ten years and reduced in intensity only because of a lack of money resulting from unemployment and of skin surface area. If this history is accurate, and there is no reason to doubt his report, the estimate is that his compulsion to attend at the same time each week, at the same cost, must have resulted in him spending £30,000 on his tattoos.

He later volunteered information regarding his unconventional sexual practices. After he had partaken in a prescribed series of rituals, he fixed to his penis at two points (underneath the foreskin and at the base of his penis) two wire electrodes which were attached to a self-styled induction coil which generated a current of up to 33,000 volts by a hand-turned crank. He claims that his aim was to achieve 'just the right type' of painful stimulation to sustain a pre-orgasmic level of excitement for as long as possible and he continues these sessions for up to 15 hours, two to three times weekly.

On occasion he has sustained severe electrical burns to his genitals. He admitted that his obsessional desire for 'just the right kind of pain' was one of his motivations in pursuing his extreme form of tattooing. His compulsive striving for perfection and completion, whether in the realm of body tattooing or in pursuing his rather extreme and dangerous sexual practices, seems to be related to his need for pain to be present, 'so that I am able to concentrate'. Only when he is satisfied that he has attained the perfection and completion that this kind of pain brings can he stop.

Although the association of tattooing and erotic piercing has been made occasionally in the literature, no link has been made between tattooing and such bizarre sexual practices, and certainly none which links obsessive-compulsive disorder with both of the above.

Sexual arousal which is specifically focused on a single stimulus to the exclusion of sexual arousal by other stimuli is very uncommon, though, as we have seen, fetishes for articles of clothing, footwear and rubber have been described, as have preferences for a part of the body (known as partialism).[28]

Brian McGuire, a psychologist from New South Wales in Australia, and colleagues report the case of a man with unusual self-directed sexual behaviours and unusual content in his sexual fantasies.[29]

The man who liked only one part of the body

This 19-year-old single man lived at home with his father, a labourer, and his sister, a student aged 17. The patient was described by his father as reclusive, spending most of his time alone in his room and rarely interacting socially with the family except at a superficial level. His parents had been separated since he was 16 years of age.

His mother had a long-standing history of psychiatric illness and is at present in a nursing home. There is no history of learning disability or psychiatric illness within the extended family although this young man was regarded as 'slow' from an early age and has received all his education at schools for children with learning difficulties, including a period at a boarding school.

The patient was unkempt in appearance, wearing torn dirty clothing, and was severely obese, weighing in the region of 300 pounds. He did not bathe or take care of his personal hygiene and he had developed ulcerated sores under the arms, above the pubis, and in the groin area. These had been present for about five years. A course of antibiotics was prescribed following a reluctantly permitted examination, but compliance was poor – he took only 12 of 20 tablets prescribed despite close daily monitoring by staff. The patient eventually claimed to have lost the antibiotics in his house.

Investigation of the poor compliance and claim to have lost the medication led the staff to discover that the sores had a functional significance for the patient and that he did not want them to heal.

Upon questioning, the patient reported that he was easily sexually aroused and habitually masturbated at least twice a day, and more often four or five times a day. Ejaculation would always occur. He reported an interest in the opposite sex and said that he often fantasized. However, the fantasy content and its accompanying behaviour never involved sexual intercourse, nor indeed any conventional sexual act. The patient's primary fantasy stimulus was that of a woman's mouth, although the fantasy never involved kissing or oral stimulation.

Rather, he imagined the woman licking her fingers or gently biting her own lips. Simultaneously the patient would put his own fingers into the ulcers/sores in his groin and/or under his arms and then lick the pus from his fingers. It appears that he ingested the pus and found both the smell and taste exciting, although he was unable to pinpoint exactly the sexually stimulating aspect of this act. He reported that the mere sight of a woman with her fingers to her mouth or lips was adequately arousing to initiate masturbation with the accompanying fantasy image and oral behaviour.

As the patient was not at all violent or aggressive, in fact was rather passive in nature, he was not considered to be dangerous. He relieved his sexual frustrations through 'soft' pornographic books and frequent masturbation with fantasy.

Counselling the patient as to the unhygienic nature of his sexual behaviour led to a reported decrease in the frequency of this behaviour, although the orally fixated sexual fantasies endured. The continuous refusal of or non-compliance with antibiotic treatment may indicate a continuing sexual functional significance of the skin lesions.

Because this patient had responded well in the past to advice counselling, this approach was chosen for dealing with his unusual behaviour. While the behaviour is unusual and has health ramifications, it is open to debate whether it should be treated as problem behaviour (or psychopathology) when it has little impact on others. Such behaviour in an aggressive or psychopathic individual would have warranted great concern because of the risk of acting out the fantasy. Female staff in contact with such individuals should be aware of the presence of the fantasies, as seemingly innocent acts on behalf of another may be construed by the patient as a sexual stimulus. In a study of the role of sexual fantasy Glenn Wilson from the Institute of Psychiatry concluded that in men fantasies are manifestations of an unfulfilled sex drive, whereas women's fantasies reflect a satisfactory sex life. In the present case, there is almost certainly a lack of sexual fulfilment as the patient has never had any sexual contact with another.

Others have suggested that some adult sexual fantasies may have been formed early in life at a time when the individual's comprehension of sexuality was primitive and was influenced by immature anxieties and needs. Again this may be pertinent for the present case, where the patient displays social immaturity, a narrowly focused image of sexual activity and a rather hazy concept of sexuality in general.

The importance of an early childhood experience in the development of fetishes or paraphilias is emphasized by the next case, which is one of autoerotic asphyxia (AEA). This is the induction of a state of brain oxygen deficiency, usually by mechanical means, to enhance sexual excitement and orgasm. Methods of inducing asphyxia include: neck constriction by ligature (the more common method), noose or sling; plastic bag over the head; inhalation of anaesthetic agents; autoerotic drowning; chest compression and use of abdominal ligature.[30]

Fatalities are reported regularly, occurring when the escape mechanism fails or the participants become unconscious through hypoxia and are unable to release themselves.[31] This sexual practice is difficult to study as it is normally discovered only when death results from the act; these individuals rarely seek professional advice. For the same reason, the prevalence of the practice of AEA in the general population is not precisely known.[32]

Estimates of death from this syndrome range from 250 to 1,000 cases per annum in the USA. Data from England, Australia and Canada indicate that 1–2 deaths per million population are detected and reported each year. But as cases are often misdiagnosed as suicides or homicides, there may be considerable under-reporting. The majority of practitioners are male, though cases involving females are known. Reported victims range in age from seven to well over 60, with the mean age of victims being around 26 years of age.[33]

The following features may be present at the scene of death (though not necessarily in every case) and partly help to differentiate the act from suicide. The body is partially suspended with a ligature around the neck and attached to a point within reach; alternatively a mechanism to restrict breathing or cut off air supply may be used; failure of a self-rescue mechanism has resulted in death; interest in bondage or other types of masochistic behaviour may be present; in most cases the victim will be nude, semi-nude or crossdressed in female clothing; sexual paraphernalia or various aids to fantasizing may be present; there is evidence of seminal discharge.[34]

Jo Johnstone, a psychosexual therapist, and Dr Rhodri Huws, a consultant psychiatrist at the Gwent Clinic for Sexual and

Relationship Difficulties, recently reported a case study of an unusual client with autoerotic asphyxia who was referred for assessment.[35]

The man who used sex to reassure himself he was alive

On first consultation, the client presented as a thin, dishevelled 28-year-old man with effeminate gestures. For more than three years, he and his girlfriend had used plastic bags to suffocate themselves while mutually masturbating. On one occasion she thought she was going to die, as he had kept the bag over her head too long and she was unable to remove it because she was bound. She then told him that if he did not stop participating in this activity, their relationship would end. He found it hard to refrain and at the time of assessment participated up to four times a day, usually crossdressing. He would tape a plastic bag over his head until he reached orgasm.

The client grew up, with his sister, in a pleasant family atmosphere. He described his mother as easygoing and affectionate and his father as old-fashioned and felt they had a happy marriage. His parents did not punish bad behaviour but instead focused on good behaviour. He described three episodes in which he had been found by his parents crossdressing, which they had ignored. He felt that they should have shown feelings of anger or revulsion and is still angry with his father about this.

He did not have bladder control until he was six years of age, and he started school wearing nappies, though he does not remember this as an upsetting time. He found school difficult in that he felt abandoned by his mother and felt inadequate compared with his peers. These problems continued into comprehensive school. He still had not made any friends, had no interest in schoolwork, and had developed severe facial acne and asthma.

He was bullied and isolated and became increasingly jealous of his sister, believing that girls had easier lives. Sexual education consisted of occasional television programmes and a biology lesson in school, but his parents never addressed the subject. At the age of eight he developed a non-sexual fixation for women's legs, and at the age of 11, following a television programme about crossdressing, he started wearing his mother's skirt.

One day he found a ladies' transparent plastic raincoat in a rubbish bin and took it home to wear. He felt good because this item of clothing was his rather than his mother's and while wearing it he masturbated for the first time. Bored one day, he slipped the sleeve of the plastic raincoat over his head, aiming to form a ruff around his neck for visual effect. His head got stuck and he began to suffocate, and while struggling to release himself he ejaculated.

Later he experimented by putting a plastic bag over his head and holding it against his throat, again producing an erection and ejaculation, and this led to the regular use of bags for asphyxiation. By this time he had left school and was at college studying car mechanics. He started to expand his wardrobe of female clothing, in particular rubber dresses and silky lingerie, and would wear these at home.

At 21, he became depressed following the end of his first relationship, which had lasted three weeks. Feeling that life was not worth living, he took three overdoses. Shortly after this he started a new relationship and had intercourse for the first time. In private, he continued to dress up and use bags, which he found more exciting and pleasurable than intercourse.

At the age of 23 years he became involved with his current girlfriend, who was then 16 years old. They started cohabiting a year later, and within weeks he involved her in his autoerotic asphyxiation. At first this was a practice of mutual pleasure, but when his girlfriend lost interest after she nearly suffocated this caused a brief separation. After a couple of months they were reunited and have not been separated since.

The client lives in a council flat with his girlfriend. He finds their relationship exciting as he feels they both like to take risks. They are unemployed and have few friends; they rarely socialize, but both maintain contact with their parents. They have sexual intercourse on average every three weeks and find this mutually satisfying. Both become sexually excited and reach orgasm, but to enhance his excitement the client uses fantasies about suffocation, and can become aroused just at the sight of plastic bags. He has a vivid fantasy life that occupies much of his time, and when he masturbates he is usually wearing female silky underwear and a dress and occasionally views himself in a mirror.

Increasingly, he has homosexual fantasies, feeling that a man would know how to sexually excite another man, but his ultimate fantasy involves a dominant woman.

Occasionally he fantasizes about death, wondering whether at the point of dying he would experience the ultimate orgasm, and equally he toys with the idea of his partner dying while having an orgasm. These are not frequent fantasies, but he stated that the more he is convinced that he is going to die, the stronger his orgasm. He has periods of depression and is poorly motivated towards anything outside of his relationship and his sexual practice and feels that his life is mundane and boring. When he first started practising autoerotic asphyxia he would remove the bag after about two minutes, but in the last six months he has increased to using the bag for over four minutes. He stated that he wanted to be so close to death in order to be reminded of the gift of life, and in spite of the danger involved he believes he is in full control and that he will not die.

This report differs from the numerous reports of deaths caused by autoerotic asphyxia (asphyxiophilia), which are mainly of solitary heterosexual men. Death is unlikely to occur if there is another participant. Although this client's fantasies were predominantly heterosexual, his recent interest in homosexuality may reflect his current partner's unwillingness to participate.[36]

Induction of asphyxia with plastic bags is increasing in incidence, the first fatality being reported in 1960. Most often the use of a bag over the head is described, but enclosing the whole body has also been reported. In 1983 one study found that 79 per cent of fatalities had used hanging, 10 per cent had used strangulation, and 4 per cent had used plastic bags. By 1995 a more recent study reported that 30 per cent of fatalities had used plastic bags, the increase probably reflecting wider availability.[37]

Some studies have noted the presence of early abuse, a finding also reported in one of the few reports of living participants, in which a history of early choking in combination with physical or sexual abuse was seen. In a study of 132 deaths from autoerotic asphyxia commissioned by the FBI in the 1980s the mortality ranged between 2 and 4 per million Americans. One hundred and twenty-seven of the fatalities studied were male, and the mean age was 26 years, with 71 per cent under the age of 30. Nearly all individuals were solitary, but in one case the victim appeared to have been a willing participant with another person.[38]

Often there is a concurrence of transvestism and bondage, though this does not appear to apply in the rare cases of female participants. Many authors stress the importance that risk be involved, and usually they describe increasingly risky behaviour over a period of time. One review found most participants to be males between 12 and 25 years and believed that the deaths were accidental. One analysis of

19 male fatalities in Canada between 1978 and 1989 suggested that none of the men showed a wish to die and that all the deaths were accidental, a finding also reported by others.[39]

A number of psychoanalytic explanations have been proposed, for instance that the use of plastic bags is motivated by an unconscious desire to return to the womb. Some therapists believe that hanging is a form of castration anxiety, occurring in situations in which the mother had breast-fed the child in such a way that partial asphyxiation had become associated with the pleasure of feeding. The constriction of the neck represents attempted penile amputation (or castration), with ejaculation relieving the anxiety by symbolizing survival.[40]

Behavioural theories include the proposal that the reason for repetitive asphyxiophylic behaviour is the ease with which orgasm is achieved; others have noted an evolution from a childhood fascination with ropes to adult autoerotic asphyxia and bondage. Some suggest that autoerotic asphyxia usually starts in adolescence as part of general thrill-seeking behaviour.[41]

Some investigators believe that most participants learn of the practice accidentally and others by word of mouth or from the media, and note that a number of autoerotic deaths have been reported after television programmes on the subject.[42, 43]

The practice of deliberate strangulation to produce sexual excitement is a lot more common than may be realized. Although it is an ancient sexual practice, first described in the Mayas of ancient Mexico, and was known among the pre-Christian Celts in Britain, the Shoshone-Bannock Indians and the Eskimos, some researchers suggest the practice has become more widespread in recent years. The middle-class link seems firmly established by the appearance of autoerotic asphyxiation in highbrow literature such as James Joyce's *Ulysses*, William Burroughs' *The Naked Lunch* and *Cities of the Red Night*, Samuel Beckett's *Waiting for Godot* and the Marquis de Sade's novel *Justine*. Erotic hanging appears in motion pictures too, such as *The Ruling Class* and the Japanese film *In the Realm of the Senses*. Victorian London even featured a social interest group known as the Hanged Men's Club.[44]

Franz Kotzwara, regarded by Bach as the best bass player in Europe, died from autoerotic asphyxia in the company of a London prostitute by the name of Susanna Hill and as a result he is known more for his bizarre sexual appetite than as the talented composer of the sonata 'Battle of Prague'. On 2 September 1791 Kotzwara visited Miss Hill, showed her his scars from past sessions of abuse for pleasure and gave her money to go off to buy some food, liquor and a rope. Upon her return he formed a noose with the rope and proceeded to hang himself, after instructing Ms Hill to cut him down in precisely five minutes. By all accounts she did as ordered but unfortunately Kotzwara could not be revived. Susanna Hill was tried for murder and acquitted, but because of the 'danger to public morality' the official court records were ordered by the judge to be destroyed. Historians have suggested that Kotzwara was probably following the advice in the pamphlet *Modern Propensities* written by one Martin Vanbutchell, an eccentric medical quack of the period. The year of Kotzwara's death was also the year that the Marquis de Sade published *Justine*, in which Thérèse helps Roland to achieve ecstatic and indescribable pleasure by hanging him briefly.[45]

Usually the body is partially hung by some kind of tight cord around the neck, frequently with protective packing to prevent bruising and attached to a point within reach of the victim. Alternative air supply restrictors include masks and plastic bags. It is usually the failure of a self-rescue mechanism which results in death. It was well known in medieval England that when criminals were being hanged they would sometimes become aroused and even ejaculate. Some autoerotics get aroused by the sensation of losing consciousness and may use this arousal as a prelude to or to accompany masturbation. The problem then becomes surviving this exciting moment, because the practitioner has to fight the temptation to keep experiencing his sexual high and stop at precisely the right moment to prevent death.[46]

Although many victims employ safety methods to release them from the asphyxiation before fatality occurs, repeatedly depriving the brain of oxygen even for small periods of time probably causes permanent but subtle brain damage. The frontal lobes of the brain are particularly vulnerable to this kind of damage, and since this is precisely the part of the brain which is used in judgement the risk of autoerotic asphyxiation is that its repeated practice is likely to reduce the victim's ability to judge when to stop strangling himself.[47]

Why do otherwise intelligent, well-adjusted people do this? Relatives and friends are often deeply shocked at the news of a death from autoerotic asphyxia as there is usually no hint before of any mental or sexual maladjustment in the victim. Psychiatrists who have seen many of these cases postulate they suffer from depression or unconscious death wishes and so autoerotic asphyxia is really a partly suicidal act even when an attempt is made to play safely.[48]

Otherwise inhibited people may finally experience release from repression (usually caused by a strict or puritanical background) only if they become giddy and delirious as a result of depriving the brain of oxygen during autoerotic asphyxia. In other words while most of us use a few drinks of alcohol to 'loosen us up' before we flirt or seduce, for some people this is not enough and they need to do something more drastic before they can become sexually aroused.[49]

Another theory is that a repressive upbringing may have drummed into someone's mind a link between pain and sex which only allows them to experience sexual pleasure guiltlessly in the presence of pain. On a primitive level bondage recreates the most constricting of environments and may be an attempt to reproduce the constriction children may experience whenever sex is discussed in a puritanical home.[50]

But the sheer amount of sexual perversity and depravity among senior public figures begs the question of whether there isn't something rather odd about the psychosexual development of our leaders. It may be that repressive, competitive, male-dominated public schools and Oxbridge produce bright but unhappy minds which can never be satisfied with the simple things in life, and constantly seek to experiment in their personal lives in a never-ending quest to escape unconscious dissatisfaction. Psychologists have found a link between ambition and a preference for risk-taking. The trouble is that as risk-takers become more successful they are usually driven to take greater and greater risks. It may be that if a successful man begins to find his career too easy and not precarious any more, he will look elsewhere in the search for thrills, and gradually turn to more and more extreme sexual perversion. The successful can also become complacent about their position in life. Soon they derive excitement from the possibility of failure; otherwise life becomes boring for them. It is precisely this kind of excitement which can kill. The following is the case of a woman who recounted to me her experience of autoerotic asphyxia.[51]

The woman who didn't know her husband

Two years ago Jane discovered the dead body of her husband in their home and was told by a CID officer he had died of autoerotic

144

asphyxia. She met Robert at a flat-warming party of a mutual friend and despite their many differences (at 32, she was seven years older than him and a senior manager in a large engineering company while he was a self-employed electrician) they immediately got on well and were married in a registry office after just five months. Jane couldn't believe her luck: he was the perfect man she had never believed she could meet, and she had resigned herself to never getting married. Her own working-class parents had had a tempestuous marriage, with her father a heavy drinker, while Robert came from a stable middle-class family. He had left school at 16 to become an apprentice builder, while she had gone to college to study business.

Before she met Robert, Jane had always suffered from periodic bouts of depression and spent a lot of time 'worrying about everything', whereas Robert never appeared to get depressed and his calm stability soon alleviated her mood swings. She had been very sensitive and would get upset by tragic news items on TV, but Robert now managed to calm her down by discussing things with her. Nothing much appeared to disturb him, and Jane felt that at last she had found a rock, an anchor in her life; he would bore their small circle of friends by going on about how wonderful marriage was.

She got on well with Robert in bed and they made love regularly with no hint of sexual perversion in his desires. The only warning she had of the future was that when she discussed previous girlfriends with Robert she found that during a short period in his life he had slept with two women in bed at the same time – a mother and daughter. Jane had been a little shocked at this, as it seemed so out of keeping with the man she knew. She remembers even saying to him 'You are describing someone I don't know.' However, Robert declared he was completely happy sexually with Jane and had no desires for the wild life he had led in the past.

They led a life of quiet domesticity, went out to work during the week and spent weekends together, with Robert doing some DIY work around the house, and Jane doing the shopping. In fact he spent so much time in with her, never going out without her, that Jane felt the need for a little time by herself. She encouraged Robert to join a local golf club, which he reluctantly did.

Then one day, three weeks before Christmas, Jane takes up the story:

'I had rung him to say don't bother picking me up from work like he usually did as I wanted to do some Christmas shopping and the traffic would be too bad. He sounded fine, and even made a little joke which was that he had found some of the special chocolates I usually bought for Christmas, and he warned me they might not be here when I got back. I went to the local shopping centre and was there for a few hours when suddenly I felt an overwhelming urge to get back home urgently. I can't tell you why I had that feeling, I had never experienced anything like it before or since, but instantly I knew I had to see him. I was in such a hurry that I got on the first bus that went by even though it wasn't the right one, but although it dropped me further from home I felt I just had to get a bus, any bus.

'I hurried back and when I got to the house I rang the doorbell. As my keys were usually at the bottom of my handbag under a lot of rubble, I usually rang the doorbell for him to open the door, but no-one came. I looked around and saw the car was still parked outside and I remember wondering "Where can he be?" Eventually I found my keys and opened the door. First I went into the living room, but he wasn't there. I then thought he's in the kitchen making some tea, so I went into the kitchen but he wasn't there either. I then thought he must be upstairs having a bath. I started going up the stairs and I remember seeing everything in very slow motion. First I noticed the trapdoor to the loft in the ceiling was ajar, and I remember thinking, why is that open? Then I noticed a towel hanging through the loft opening and I remember thinking, what is that doing there? Then I saw Robert, naked, hanging from the towel. The shock just blew my mind. I didn't go any further up the stairs. I went down to the phone and called an ambulance and then I called my parents and then his parents. Apparently they said I was talking in a very matter of fact monosyllabic way – I said to his mum, "I think you should come over, Robert has hanged himself." His dad came to the phone and said, "I don't think this is very funny." I said, "I am not joking."

'When the ambulance and the parents came they said to call the police. I couldn't stay in the house and was out in the garden when the CID officer came out and told me it wasn't suicide. He said he had seen a lot of cases like this before and he was getting sexual excitement from strangling himself only it had gone wrong. Robert had used a towel to cover the rope so that the rope wouldn't leave any marks on his neck, which you wouldn't do if it was a suicide, and the beam around which the rope was hung showed evidence that he had done this many times before. He had moved a table and carefully cleared it so that he could stand on it and had had a clock by him so that he could time himself. He had used a special knot they all usually used, so that he could release it quickly, but obviously things had gone wrong. When I said it can't be true, he wasn't like that, he wasn't a pervert, the police officer said, the wife never knows.

'The coroner agreed that this was a case of autoerotic asphyxia but I have always had a nagging doubt as this final image of him was so fundamentally different to what he was like in real life. Despite a couple of years of counselling I still cannot come to terms with this because it was clear none of the counsellors had ever met anything like this and they couldn't really deal with it. I have not met anyone else who has gone through this and I need to meet someone like that who I can really talk to and who will really understand what I have gone through. I am still so perplexed that something so monumental could have been going on without me knowing. I am in another relationship now, but I could never marry again, or even make a complete commitment to anyone else, as I now feel I have had the rug pulled out from under my feet in such a fundamental way. I can't ever go through that again. I am much more held back now in any kind of relationship, and although I used to get depressed before I met Robert, since all of this I now get violent manic depression mood swings, so now I go high as well. I am on tablets which have more or less cured it, but the problem is this is the most isolating form of bereavement, because in every other case of death everyone knows someone else who has gone through the same thing, so you can talk about it with them, but in this case it is difficult to find anyone else who will admit to going through the same thing. There is such a stigma attached to it. His parents are deeply puzzled but they are so ashamed they won't talk about it and now his father won't have his name even mentioned in his house. You see, everyone thinks it was suicide, they think he was in despair, but they don't know the truth, that it's me who is really in despair. I am so angry with him that if he came back now, I think I would kill him.

'I think this is the biggest betrayal of all, because we were always thinking of each other before. I remember that I gave up smoking because he asked me to. I remember his saying, can't you stop smoking, can't you think of me? Now I think, was my marriage at all meaningful? It has left so many things unresolved, that you go backwards and forwards on yourself all the time. I mean, where did he hear about it in the first place? Did this all date from the time he was leading his wild life with this mother and daughter?

'I think the human psyche can deal with almost everything, except not knowing what it is dealing with.'

Practically all research to date in the area of perversion has been undertaken on male patients and there is no doubt that symptoms of perversion are noted much less often in women. Perhaps female analogies to voyeurism, frottage (the act of obtaining sexual pleasure by rubbing against another person, usually a stranger, in a crowd), exhibitionism and paedophilia are much less likely to be reported because the male 'victims' might not perceive themselves as having been 'victimized'.

In relation to sexual practices, one of the few but not infrequent ways that women come to the attention of doctors is the situation when a vibrator is inserted too far into the vagina to be retrieved. B. R. Burg, writing in the *Journal of the Royal Society of Health,*[52] warned, 'The trapped vibrators present particular hazards. After they have been inserted past the point of recovery, they usually cannot be shut off. It is often hours before the injured summon sufficient will to go to the hospital and in that time the constant vibration can cause considerable discomfort or pain, particularly if the vibrator has been equipped with long-lasting alkaline power cells rather than ordinary batteries.' They just keep going and going. Rarely has such a good argument been mounted for buying a less expensive product.

Data suggests that women very rarely commit aggressive sexual offences or exhibit patterns of rape, nor do females often take the sexually active role in incestuous activities. Except for sexual masochism, where the sex ratio is estimated to be 20 males for each female, the other paraphilias are almost never diagnosed in females.

To date, attempts to provide an explanation for this – such as references to the greater cultural flexibility for the expression of female sexuality – have not been very convincing. Psychoanalytic explanations – which basically theorize that the early processes during which female sexual identity is developed are less affected by traumatization than is the case for men – are not consistent with the most recent conclusions of infant and small child research.

A more modern approach, going beyond that of Freud, and one which is quite widespread in clinical work, is the construct of the 'perverse plug' introduced in the 1980s where perversion is basically understood as a type of repair mechanism. Perversion is viewed psychologically, first and foremost as a function. This function can best be described as a filling, as a plug, as an object which closes the gap created by a maladjusted development. Thanks to that plug, a balance is made possible. For men, this 'plug formation' affects sexuality first and foremost.

Almost 70 years ago, the American psychoanalyst Karen Horney,[53] in her criticism of Freud's concept of penis envy, made the astute observation that 'femininity' was in no way to be understood only as a poor substitute for 'masculinity', with motherhood and the desire for children being inadequate compensation for the never-received penis. She asked:

> And motherhood? And the blissful feeling of carrying new life inside yourself? And the tremendous joy of ever-increasing expectation in the appearance of new life? And the happiness when it's here at last? And when you hold it in your arms for the first time? And the profound, lustful satisfaction from nursing? And the joy of infant care?

Although it is evident that Horney is describing a mature adult woman here – in contrast to Freud, who studied young girls and their infantile genital organization – she makes it clear that reproduction involves more than the biological process of conception, pregnancy, birth and breastfeeding. Reproduction presents opportunities for interaction between mother and child on various realistic levels as well as in the realm of fantasy and imagination. For example, in reality the child is nursed and the mother is similarly satisfied ('profound, lustful satisfaction'). An example of fantasy in the mother–child relationship would be that the expectant mother is looking forward to an imagined reality ('the tremendous joy of ever-increasing expectation in the appearance of new life'). This leads to the following question: might the irrationality that we so often see in the sexual area among men, for women be situated in the reproductive area of their sexuality?

Dr. K. M. Beier of the Institute for Sexual Medicine in Berlin suggests an illustrative case from history which elaborates the idea that there is a female version of perversion but that this manifests itself most in disturbed relationships with offspring.[54]

The woman who manifested perversion in her relationships

Aurora was born in 1890 and is believed to have died in December 1955 in a psychiatric hospital in the Spanish village of Ciempozuelos.

On 9 June 1933, at approximately 8 a.m., she shot and killed her sleeping 18-year-old daughter Hildegart, with four bullets at point-blank range. She subsequently turned herself in to the authorities and after a spectacular trial she was sentenced to 26 years and 8 months in prison. After only a year and a half, however, she was transferred to a psychiatric hospital. The reason for the intense degree of public interest in this unusual case was that Hildegart Rodriguez had possessed genius-level intelligence and immense writing talent, and she had become a significant figure in public life.

As Vice-President of Spain's Socialist Youth Group, the volunteer General Secretary of the League for Sexual Reform, and the author of several brochures and numerous articles in the daily newspapers, she had fought with keen intelligence for the emancipation of women and for the realization of socialist societal models. A highly talented woman, she was attaining significance in the political life of Spain during the pre-Franco era; more than anything, she was a bastion of hope for women.

Aurora was the third of four children in a middle-class household in a large port city in north-western Spain. Her mother had studied to be a teacher but had never practised her profession; her father was an attorney and procurator at court. As was customary practice for girls at the time, Aurora's playful activity was limited. Her mother was reportedly dominating, impatient, hard, often in a bad mood and unable to empathize with others. In contrast, Aurora's father was passive and acquiescent.

Sexuality was laden with disgust and feelings of shame for Aurora. She had observed her sister engaging in premarital sexual activity and, as she later admitted to the judge, was deeply disturbed and disgusted by it. Her sister became pregnant and a wedding had to take place quickly. However, shortly after the birth of her son, Pepito, Aurora's sister wanted to share in the adventurous life of her husband, a textile dealer who was often overseas. She abandoned the child, leaving it with 11-year-old Aurora because the grandmother was uninterested.

Aurora built up a closely emotional, 'compensatory-motherly' relationship with her nephew, carrying him on hour-long walks, protecting him from the impatience and lack of understanding on the part of adults, singing him to sleep at night and playing him pieces of music composed for children on the piano. Under Aurora's guidance, Pepito became a child musical prodigy; he could play the piano at the age of three and was soon giving his first concerts. At that point, the child's parents regained interest, decreed that it was time for better teachers, and Aurora was no longer needed.

She had considered her nephew 'her work', and the loss of him was very painful; the separation was a traumatic event in her life. In the same year that her mother, who was perceived as impatient and depressive, died, Aurora had her first menstrual period. This lowered her self-esteem: she felt like a second-class citizen. She eventually became financially independent and occupied herself incessantly with social theories, all of which were centred on equal rights for women. At the age of 23 she announced in the city's newspaper that she was desirous of becoming pregnant, that the father of the child she wanted to bear should kindly reply, but that she was determined neither to marry nor to enter into a marriage-like relationship.

Later, she told the court that she was looking for a 'physiological colleague' for her second big work; her 'life's work', her own child this time. She was happy when it turned out to be a girl, as she had hoped. She named her daughter Hildegart, 'Garden of Wisdom'. Aurora considered almost everything about how children were customarily dealt with to be wrong and attempted to give her daughter a unique upbringing. She rejected both baby talk and pre-conceived toys. From the day of her daughter's birth, Aurora talked to her as if she were an adult. She explained the alphabet and multiplication tables to her daughter – no matter if she understood them or not. At the age of two, Hildegart received a typewriter, and only one year later (by way of appropriate proof of performance) received a nationally recognized certificate of typing competence.

She began school before her sixth birthday. After a week, she was promoted to second grade; six months later, she skipped another grade. Hildegart began to study law at the age of 13, because Aurora considered this crucial for her daughter's later political career and had successfully petitioned the Education Minister for a special permit. At that time, Hildegart was already writing articles for socialist newspapers that dealt with the liberation of women, sexual hygiene and the role of young people in the coming transformation of society.

According to Aurora, Hildegart's personality changed at the age of 18. Suddenly, she wanted to choose her clothing and her jewellery herself. She also fell in love and received an offer of a scholarship to study abroad. Aurora felt pushed to the sidelines. 'Strangers took possession of my daughter,' she later told the court. Shortly before

Hildegart's journey to London, which she was to undertake without her mother to begin studying with Havelock Ellis, the renowned British sexologist, she was shot to death in her sleep by Aurora.

Aurora explained to the court that, in her opinion, Hildegart had no right to take such a step towards independence. She had her mother to thank for her life, for the favourable and even ideal conditions of her life, and for her knowledge and her abilities. Hildegart was to fulfil an assignment, even if the price was giving up an independent identity. Hildegart was her mother's 'work of art' and Aurora was the 'ruler' over life and death: she had given life, and she could take it away. For Aurora, even a slight modification of the relationship as constructed by her was out of the question. However, since a change in the relationship had to take place, it seemed to Aurora that the physical destruction of Hildegart would be less painful than having to accept her daughter's move to London. Through the death of her daughter she was able to avoid her own breakdown.

Of course, the concept that a person can use any function – including mothering – to play out previous conflicts is nothing new. Nor is the idea that a child can become a self-object for a woman. But this case suggests that unlike the mechanism for self-esteem regulation in males as a basic component of perversion, a functional stabilization of the female self-concept seems more likely if conflict drives were to be focused on reproductional aspects and not on sexuality.

WHEN SEX AND MADNESS COMBINE

One of the great difficulties of understanding and classifying perversion is that sexual life, being private and taboo, is very difficult to discuss and compare with standards widely prevalent in society. So our sexual lives remain as mysterious to us as to others because we have so few reference points. There is a particular problem with perversion because the embarrassment involved means it takes a lot of courage for sufferers to talk frankly with professionals about their problems. So suspicion is naturally raised when someone seems to want to describe graphically and in detail their sexual habits to a wide audience. Yet there is a group of people – psychiatrists might refer to them as hysterics – who appear to have a new kind of perversion: the desire to be perversely open about their intimate lives.

The following case was reported in the academic journal *Contemporary Hypnosis*, because its author, Dr Michael Heap of the Centre for Psychotherapeutic Studies at the University of Sheffield, was involved as an expert witness in the civil case from which it arose.

In this extraordinary case a man claimed to have begun suffering overwhelming urges to make love to his furniture and domestic appliances, supposedly after taking part as a volunteer in a stage hypnosis show put on as an entertainment at a seaside hotel he was staying at. In the months and years following the show he began to report an unusual gamut of weird sexual symptoms and other difficulties which received a range of medical diagnoses from his doctors, including clinical depression, post-traumatic stress disorder, schizophrenic-related disorders and paranoid psychosis.

However, it is clear from the report of the case in the journal that Dr Heap himself is sceptical about these diagnoses. So among other issues this case illustrates that often in psychiatry and psychology there is much more controversy over the precise diagnosis than there is in the rest of medicine.

The two psychiatrists who represented the plaintiff in the case were convinced that his problems had been caused by the stage hypnotist's suggestion that the volunteers in the show would feel extremely sexy when they went to bed that night. In particular they believed the 'victim' had probably not been properly taken out of the hypnotic trance at the end of the show and as a result continued to be influenced long after the show was over by the hypnotist's commands.

Cases like this are intriguing because they go to the core of the controversy over precisely what kind of mental state is induced by hypnosis. If, as stage and media hypnotists frequently claim, the state they induce is a special and unique one, in which the participant is not colluding with the hypnotist by willingly going along with the game-playing required in stage shows, then hypnosis is indeed potentially dangerous. However, many psychologists and psychiatrists argue that even under hypnosis we can control our behaviour, and if we appear to do the bidding of the hypnotist it is entirely because we choose to do so.

So hypnosis presents a conundrum, for it appears to be a state where we agree to give up our free will, but we should be able to take it back again. But suppose, even if that is the case, that a subject fervently believes he has lost his free will to the hypnotist – then in a sense he may indeed have lost control because he believes he has. Yet if he had a different understanding of the hypnotic situation, he would be able to take back control.

In this case the doctors appearing as expert witnesses asserted that the plaintiff had been traumatized either by his experience on the show itself or by subsequent events when he was indulging in sexual behaviour with his home appliances.

The author of the original case report, who appeared for the defendant and whose views need to be viewed in that light, considered that the victim was clearly manufacturing his claim of affliction with unusual sexual compulsions. The term used to describe this situation is malingering. 'Malingering' has a very precise meaning in psychiatry: the key point is that not only are you making your symptoms up or pretending to have them, but you do so with a clear intent in your own mind. In this court case the intent was probably to obtain a large legal settlement from the hypnotist for damaging the victims' health.

However, in many cases where doctors believe symptoms are being manufactured the reason for producing them may not be clear in the patient's own mind. It may be that the symptom serves a function related to emotional or relationship issues in the patient's life which remain obscure to observers like psychiatrists. This is probably the situation with disorders like Munchausen's syndrome (which we discuss in a later chapter), where patients wander the country trying to gain admission to hospital, yet with no obvious financial or other motive. This group of disorders is called 'factitious', and Dr Heap who reports this particular case considers the more long-lasting problems as belonging to this category. So there was clearly a lot of disagreement between rival experts in the prosecution and defence camps. Even though the precipitating incident had occurred more than four years before the case came to trial, these disputes could not be resolved.

Since the case was funded by thousands of pounds of public money, it is important to the rest of society that distinctions between malingering, factitious disorders and real illness should be made precisely and accurately despite the absence of available objective tests.

All the names are changed in Dr Heap's original case report, and he refers to the case as 'Norman versus Byrnes'.[55]

The man who had sex with his furniture

In 1993, Mr Norman took part in Mr Byrnes's stage hypnosis show at a seaside hotel. At some point in the show Mr Byrnes offered to help Mr Norman give up smoking. Among other things, he gave him a post-hypnotic suggestion that from then on cigarettes would taste foul (or, as Mr Norman claimed, would smell like 'cow manure' or 'cow shit').

In a later stunt, Mr Byrnes suggested to his volunteers that, as they were sitting in their chairs, they would feel more and more sexy. He then hit his microphone repeatedly, calling out 'ten times more sexy . . . 20 times more sexy . . .' and so on.

According to the defendant (the hypnotist) and his witnesses, Mr Norman participated with gusto and became quite carried away with the idea that he was becoming more sexy, to the extent that he stood up and made thrusting movements behind the chair. (Mr Norman said that Mr Byrnes – who denied this – actually said 'Fuck the chair!' and in court he claimed that his penis became stuck in the back of the chair while he was doing so.) Mr Byrnes then suggested to the participants that when their heads hit the pillow that night they would feel 70 times more sexy than they did at that moment.

Mr Norman alleged that when he resumed his place at the bar at the end of the show, the smoke from cigarettes smelt like cow manure. He further claimed that he made a nuisance of himself by accosting other smokers and complaining to the landlord. Mr and Mrs Norman both stated that when they returned home that night and went to bed, as soon as Mr Norman lay down he started shaking violently and bouncing up and down. Mr Norman claimed that he was having sexual intercourse with the mattress, and that he found it sexually attractive. He continued simulating intercourse with the mattress and the other contents of his bed, with the exception of Mrs Norman. The exclusion of Mrs Norman was not apparently picked up on in the case report but would have had some significance to a psychiatrist sceptical about the precise state Mr Norman was in.

Mr and Mrs Norman also related that his penis had become 'gigantic'. At some point Mrs Norman decided to have a cigarette. When she lit it her husband immediately felt sick and ran to the bathroom, coughing violently. After some time he returned and resumed his sexual activity. Throughout the night Mrs Norman could only subdue him by blowing cigarette smoke at him, where-upon he would rush to the bathroom and be sick.

They agreed that all this went on unceasingly from 1 a.m. to 5 a.m. He then slept until 10 o'clock, after which he was fine that day. For the next three days Mr Norman was relatively well during the day and spent the evenings drinking at the same hotel. However, during the nights his behaviour continued to be disturbed and he had the same uncontrollable urge to have sexual intercourse with his furniture and domestic appliances. As well as his bed, articles that were allegedly the objects of his sexual interest included the bedroom ceiling, an armchair, various ornaments, the bath, a tumble-drier (at least while it was in the act of tumbling) and the ambulance that came to take him away. (On two of these nights he was taken to the local accident and emergency department.)

During this time Mr Norman's family made a video of his disturbed behaviour. Five days after her husband's stage hypnosis, Mrs Norman went to see a solicitor. Two days later Mr Norman went to see his doctor. This order of priority might also be regarded with some significance by a psychiatrist considering whether malingering is involved.

Mr Norman's doctor prescribed him antipsychotic medication, which is usually prescribed for serious behavioural disturbances caused by psychotic illnesses. Several days later, his doctor 'performed hypnotherapy on him to remove the post-hypnotic suggestion'. This seemed to be successful. However, about three weeks later Mr Norman was referred to a psychiatrist because of his depression, delusions and violent behaviour.

Meanwhile, he continued to have hypnotherapy from his doctor, who had received training from the British Society of Medical and Dental Hypnosis.

The psychiatrist saw Mr Norman about four months after the stage hypnosis show. Several days before the appointment, Mr Norman had been the subject of an exorcism in a local church. This was conducted by his general practitioner. In his report to the court the psychiatrist states that Mr Norman was now cheerful, calm and relaxed, and apparently normal. The psychiatrist ascribed Mr Norman's problems to Mr Byrnes's failure to take him out of the hypnotic trance. He considered that the exorcism had been successful in taking Mr Norman out of the hypnotic state.

Things went quiet for several months, and Mr Norman received no medication or treatment until early 1994. (In court, Mrs Norman claimed that during this period her husband had tried to convince himself that he was better, but he was still troubled by inappropriate erections in response to inanimate objects.)

Here I would like to mention, without further comment, the fact that in early 1994 media attention was being given to a number of sensational claims concerning the adverse effects of stage hypnosis. Mr Norman was then re-referred by his doctor to the psychiatrist, this time with problems of agitation and some difficulties in his short-term memory, neither of which had responded to hypnotherapy. The psychiatrist concluded that Mr Norman had significant depressive symptoms and prescribed an antidepressant. He continued to monitor his progress and in a report dated 12 months after the show he diagnosed him as having post-traumatic stress due to his experience of stage hypnosis. In a later report, towards the end of 1994, he diagnosed Mr Norman with severe post-traumatic stress disorder and a moderate depressive illness, both caused by his experience of stage hypnosis.

Mr Norman's solicitors obtained further expert witness testimony from a Dr James, a consultant psychiatrist. Dr James relied on medical reports and on witness statements by Mr and Mrs Norman and made several allegations of negligence against Mr Byrnes. First he asserted that Mr Byrnes's volunteers were told to simulate copulation in public.

There is an assumption by the original psychiatrist, Dr James and Mr Norman's doctor, based on Mr Norman's testimony, that Mr Byrnes asked his volunteers to do this. Mr Norman's doctor goes so far as to maintain in a letter that his client had been given the post-hypnotic suggestion that he would make love to a tumble-drier and to his bed, something which Mr Norman himself never claimed. In fact, witnesses for the defendant, and Mr Byrnes himself, merely said that the participants were told that they would feel many times more sexy, as they sat in their chairs, and they would do so that night.

Second, throughout his report Dr James insists, on the basis of Mr Norman's testimony, that Mr Byrnes did not cancel various suggestions or post-hypnotic suggestions. He states how they should be cancelled and intimated that Mr Byrnes should have cancelled instructions for each suggestion to each person individually. Moreover, Dr James implies that Mr Byrnes was further negligent in not checking afterwards that the suggestion was indeed cancelled.

I should point out here that the notion that Mr Byrnes did not 'terminate the trance' or issue a general 'removal of suggestions' edict at the end of his performance was simply assumed by the three doctors on a reading of Mr Norman's statement. Mr Byrnes described to me a protocol that he uses at the end of each performance. He alerts the participants and recites a general reversal of all suggestions and post-hypnotic suggestions, in accordance with the Home Office guidelines that were in existence at the time. He had witnesses to support his assertion.

Dr James also accused Mr Byrnes of negligence in two subsequent interactions with Mr Norman. In response to an answerphone message from Mrs Norman, Mr Byrnes telephoned Mr Norman and reassured him in some general way that he was no longer hypnotized and that he would feel better. Then, at the suggestion of Mr Norman's family and the staff of the local accident and emergency department, Mr Byrnes visited Mr Norman at his home.

He attempted to reassure him and to remove the alleged ill-effects of the stage hypnosis experience by further hypnotic suggestion. Mr Byrnes found Mr Norman to be co-operative, relaxed and they parted on pleasant terms. Mr Norman reported that he was terrified of Mr Byrnes; he thought he was going to kill him, and that Mr Byrnes attempted various procedures to re-hypnotize him but none worked. Dr James's charge against Mr Byrnes was that he did not take enough trouble to establish what the exact counter-suggestion should have been to dispel the post-hypnotic suggestion under which Mr Norman was behaving when having sex with his furniture and domestic appliances. Mr Byrnes was negligent in not summoning a person in whom Mr Norman had confidence, such as his own doctor, to attend the 'wiping-out-of-the-suggestion' ceremony. The assumption here is that the presence of Mr Norman's doctor would in some way render the counter-suggestion more potent. Thus, one supposes, Mr Norman would have been spared his subsequent four years of apparent mental illness.

When one considers these serious allegations one cannot help recalling some variation of *The Sorcerer's Apprentice*. Dr James casts Mr Byrnes in the role of an inept would-be wizard whose task it is, under the stern eye of a properly qualified master wizard, to discover the best counter-spell or incantation that would lift the evil curse with which he had previously and inadvertently bewitched Mr Norman.

When Mr Norman was interviewed, there seemed to be no limit to the symptoms that he was prepared to disclose. Indeed, the accounts given by him and his wife became progressively more dramatic and inconsistent as time went on. They include inappropriate and uncontrollable sexual arousal and behaviour, taking a bath in the sink (an account of which was given by Mrs Norman on television), uncontrollable verbal and physical aggression, regression to childlike behaviour, severe anxiety, confusion, fear of losing control in public, sleep disturbance, nightmares, blackouts, cessation of breathing, depression, suicidal thoughts, auditory and visual hallucinations, delusions, thought disorder, manic episodes, paranoia and loss of visual imagery.

Mr Norman was persistently described as a 'puzzling case' and perhaps it is not surprising that his case was mentioned in parliament as an illustration of the potential harm of stage hypnosis.

Even at the trial, Mr Norman's disclosure of yet more bizarre symptoms continued. He claimed that he was visited every night at 11.20 p.m. by another person who encouraged him to speak profanely, at which time he would see Mr Byrnes's head in place of his wife's. He even proclaimed that he saw Mr Byrnes's head on top of the shoulders of every man in the courtroom. Indeed when the psychiatrist came to give his testimony he announced that, having observed Mr Norman in the witness box, he had updated his diagnosis to major depression. The psychiatrist was asked to submit a further report and later claimed that Mr Norman had exhibited thought disorder in the witness box.

During his cross-examination Mr Norman was obliged to authenticate himself on two fronts that were incompatible. First, he had to convince the court that he was a man with a severe mental illness. To this end he described an ever-increasing multitude of bizarre symptoms which are collectively not seen in psychiatric practice. Indeed, the more symptoms, the less likely it seemed that he was experiencing them. Second, he was required to defend himself against a prolonged verbal tirade against his honesty and integrity and to justify inconsistencies and anomalies in his account of his previous work record (or, as it turned out, lack of it) and his alleged mental problems.

Mr Norman was most probably a man mimicking a mental illness and insofar as his claims about the immediate after-effects of his stage hypnosis were concerned, he was obviously malingering, basing his allegations on popular misconceptions about the nature of hypnosis. Indeed a witness for the defence who took part with Mr Norman in the stage hypnosis act was ready to testify that Mr

Norman, in the days and weeks following, had been preoccupied by his claim and had talked about it unceasingly, and the possibility of his receiving enormous compensation. The witness claimed in his statement that Mr Norman put pressure on him to make a similar dishonest claim. This witness and others would testify that Mr Norman's behaviour immediately after the show, when he lingered in the bar drinking, was normal.

There was the possibility of classifying Mr Norman's further problems in the category of factitious disorder. In the case of both malingering and factitious disorder, the person deliberately feigns physical or psychological symptoms. However, while malingering is associated with some obvious gain, such as monetary compensation or exemption from an onerous duty, in a factitious disorder the person has a compelling psychological need to be perceived as ill.

The court hearing ran for more than four days. Notwithstanding the extraordinary revelations concerning Mr Norman's post-hypnotic sexual proclivities, including at one point his bawling out 'I fucked a washing machine!' and 'I tried to shag the ceiling!' (to which the opposing barrister enquired as to whether he was 'arching his back and had an erection'), the proceedings were attended by his four children, the youngest of whom was 14.

On the fifth day the trial collapsed because Mr Norman's financial backer withdrew. Mr Norman had already had his legal aid revoked on a technicality – namely that any compensation that he was likely to be awarded would be offset by the mandatory repayment of the considerable welfare benefits he had received while being unavailable on the job market.

This story begins in a hotel bar in a rundown seaside resort in which people felt obliged to act out ridiculous roles to satisfy the demands of the situation in which they found themselves. And this is exactly how it ends, more than four years later: in a provincial English county court, complete with men dressed in black cloaks and wearing grey wigs.

If stage hypnosis is about playing a role for the benefit of the audience and the hypnotist, then this role playing goes on more than we may consciously realize – from courtrooms to doctors' surgeries.

5

THE DELUSION OF LOVE

This thing of darkness I acknowledge mine.
The Tempest, V i, 274–5

Falling in love is sometimes jokingly seen as tumbling into the grip of a form of madness. However, sometimes love causes extreme suffering as well as bizarre or dangerous behaviour, and so these forms of love enter the domain of the psychiatrist. Different types of 'pathological love' have attracted increasing interest because of prominent cases.[1]

The following disturbing case was reported by Dr Albert Roberts of the School of Social Work, Rutgers University in the USA, with a colleague, Dr Sophia Dziegielewski.[2]

The woman pursued by a 'friend'

Jill arrived for her appointment with her social worker and upon entering the office she slumped down in a chair as she began to describe her desperation over recent events. According to Jill, she had met John, the cousin of a co-worker, at a Christmas party. Although Jill, aged 36, was considered to be successful in her career in management, she admitted that she felt uncomfortable with the dating process. John, who was 39, seemed interesting to Jill, and she was pleased when he invited her out the following evening.

From the moment they met they seemed to get on beautifully. Jill could hardly believe the interests that they had in common and John seemed in tune with Jill's every word. Unfortunately, according to Jill, this was the beginning of a two-week nightmare.

Jill had left town for several days and when she returned home, she found numerous messages on her answering machine from John. He sounded very upset and angry, stating something about being kicked out of his apartment. Before Jill could respond to the messages, John was knocking at her door.

When she greeted him, he looked dishevelled and it was evident he was upset. John informed Jill that he had been mistakenly evicted from his apartment and just needed a place to stay for the night. Jill said that she felt sorry for him and agreed to let him spend the night on her couch. Later that night, John joined Jill and they engaged in 'protected' intercourse. Afterwards, John seemed angry and when Jill asked what was wrong, he said that he was disturbed by Jill's actions. He expressed concern that her requirement that he use a condom put an artificial barrier between them, which decreased his pleasure and made him feel that Jill did not trust him. Jill stated that John's 'uncanny way of turning things around' left her feeling confused and guilty.

In the morning when Jill left for work John agreed that he would call her that evening to let her know where he was staying. When she came home that night John was still there and had cooked dinner for her. His explanation was that he could no longer stay with his friend as planned and was in the process of making alternative arrangements.

John spent the night at Jill's flat again but this time Jill locked her bedroom door and 'nothing happened'. The next morning Jill's car would not start and John volunteered to repair it. After this Jill insisted that he leave. John became very excited and angry and mentioned possibly hurting himself (she quoted him as saying 'I could blow my brains out over this') because of her rejection. When the caretaker of the building stated that he was going to call the police John left immediately. The caretaker later told Jill that John was seen working on her car before she returned from her trip. Jill also recalled messages left on the answering machine from John, when he described seeing her having lunch with a male co-worker.

The next day Jill heard from John's cousin that John had boasted of how pleased he was finally to meet Jill and that he knew from the first time he saw her how special she would turn out to be. When Jill arrived home that day John had again left numerous messages on her machine. Some were begging her to reconsider while others cursed her behaviour. Jill took the tape to a friend who was a police officer but was told that there was not enough evidence to do anything with the tape. When Jill mentioned that she believed John had tampered with her car, again she was told that nothing could be done – especially since she had given him permission to work on it.

After she had returned home that night, John again came to her door and hollered and banged on the door so loudly that the police were called. John told them that he was staying there and that Jill had just thrown him out. The police told John to leave peacefully and said that if he did not, charges would be filed. John left as instructed.

The next day at work Jill was horrified to see John approaching her office. He walked straight up to her and asked her very quietly, 'Can we please talk about all this.' Jill feared agitating him and agreed to go outside. He told her that he just wanted to see her again and give their new relationship a second chance. Wishing to avoid a confrontation at her job, Jill told him to call later and they would discuss it.

Jill decided to turn to the social worker for help. She was at a loss and feared if she did nothing, or became complacent in the relationship, it would only get worse.

This case seems to be easily categorized as an example of 'stalking', a phenomenon that has gained centre stage in the media recently. However, as we will explore in this chapter, the possible explanations and dynamics of what is going on here are a lot more intriguing and complex than the simple media diagnosis allows.

One possibility is that John is suffering from erotomania, the delusional belief that another person is in love with you but for some reason is denying this emotion. The job for the stalker is to get the victim to acknowledge this love. The denial of the awful possibility that you are not really loved by the person you desire drives much common behaviour. For example the mistress who fervently believes that the man she sacrifices her own long-term security for would leave his wife for her, but for his loyalty to the children. Here the mistress has had to come up with a reason why her love is not fully reciprocated.[3]

Another possibility is that John suffers from a personality disorder which means his personality or a core part of his character is such that his expression of emotions is socially inappropriate. For example, individuals with histrionic or hysterical personality disorder exhibit a pervasive pattern of excessive emotional reactions and attention-seeking behaviour. Based on what we know of John, he certainly appears to self-dramatize and theatrically exaggerate his expression of emotion.[4]

Obsessive-compulsive behaviour has also been noted in stalkers, and these individuals are driven by recurring and relentless thoughts and actions related to the stalking behaviour. (In this case John appears driven to get Jill to acknowledge a more intense relationship than there actually was.) There is also an element of addiction to much stalking in that the activity itself becomes addictive. Stalkers have reported that their pursuit behaviours provide excitement and in a bizarre sort of way challenging entertainment.[5]

THE MADNESS OF LOVE

The delusional belief that one is loved is the defining characteristic of a psychiatric disorder clinically described by French, German and British doctors in the 1920s and termed Erotomania. This delusional disorder has a prevalence rate of approximately 3 in 10,000 in the general population, and is a rare disorder even in psychiatric samples, representing only 1 to 2 per cent of inpatient admissions.

Although most individuals with this disorder are not violent, approximately 10 per cent of individuals who stalk have a primary diagnosis of erotomania, and rates of violence among stalkers average 25 to 35 per cent. Homicide rates among stalkers appear to be less than 2 per cent. In a review of 10 studies of obsessional followers involving 180 subjects, psychiatrist Dr J. Reid Meloy of the University of California–San Diego, a world authority on stalking, found that if violence occurred, the target was the object of 'love' at least 80 per cent of the time.[6, 7] The next most likely target was a third party perceived as impeding access to the object. Dr Meloy referred to this latter behavioural phenomenon as *triangulation*, and has developed a psychological explanation for its occurrence. The following case illustrates this pattern of violence.

Dr Meloy recently reported a case of homicide by a 29-year-old male with erotomanic delusional disorder and various personality disorders. Following a month of pursuit of a female stranger with whom he had conversed briefly in a local bar, he attacked the automative plant where she worked, delusionally believing that she was at imminent risk and needed to be rescued. One plant manager was killed and two police officers were wounded. The case illustrates triangulation, where rage against the rejecting object is displaced onto a third party, who is then perceived as impeding access to the victim.[8]

Triangulation is also present in jealousy, whether delusional or not, but then it is motivated by perceived competition for the love object.[9]

The psychodynamic understanding of triangulation is complex, and is grounded in two components when erotomania is present: the role the defence of projection (and thus paranoia) plays in the disorder; and the narcissistic psychopathology common among erotomanics, usually evident in their hubris or martyrdom.[10]

Erotomanic individuals project the impulse to love onto the object, and experience it as coming from within the object. They are the ones attracted to the target but they deny this to themselves and imagine that love for them is coming from the target, which protects them from having to own up to their own feelings of unrequited love. They are extremely sensitive to rejection, when it occurs, defending against their consequent feelings of humiliation with rage and a desire to damage or utterly devalue the object of pursuit. This diminishes envy of that which cannot be possessed, and may satisfy certain primitive talionic impulses (an eye for an eye). Destruction of the rejecting object may also restore the delusional and idealized narcissistic linking fantasy to the object – for instance, a conscious belief that they are destined to be together in a perfect, usually non-erotic union.[11]

In triangulation, however, the psychodynamic process has an added step. In order to protect the delusional and narcissistic link to the object, the rage felt in the midst of rejection is displaced and projected onto a third party. Now an otherwise neutral person or group poses an imminent risk to the object of pursuit, and sometimes to the erotomaniac himself. A paranoid pseudo-community is created in the mind of the perpetrator, and thoughts turn to fantasies of rescue. Rejection has become protection. This paranoid magnification intensifies fear and anger and becomes a substitute for actual, affectional bonding love.[12]

Fantasies of rescue in erotomanic delusion may be the psychotic basis for acts of violence that are planned, purposeful, emotionless and quite lethal. This strange form of 'pathological love' was first described in the 1920s by the French psychiatrist G. G. de Clérambault.[13] He called the phenomenon he had discovered '*psychose passionelle*' and published five cases of what has become known as De Clérambault's Syndrome or erotomania. It usually consists of a woman's sudden conviction that an older, unattainable man of high social status is in love with her. Often the man is a public figure: an actor, a politician, a millionaire or even a member of the royal family. Classically the condition has a sudden onset, the delusion appearing out of the blue with no background of previous similar beliefs or fantasies.[14]

The fundamental assumption made by the woman suffering from erotomania, according to Dr Clérambault, is that it is the man 'who started it all and who loves most or who alone loves'. She interprets all his subsequent actions as subtle and secret signs of his love for her, like fleeting exchanges of looks or the clothes the man wears, all of which the woman believes hold special significance for her. In reality they actually have no relationship to her at all, as the man is frequently unaware of the woman's existence. Whether or not he actually comes into contact with her is immaterial to the sufferer, who is content for a while to observe her lover from afar. Up to this point the syndrome may be considered innocuous but then things tend to take an ominous turn, as the woman often begins to feel that the man by his 'amorous persistence' merits love in return.[15]

This syndrome of the delusion of being loved is also known as *amor insanus*, delusional loving, old maid's insanity, and *melancholia érotique*. Erotomania should be distinguished from other forms of pathologic love. Excessive desire for coitus is termed nymphomania in women and satyriasis in men. The phantom lover syndrome is the delusion of being visited by a secret lover who does not exist. Obsessional love is more common than erotomania; in this syndrome the patient is just as obsessed with the love object but does not harbour the delusion that the object reciprocates this feeling. The term 'erotomania' first appeared in 1640, although cases fitting this description can be found in medical literature dating back to Hippocrates.[16]

De Clérambault distinguished between pure erotomania, when the syndrome occurs alone, and secondary erotomania, when it occurs in association with another psychiatric disorder.[17] Since the essential component is the sudden onset of the conviction of being in amorous communication with a person of much higher rank who was the first to fall in love and the first to make advances, the delusion fulfilled the psychological demands of sexual pride that life had failed to provide. This meant the disorder could be explainable and understandable in psychological terms, so there might not be a need to resort to biological brain dysfunction to account for it. Kraepelin, a German psychiatrist, hugely influential at the beginning of the twentieth century, suggested that the delusion served as a 'psychological compensation for the disappointments of life'.[18]

In erotomania the patient may deny the 'beloved's' marriage or consider it invalid, and although she may acknowledge that the 'lover's' behaviour is contradictory to her belief, she chooses to ignore or misinterpret this. De Clérambault pointed out the strong sexual craving present in many of these cases.

Erotomania has been known since ancient times, with one case being recorded by Plutarch.[19]

In the last 75 years there have been increasing reports of erotomania occurring in both men and women, young or old, sexually and socially active or isolated, and heterosexual or homosexual. Classification of the syndrome has been controversial, with some authorities maintaining that erotomania is usually a component of a more generalized disorder, frequently paranoid schizophrenia or manic depression.[20] What hasn't changed since the disorder was first described is psychiatrists' concern with the great potential of this syndrome for prompting extraordinary and violent behaviour. In 1979 Enoch, Trethowan and Barker in *Some Uncommon Psychiatric Syndromes* noted some of the various implications of the disorder.

> The patients may bring chaos into the lives of their victims who usually give them no encouragement whatsoever. They may bombard them with letters, telegrams, and telephone calls without respite, both at home and at work and for long periods of time . . . These patients may even be dangerous and wind up making an attempt on the life of their victim or members of his family. This is particularly liable to occur when the patient reaches the stage of resentment or hatred which replaces love, after repeated advances are unrequited. They may thus require prolonged hospitalization to prevent them from carrying out threats which are contained in their letters.

Here are a few sample cases that demonstrate the kind of violence associated with this delusional disorder:

In a case which gained national notoriety in America, a 35-year-old Californian man was arrested after he became convinced that a daughter of a former President of the United States was his lover. He repeatedly approached her in person and sent her a series of love letters. They were of course perfect strangers and the courts eventually became involved, as is the usual pattern with cases of erotomania. Despite the judge's warning to desist from annoying the woman, the man phoned repeatedly from jail. He was finally transferred to a psychiatric hospital. He maintained throughout that they were both in love.[21]

In another case dating back to 1988, Richard Farley shot his way into a Californian electronics firm, killing seven people and wounding three others, including Laura Black, the young woman who was the object of his delusional love.[22]

Still in the United States, a 36-year-old woman became convinced that television newsmen were romantically involved with her. She repeatedly telephoned them, and in response to complaints the Sheriff's Department threatened to remove her telephone. Her father eventually disconnected the phone whenever he left the house. One day she went to the home of a television newscaster whom she had never met and announced that they were going to be married. She then attempted to evict the newscaster's wife from the home. The police were summoned and the woman was taken to a psychiatric facility.[23]

A 44-year-old farmer was arrested and charged with breaching a court order to stop harassing a famous singer. He had followed her around the country pestering her with unrequited attempts to win her hand. He was ultimately found incompetent to stand trial and confined for an indeterminate period of time to a mental health centre.[24]

Psychiatrists Dr Stephen G. Noffsinger and Dr Fabian M. Saleh at the Northcoast Behavioral Healthcare System in Northfield, Ohio, recently reported the following case of a man who held delusions of an erotic nature about female TV newscasters.[25]

The man who was in the news

Mr K., an inpatient in a state psychiatric facility, believed that local and national newscasters spoke directly to him and controlled his thoughts. Mr K. wished to impregnate several local female news-casters. He also believed that one specific local newscaster had killed his brother and was also conspiring to kill his father. Mr K. wished to kill this newscaster in retribution for the perceived killing of his brother and to prevent the newscaster from killing his father. Previously, Mr K. had approached the office of a local television station to verbalize his grievances to the newscaster but peacefully left the premises when confronted by security staff.

Clinicians contacted the potential victims in the hope that their knowledge of the risk could prevent a violent act. The clinicians sent them a letter outlining the nature of Mr K.'s delusions and the risk factors involved, with an invitation to meet. Mr K. was fully informed of these communications and agreed to the release of the information. The clinicians considered arranging a meeting between Mr K. and the newscaster at most risk but this option was dismissed because of the concern that personal contact could intensify Mr K.'s delusions.

After the disclosure, several local newscasters contacted hospital administrators with questions about potential risks. The newscaster especially targeted by Mr K. was alarmed when informed of his homicidal intent. Management staff at the newscaster's station con-sulted the network's legal counsel and hired an independent forensic psychiatrist, who monitored the case.

Schizophrenic patients may incorporate television programming material into their delusions, may believe that they are on television themselves, or may think they are the topic of television pro-grammes.[26] The prevalence of ideas of reference about radio or television personalities is believed to be low. 'Ideas of reference' is the term given to the mistaken belief that something totally irrele-vant to you has a deep personal significance. A typical example would be the sense that a newsreader is directly addressing you per-sonally or that an advertising hoarding is referring to you specifically. Significant risks occur when psychotic patients develop ideas of reference and paranoid delusions about television personalities.

As a result of previous legal precedent in the USA, clinicians have a legal duty to take reasonable steps to protect the potential victims of their patients.[27] Disturbingly, they rarely discharge their duty to protect potential victims in the manner specified by law, fearing that the treatment relationship will suffer.[28]

It is noticeable that although erotomania was originally described as a disorder of women, most modern cases involve men. One reason for this may be that men are more prone to aggressive behaviour than women so it is not surprising that men suffering from erotomania are more likely to act on their delusions in a violent way. This is especially so when love is unrequited. However, shifts in sex roles in society since De Clérambault first described the syndrome might also affect its distribution among men and women. Women are increasingly perceived as powerful and successful figures and possibly more likely to attract grandiose romantic fantasies than ever before.[29]

Whatever the explanation, does this disorder have the potential to tell us something about romantic love? One striking element is the persistence of these patients in the pursuit of gratification of their emotions. Despite all the obstacles placed in their way, including imprisonment, they continue to live out their obsession. Even in the face of strong opposition from their quarries, they cling to their notions of love.[30]

Perhaps this illustrates an important aspect of love, which is its addictive quality. There are many similarities between the power of this addiction and that of drugs. They are often so close that biochemical theories have been invoked by researchers. Scientists involved in this work have included doctors at the New York State Psychiatric Institute. They argue that love brings on a giddy feeling not dissimilar to the high of drugs like amphetamines. The craving for romance is like the craving for a particular kind of high, and the crash that follows a break-up has similarities to the depression experienced by addicts following drug withdrawal. In fact a substance related to amphetamine has been found to be produced by the brain, called phenylethylamine (PEA).[31] One speculation is that love feelings are similar to amphetamine highs because the brain of a person in love produces this intoxicating substance. The variety of emotions produced by mood-manipulating drugs include, among the 'highs', euphoria, excitement, relaxation, spiritual feelings and relief. Among the 'lows', anxiety, panic attacks, pain and fear are also produced by both.[32]

Some of the drugs used by doctors in the treatment of depression include those known as monoamine oxidase inhibitors or MAOIs, and these may inhibit the breakdown of PEA in the brain. This has kindled speculation that a drug derived from these principles may be developed for 'stabilizing' the 'lovesick'. Those suffering from unrequited love go into a state resembling drug withdrawal, these researchers suggest. This may explain why this state is accompanied by a craving for chocolate, among other foods, as chocolate contains PEA.[33]

While the dangerous potential of illicit drugs is widely acknowledged in our society, it seems a more common and equally destructive addiction lurks within all of us in the form of these pathological loves. Perhaps one obvious cure for love's incessant obsessive quality so far neglected by psychiatrists is marriage.[34]

The other notable theme running through cases of erotomania is the high status of the recipients of the patients' attentions. Often ordinary people's fantasy lovers have special talents or characteristics. This may illustrate a common need for our loved ones to live out an undeveloped aspect of ourselves. In other words, we live vicariously through their accomplishments, which are often in an area which we would like to develop ourselves. Lack of ability in some aspect of life is an important cause of unhappiness, and one way we seek to compensate for this is to find success through our mates.[35]

Another theory is that since most sufferers seem to be lonely, isolated individuals who have not been very successful in love, the delusion that an unattainable celebrity has fallen in love with them elegantly compensates for and explains their single status to others: 'The reason my love is not with me today is that she is playing in the singles final at Wimbledon . . .'[36]

Yet another theory is that when we fall in love we tend to do so with a distorted fantasy image of our partners, usually a rather idealized version of the reality. One result of the media explosion of the latter half of the twentieth century is that we have more information than ever before about the successful in our society. This only serves to emphasize the differences between the famous and the anonymous and those in the limelight may be more vulnerable than ever before to the attentions of those suffering from erotomania. Perhaps the media even play a role in creating erotomania. Many sex scandals of the future may be the result of a public figure becoming beguiled by the attentions of an erotomaniac.[37]

Whatever the trends of the future, and the speculations of the present, it is worth remembering that despite all our problems with love, these difficulties are far from new. In the first century BC Cicero remarked: 'Omnibus enim ex animi perturbationis est profecto nulla vehementior. Furor amoris.' ('Of all the emotions, there is none more violent than love. Love is a madness.')[38]

The central problem with delusions of love is that in the vast majority of cases patients have no demonstrable biological abnormality or disease of the brain. This has led to a debate within psychiatry as to whether this is a psychological or an organic problem.

Dr Alan Anderson and colleagues from the Departments of Neurology, Surgery (Emergency Medicine), and Psychiatry of the University of Colorado Health Sciences Center in Denver recently reported a fascinating case of erotomania where the cause appeared to be a definite brain injury.[39] Even though the advances of the erotomaniac are unexpected and unwanted, any denial of affection by the object of this delusional love is dismissed by the patient as a ploy to conceal the forbidden love from the rest of the world.

The woman whose brain fell in love

The case involves a 48-year-old Korean-born woman, aged 39, who began to experience headaches and alteration of consciousness. A brain scan showed extensive haemorrhaging into the brain due to weakness in the arterial wall (an aneurysm). Following brain surgery the patient recovered and was able to return to work after several months.

Four years after the hospitalization, the woman was treated for depression and was heard to comment about a romantic relationship that was 'not working out'. It became evident she believed that a physician at the hospital where she worked was in love with her. She based this belief on the 'special' look he had given her in the hospital cafeteria. There was no known prior contact between the patient and this physician. He denied any romantic inclinations, but the patient persisted in her belief. She sent gifts, made phone calls and visited the office where he practised. This behaviour continued despite ongoing psychotherapy, treatment with antipsychotic medication and a restraining order. After multiple violations of the restraining order, she was committed to a psychiatric hospital.

On admission, she steadfastly held to her belief that the physician loved her and would return her affections if he were not constrained by his job and family. She complained of recurring depressive symptoms with fleeting suicidal tendencies and dull, diffuse headaches.

She had some difficulty maintaining a coherent train of thought, but her memory was intact and she spoke normally in both Korean and English.

However, the patient reported vivid memories of three near-death experiences. The first occurred when she was eight years old; the second near-death experience occurred with a pill overdose at age 21, and the third with her ruptured aneurysm. She repeatedly stated her belief that God had worked through American doctors to make her live.

Dr Anderson points out that the rupture of aneurysms such as these is usually a neurologic catastrophe associated with high morbidity and mortality. Psychiatric symptoms among survivors of such brain haemorrhages are common; although psychotic or delusional symptoms are rare, most patients manifest depression or anxiety. In this case, erotomania developed from a bleed into the brain and persisted despite treatment for five years.

Dr Anderson found that while the vast majority of reported cases of erotomania appear to have no observable biological abnormalities of the brain, there are also cases associated with neurologic and medical conditions. At least 29 such cases in addition to Dr Anderson's suggest an association with demonstrable brain abnormalities.[40]

Erotomania associated with pregnancy has also been reported and there is a report of a woman who developed an erotomanic attachment to the physician who performed her abortion, raising the question of an association with either the hormonal changes of pregnancy or the psychic trauma of the procedure as the trigger for the delusion.[41] Another description is of a pregnant woman with no psychiatric history who developed the delusion that her obstetrician was in love with her and was communicating with her through psychic messages. This persisted for over three years. The report states that following treatment with antipsychotic medication the patient refrained from contacting the physician for 18 months.[42]

Demented patients with erotomania have also been reported, for example a woman with Alzheimer's disease who had the delusion that a young maintenance man at her apartment was in love with her.[43] Oddly the delusion faded as she became progressively more demented. One woman with dementia caused by repeated multiple strokes had the erotomanic delusion that the Prince of Wales had proposed marriage. She also held the belief that she had been married and separated from the former Israeli Prime Minister Shimon Peres.[44]

In yet another case a man with a progressive neurologic illness that was probably of a dementing type developed the delusion that an English princess was in love with him and that they were to be married. This belief was based on special signs he claimed to receive from the photocopy machine he used at work.[45]

In patients with erotomania, there is a fundamental mis-interpretation of another person's intent. The erotomaniac perceives a look, a gesture or a spoken or written word as containing a special and unique meaning. This disturbed perception is clearly more complex than simply mistaking someone's expression; it may involve the partici-pation of widespread cerebral networks. The right brain is associated with emotional expression recognition in others, so dysfunction here could explain the tendency for erotomaniacs to be convinced they know the true feelings of the person they are pursuing.[46]

A striking feature of erotomania is the duration of the delusional belief, which may persist for decades in the absence of reinforce-ment. This belief is abnormal in its initial formation, in its resistance to testing for external validation and in its failure to vanish when shown to be incorrect. These features imply that brain dysfunction contributes to the syndrome. Erotomania may therefore represent an opportunity to investigate the cerebral operations involved in the formation and persistence of delusional thinking and the represent-ation of emotional function, like love, in the human brain.[47]

IS STALKING JUST ANOTHER FORM OF OLD-FASHIONED LOVE?

A modern variant on old-fashioned love – obsession, now termed 'stalking' – has rapidly gripped the popular imagination, partly because some of the facts are so sensational. For example a US study of the enclosures sent in mail to Hollywood celebrities and US Congress members included syringes of blood and semen, a bedpan and a coyote's head.[48]

While we are used to the idea of celebrities being stalked, there are many more obscure and unusual victims, for example the in-carcerated armed robber who received considerable media exposure and as a result became inundated with letters from adoring women. One became so persistent, even flashing her genitals at him during a

174

non-contact prison visit, that the inglorious victim had to appeal through his lawyer for the 'hero worship' to stop.[49]

The adolescent grip of first love can induce many to consider sacrificing everything for their infatuation, but the central difference with stalkers is that, unlike other immature lovers who usually hanker for their loved one in silent anonymity and are exquisitely sensitive to the slightest rebuffs, the obsessive follower never takes no for an answer and openly persists with increasingly outrageous behaviour despite the obvious distress they are causing the object of their so-called affection.

Research into obsessive followers of the non-famous produces the following profile: their average age is 35, most are unemployed, 60 per cent have had previous psychiatric treatment, one in seven is married at the time of their pursuit and many have never had a serious close relationship and have very poor social skills producing extreme isolation.[50] Yet none is below average in IQ, hence their resourcefulness and the frequent inability of victims to elude pursuit. (Stalkers have posed as police officers to obtain addresses from automobile records departments and decoded unlisted telephone numbers of victims by using telephone installation equipment).[51]

But while the fascination with stalkers focuses on their relentless pursuit, the key to their pathology is the immense disparity in status between pursuer and victim. In most relationships our expectations about who might find us attractive govern those we try to woo, so we tend to end up with partners who are perceived to be of similar attractiveness. Stalkers in contrast target potential mates who are usually way out of their league, and this tells us a great deal about what stalkers think about themselves. It is obvious that they have a grossly unrealistic view of their own desirability.[52]

This conviction of their own allure produces the mistaken belief that if they persist for long enough the other party will simply come round – or that the victim actually does fancy them and they are just playing hard to get. However, once they become convinced they are being teased this unleashes grave hostility.[53]

Their grandiose sense of self also has to try to resolve the small problem of their lowly station, perhaps by seeking to obtain someone of higher social status as a trophy to prove they really are more special than the world has found them to be. They treat their victims more as objects to be possessed than as people to be cherished.[54]

But these pretensions to grandeur are really a defence against loneliness (I'm single because no-one is good enough for me) and so stalkers are likely to be hugely hurt by rejection. This then leads to outrage that anyone should dare to reject them, and an anger which is then directed at their victims. They make sure their intended feels sorry for ever having had the temerity to say no. The need to predict the dangerousness potential of the stalker from early innocuous signs like love letters is urgent. The fatal error most victims make is to underestimate the disturbance of mind involved and to try to reason with their pursuer in the early stages of the obsession. As previously mentioned, this kind of contact is misconstrued and merely serves to exacerbate the delusion that the quarry is 'playing' hard to get.[55]

Psychiatrists find the most worrying earliest signs relate to correspondence over periods of one year or longer, the writing of more than 10 letters and the presence of two or more geographically different postmarks on envelopes.[56] These are all signs of preoccupation, for if you can still find the time to send mail even when far away from home, something is clearly preying on your mind.[57]

But the problem of embarking on the scientific study of a behaviour that is as yet not properly defined can make objective study appear ponderous. For example, an attempt to 'operationalize' the definition of stalking so that scientists can agree on what is being studied means the definition in some research papers is cumbersome and can appear oddly unfeeling to victims. Nobody would want to advise a terrified victim who has had a man standing outside their house looking up at the window on nine consecutive nights that, according to the academics, there was another night to go before he or she could lay claim to being stalked.

Another issue is whether the celebrity stalker is really a completely different phenomenon to the more common stalker of the obscure victim. Examples include the spectator who stabbed tennis star Monica Seles in Hamburg and another whose attachment to Seles led to his taunting of Steffi Graf at Wimbledon, having followed her from Paris. These cases share similarities with but also show important differences from the more 'ordinary' stalker, as exemplified in the case below.[58]

Claire Burke Draucker of the School of Nursing, Kent State University in Ohio, USA, reports the following case of a woman who was stalked for three years by a near-stranger. This case report is important because despite media interest in the phenomenon of stalking and the prevalence of the problem in the United States, its acute and long-term effects on the lives of those targeted have not been adequately determined.[59]

The woman who tried to help her stalker

'Mary' is a woman who participated in a research project Dr Draucker conducted on sexual assault. During an interview about a rape she had experienced years earlier, she began to discuss a more recent incident of stalking. Dr Draucker was struck by the terror the woman had experienced at the hands of a man she hardly knew, and the degree of disruption in her life that the stalking caused.

As they spoke, Mary drew parallels between the effects on her life of the rape and the stalking. Although she had not planned to discuss the stalking during the interview, her experience seemed very pertinent to a project dealing with the victimization of women. She expressed a willingness to have her story told so that nurses and other mental health professionals could become more aware of the potential impact of stalking on a woman's life.

Mary was working as an accountant when she met Harold, a middle-aged executive, while preparing his taxes. During the course of their business dealings, Harold began to reveal to Mary how unhappy he was with his life because he had no friends and was lonely.

Mary stated that she initially got 'sucked in' to listening to his problems because she felt sorry for him. Harold's behaviour soon began to turn 'really strange'. He began following Mary, calling her at home, and leaving little gifts for her. He would rummage through her rubbish and bring her exact replacements of things she had discarded. He also began to call her frequently. At one point, he planted a device to record her phone calls and replayed tapes of her conversations with other people on her answering machine.

After Harold recorded a conversation Mary had with a male friend during which they discussed Harold's strange behaviour, Harold became hostile. He left a copy of that tape in Mary's mailbox and threatened, 'I know what you have done, and you will pay . . .' Harold would leave signs in front of Mary's home that were alternately amorous ('You are loved') and hostile ('A bitch lives here'). He would also plant such signs in front of the homes of her family members. He would follow Mary's car and park near her house for hours, waiting for her to come out. He threatened to 'get' her young daughter. On several occasions he scattered nails on her driveway. He even rented cars so that he could follow Mary anonymously. At one point, Harold actually entered her residence.

Harold had also been stalking Jane, Mary's business colleague. The pattern of stalking behaviours was particularly difficult for Mary. Harold would 'lay off' for a while, just long enough for her to relax. He would then start his pursuit again, often by sending a greeting card to her on a special occasion, such as her birthday.

Mary changed jobs, bought a new car and got an unlisted phone number. At one point she moved to a house on a private road to prevent Harold from driving by at will, which he did nonetheless. She had to go to her child's school and insist that she be the only one to pick up her daughter. She worried about her parents' safety. Mary experienced intense anxiety and fear and had frequent nightmares. She was convinced that Harold would injure or kill her or her child.

Mary consulted a behaviour modification specialist, who recommended that she have no contact with Harold and refuse to acknowledge any correspondence. Mary took the expert's advice. Harold's pursuit did, in fact, intensify before temporarily subsiding. Mary believes Harold finally stopped stalking her only because he found someone else to pursue. She summed up her experience: 'It is hell. It's pure hell. And I went through that for three years.'

The stalking had an enormous effect on Mary's life. She explained that being stalked was more emotionally intense than being raped because the stalking 'just kept going on and on and on and on'. She stated, 'It's the same feelings of being violated and someone watching you and knowing what you're doing and the thing that gets me the most, the thing that bothers me the most, with both incidents, is that I had to change my life for this person . . . [The rapist and the stalker] were the ones that were violating me, yet I was the one [who] had to change my entire life because of it. It made me so angry.'

Little research has been conducted to determine the effects of stalking on individuals who have been targeted. However, an Australian study of 100 stalking victims (83 female and 17 male) found reported stalking behaviours included: repeated unwanted telephone calls (78 per cent of the participants), letters (62 per cent) and unsolicited material (50 per cent), direct approaches (79 per cent), physical surveillance (71 per cent), and property damage (36 per cent).[60] Fifty-eight of the participants were threatened, and 34 were physically or sexually assaulted. The stalking incidents lasted from one month to 20 years.[61]

Many participants made major changes in their lives (such as changing or stopping their employment, or changing residence) in response to the stalking. They also reported increased levels of anxiety (83 per cent), intrusive recollections and flashbacks (55 per cent), suicidal ruminations (24 per cent) and symptoms of post-traumatic stress disorder (37 per cent). In another recent study a significant portion of the sample (83 per cent) indicated that their personalities had changed as a result of the stalking. Many reported becoming more cautious, paranoid, easily frightened and aggressive.

Other research confirms that possible responses to stalking include post-traumatic stress symptoms, traumatic depression and suicidality. Crisis interventions for victims of stalking are similar to interventions for victims of other types of traumas.[62]

Surveys have found the following three strategies are the ones most often used to cope with stalking: ignoring or hanging up the phone, confronting the stalker and changing one's schedule to avoid the stalker. Women were most likely to ignore the stalker, and men were most likely to confront the stalker.[63]

The problem is that there is very little research on what is actually the most effective way of dealing with stalking. The standard advice from stalking experts is that, because law enforcement officers are unable to provide protection at all times, clinicians should emphasize that stalking victims are ultimately responsible for their own safety and must be proactive in improving the physical safety of their environment (e.g. obtaining a home security system, minimizing personal exposure to the stalker).[64]

Battered women are extremely likely to be stalked by partners or ex-partners when the woman attempts to end the relationship.[65] These particular women are at greatest danger of homicide or severe abuse at the time of separation. Because men who batter are likely to stalk their ex-partners at this time, experts suggest short-term interventions for women who are leaving violent partners. Battered women who are being stalked should anticipate and prepare for an escalation in violence. They should be prepared to hide, involve police or get out of town.

Women who are harassed over the telephone are usually advised to get an answering machine to screen calls and record messages. They should have the telephone company trace the calls, and obtain a caller identification device to verify the harassment. The importance of documenting each stalking incident is stressed, as is retaining all physical evidence (audiotapes, letters, gifts). Because any contact serves as intermittent reinforcement, clients should avoid all personal contact with the stalker. Even negative contact in the form of telling the stalker 'to go away' is in fact seen by the stalker as positive encouragement to continue his pursuit. Why this should be, we discuss later, but it is a vital point and accounts for why victims often encourage their stalker without meaning to.[66]

A third party should inform the stalker that the pursuit behaviour is unwanted and must stop immediately or the police will be contacted. Police should be called when there is more than one unwanted intrusion that results in anxiety, fear or anger. Early intervention is emphasized because this is more likely to stop the stalker developing the belief that he may get somewhere if he persists. So knowing what to do must relate to some extent to what is going on in the mind of the stalker and this is an issue on which there is much popular misunderstanding.[67, 68]

One way of classifying and so beginning to understand stalking is to focus first on the relationship between the stalker and the victim, and then to decide on a simple division between psychotic and non-psychotic stalkers. Finally it is important to include what motivates and sustains the behaviour. The following typology of stalking has five categories and was pioneered by an Australian expert in stalking, Dr Paul Mullen.

THE REJECTED STALKER

The rejected stalker pursues an ex-intimate, usually a previous sexual partner, but just occasionally a family member or close friend. The rejected stalker usually claims to be seeking a reconciliation though occasionally will acknowledge that he or she is motivated by a desire for revenge. In practice, those behaviours aimed at reconciliation and those aimed at vengeance often coexist, producing a fluctuating mixture of appeasement and aggression. The stalking probably occurs because it maintains some semblance of a relationship with the lost intimate, and because it offers a vehicle for the stalker to vent his or her rage at lost hopes and disappointed expectations. It is with this type of stalker that connections to prior domestic violence may be found.

THE INTIMACY SEEKER

The intimacy seeker's stalking is aimed at realizing a relationship with someone who has engaged his or her affections and who is often mistakenly believed already to reciprocate that affection.

Intimacy seekers are convinced they are destined to establish a loving relationship with the target. They are oblivious to the victim's feelings and in practice often reinterpret even the most blunt of rejections as a positive response. This type of stalker is drawn almost exclusively from those whose lives have been bereft of intimacy and the stalking is sustained because it maintains a semblance of a relationship and provides hopes and dreams of eventual union. From the ranks of the intimacy seekers come the star stalkers.

THE INCOMPETENT SUITOR

The incompetent suitor is also seeking a relationship, but in contrast to the intimacy seeker is not in love, merely looking for a date or attempting to establish initial contact. These individuals usually lack basic interpersonal, let alone courting skills but despite this they often evince a remarkable sense of entitlement to a relationship. They appear uninterested in the other's wishes in the matter, repeatedly pestering and harassing their targets. This type of stalking is rarely sustained, presumably because it provides few satisfactions. This stalker usually gives up after a matter of days or weeks. Unfortunately, they are prone to repeat the behaviour with a new target.

THE RESENTFUL STALKER

The resentful stalker aims to frighten the victim. The stalking emerges out of a desire for retribution for some actual or supposed injury. Resentful stalkers usually feel justified in pursuing their target and not infrequently present themselves as victims fighting back against injustice and oppression. The stalking is frequently sustained by a self-righteous commitment reinforced by the satisfaction obtained from the sense of power and control which the stalking provides.

THE PREDATORY STALKER

The predatory stalker stalks preparatory to launching an attack, usually sexual in nature. The stalking is a combination of information-gathering, rehearsal in fantasy and intrusion through surreptitious observation. The stalking is a means to an end, the end being the assault, but is sustained by the gratifying sense of power and control, often augmented by the pleasures of voyeuristic intrusions.

Stalking still tends to be regarded in Europe as an American problem largely confined to 'Hollywood stars', not a real issue for ordinary folk outside the States. But stalking emerged dramatically in the English-speaking world at the end of the twentieth century partly because particular types of harassing behaviour were indeed becoming more common and more obviously disturbing to a wide range of individuals.

A point almost completely ignored by the media, who prefer to focus on celebrity or 'star stalking', is that stalking has emerged as an issue today largely because of the changing status of women. Evidence for this comes from the National Violence Against Women (NVAW) Survey, a random telephone survey in 2000 of 8,000 women and 8,000 men in the United States, which was the first national study of stalking.[69]

Stalking is often a variant of the domestic violence cycle. In the NVAW survey, 59 per cent of the female victims were stalked by a current or former partner; about half of these women were stalked while the relationship was intact. Of those women who were stalked by an intimate partner, 81 per cent were physically assaulted, and 31 per cent were sexually assaulted.

Basically what has happened is that the rise in women's economic and social power has meant that more of them have been able to leave unsatisfactory men than ever before. Those who unilaterally end relationships have probably always run the risk of becoming the target of harassment from the ex-partner.

Establishing stalking as a universally condemned criminal activity is in part about society acknowledging that women are not the chattels of their male partners, that relationships can and do end, and women as well as men have a right to say 'no, this is enough'. Stalking is created by the tension between a declining tradition concerning the permanence of marriage and women's place in such unions and an emergent set of values around women's right to independence and equity.[70]

There was an increasing concern in the 1980s with the persistent pursuit of women, usually by ex-partners. Such behaviours were described at the time as obsessive following or psychological rape. Despite the best efforts of the women's movement, little public attention was paid to such harassment. But then in the late 1980s and early 1990s the American media became intensely interested in what initially appeared to be a totally unrelated phenomenon: the persistent pursuit of the famous. This they termed 'star stalking'. The stalking and eventual murder of actress Rebecca Schaeffer by a disordered fan provided the paradigm example. The extraordinary success in 1987 of the film *Fatal Attraction* further fed an emerging fear of being pursued by a disturbed individual who has become obsessed with you.

Star stalking occurs because of the avidity of the famous for public exposure and their desire for protection from that myriad of strangers who form their audience. This conflict was mirrored in the audience, who wanted to know more and to see more of the famous, but at the same time were becoming critical of the methods used to appease their own hunger.

The paparazzi are our agents in stalking the famous and we, the audience, are in conflict about the results of our own intrusive curiosity. The death of Princess Diana in 1997 was at first roundly attributed to 'stalking' by paparazzi photographers – and since these photographers were merely serving the public need for such photographs, this extended the concept of stalking to the audience in general, rather than to a few disturbed individuals.

For the first time the audience had been put in touch to some extent with what the isolated stalker feels in his frustration to get near to a longed-for object who appears to taunt, tease but finally reject.

The social distance which now exists between people is problematic for isolated individuals who are disadvantaged interpersonally and often economically. The social skills required to negotiate the transition from stranger to acquaintance, and from acquaintance to potential partner, are hard to attain in a fragmented, fearful society.

But stalking is in fact a new word for an old behaviour. People have long been exposed to being harassed. Dante shadowing Beatrice for years on end and Petrarch showering Laura with 364 daily poems were not regarded as a scandal, but as a romantic ideal. They were men constructing images of the beloved which took no account whatsoever of the real women who were the object of their passion. Dante and Petrarch continued their persistent intrusions ignorant of, or indifferent to, the preferences and reactions of the women. Such behaviour nowadays would be more likely to be condemned as stalking than idealized as romantic love. But the transformation from acceptable, or even admired, forms of social interaction, albeit one-sided in their nature, required major shifts in the cultural assumptions of societies, particularly about the relationships between men and women.

The bulk of stalkers will desist under the threat of prosecution but abstinence is often assisted by an appropriate supportive yet directive therapeutic relationship. Understandably, some therapists may be reluctant to take on for long-term therapy someone with a prior history of stalking, fearing that they themselves might be stalked.

YET ANOTHER NEW PHENOMENON: DELUSIONS ABOUT BEING STALKED

The first ever case of false stalking claims was reported in 1984 when a middle-aged US woman was supposedly terrorized for four years by a mysterious stalker called 'The Poet', so named because of the rhyming threatening letters she received from him. She claimed a butcher's knife arrived from him at Christmas, he apparently cut her telephone line, threw concrete blocks at her home and even abducted her, stabbing her in the back.

When she was found mailing letters from 'The Poet' among her own correspondence, she confessed there never had been a Poet, and she had even cut herself to add credibility to her story.

The motivation in this case remains to this day mysterious, even to the investigating psychologists, but the speculation was that attention-seeking, the only way for an isolated individual to obtain sympathy, often drives this bizarre behaviour. This has long been thought to be the motivation in the small group of patients who dedicate their lives to pretending to have physical illnesses. For example there are cases on record who feign having breast cancer: they lose weight, shave their heads to simulate hair loss and join cancer support groups, but are perfectly physically fit.

Understanding this phenomenon is becoming more urgent as a new set of disorders has now joined illnesses like cancer, which used to be a favourite amongst those who set out to dupe doctors. The latest problem has uncovered a new breed of 'pseudo-victim' and the diagnosis appears to be what is now called 'false victimization syndrome'.

In another famous US case a woman filed 60 complaints over six months including discovering her underwear in her house with red hearts drawn on it in lipstick, break-ins at home, and finding blood-soaked teddy bears positioned above her garage entrance so they would fall on those closing the door. One was found in her baby's crib.

After several press conferences held by the victim where she complained about the lack of interest of the local police, she was caught on videotape placing a teddy bear in her garage. The motivation turned out to be an attempt to make living in her house so uncomfortable it would force her reluctant husband to agree to move.

A famous celebrity false stalking case occurred in Los Angeles in 1995 when Cyndy Garvey, the ex-wife of a famous baseball player, reported a number of stalking events to the police. After many phone calls to the police pleading for help, she presented to them with a black eye and damaged nose. It later emerged she had in fact been harassing her ex-husband and an ex-boyfriend. She confessed later she manufactured the stalking incidents to target, and so obtain revenge on her ex-boyfriend.

This turns out to be a common motivation – to inflict vengeance on an uninterested suitor who ended a relationship desired by the victim; to punish the rejecter. Alternatively an ex-boyfriend may be galvanized into protecting the victim from a mysterious anonymous threat, and so fictitious claims of being stalked can reignite or at least reconnect the stalker with someone who otherwise would not have come back.

Studies in the early 1990s from the Los Angeles Police Department Database (California, with more celebrities per square mile than anywhere else on earth, is also the world's stalking capital) had previously suggested that one in 50 cases of stalking was really a false allegation. But research published in the *British Journal of Psychiatry* in 1999 by Australian psychiatrists Dr Michele Pathé and colleagues suggests that nearly 10 per cent of stalking claims may be fictitious.[71] None of the 12 individuals in Dr Pathé's research, who falsely claimed to be victims of stalking, were in a stable intimate relationship, a stark contrast with the true victims the Australian doctors saw in their specialist clinic. This strongly suggests that it is the search for help and support from others which drives the need to claim you are in danger.

Psychiatrists observe that true victims of stalking are usually embarrassed by their situation and would rather not draw attention to themselves, in contrast to 'pseudo-victims', who maximize the enlistment of assistance from others. Genuine sufferers are often reluctant to notify the authorities of their problem, fearing this might exacerbate their predicament, while false victims assuredly, even gleefully, come forward.

Another clue as to what is really going on lies in the rhythm over time in the way incidents are reported. Pseudo-victims tend to generate more crime complaints whenever it seems others might be losing interest in the case. But in three of the 12 cases reported from Australia, the victims had suffered genuine stalking in the past, and had become hypersensitive to possible recurrence, seeing stalking in the blameless actions of others. In six of the cases Dr Pathé describes, the causes of the false claims were in fact paranoid delusions about being followed which the psychotics had incorporated into their fantasy life, perhaps because paranoia about stalking is currently so widespread.

Ironically, in one case reported to Dr Pathé, the false victim of stalking was in fact a stalker themselves; the false claim seemed to be an attempt to pre-empt their victim's complaint. This echoes another bizarre case from the US where a stalker took out an injunction against their victim, to stop them following the stalker! But this begins to make psychological sense if you see stalkers as so obsessed with their victims that they are unable to get thoughts of their quarry out of their minds even when they may want to. In a sense they feel trapped by their targets.

But however complex the problem of telling the genuine from the false in the weird world of stalking, one salient fact is incontestable: the time and energy devoted to investigating false claims take away precious and increasingly meagre resources from genuine crimes and victims.

But even when the authorities suspect they have a pseudo-victim on their hands, the problem of how to confront the issue with the perpetrator can lead to a reluctance to acknowledge false victimization, even when the evidence is overwhelming.

Dr Pathé and her colleagues suggest a 'sympathetic' approach which acknowledges that false victims in most cases are distressed and disturbed individuals. Dr Kris Mohandie, a police psychologist at the Los Angeles Police Department who specializes in false victimization stalking syndrome, explains that their approach is to state clearly to the 'pseudovictim' that 'events did not occur as you told us'. But they then allow a face-saving exit for the perpetrator by portraying the falsehood 'sympathetically' as a 'cry for help'. After all, seeking a victim role as the only way of achieving a meaningful sense of personal identity suggests that something fundamental has gone wrong somewhere in their psychological development.

But maybe the cause also partly lies in a society so enmeshed in the cult of celebrity that anyone who is anyone must have their own stalker – now the ultimate status accessory. In this same society, assuming the victim role is becoming the only way to get any attention.

6

DELUSIONS OF THE BODY

Orandum est ut sit mens sana in corpore sano – Your prayer must be
for a sound mind in a sound body.

Juvenal (60 BC), *Satires* X, 356

In Southeast Asia a special disease has been known for many years, where acute anxiety is generated by the strong belief that the patient's sexual organ will retract into the abdomen and that the complete disappearance of the organ will result in death. It has become known as koro, and it occurs in single cases as well as in epidemic proportions in different Southeast Asian cultures (South China, Malaysia, some areas in Indonesia).[1]

As the term 'koro' has cultural connotations (it is a Malaysian–Indonesian word meaning turtlehead), some psychiatrists have proposed instead the introduction of the term 'genital retraction syndrome' implying the universal nature of the syndrome rather than making it specific to a particular culture.[2]

It was first documented in the West in 1895 but was described in Chinese in the *Yellow Emperor's Book of Medicine* as early as 3000 BC.[3] It affects mainly men, since it relates to the penis, although it has also been recognized among women, who feared the involution

188

of their labia, vulva and breasts. In men, the syndrome is accompanied by a terrible and encompassing fear that when the penis disappears completely he will die.[4]

The symptoms can be accompanied by bodily sensations and different – mostly mechanical – methods are applied by the patient to prevent his sexual organ from disappearing. The generally accepted view is that koro is a psychogenic disorder related to Far Eastern cultures, appearing in cultural environments where Chinese medical views and the Chinese folk beliefs and superstitions about sexual life are prevalent.[5] Koro epidemics have reportedly occurred among the Chinese population in Singapore, and have been reported in Thailand and India, which have very different cultural backgrounds from the Chinese. The last incidence on record was an epidemic in South China in 1984–5.[6]

When a koro epidemic hit Singapore in July 1967, of the 536 cases that were then seen by medical professionals 521 were men and only 15 were women (less than 3 per cent of the cases).[7] Epidemics of koro have also been reported in West Bengal, India, in July 1982 and in north-eastern Thailand in November 1976.[8]

During the epidemic of 1982 in India well-intentioned parents who were concerned that their son's penis was shrinking tied a strong thread to the foreskin of the penis. That thread was then tied to another thread which had been tied around the boy's waist. Consequently, painful ulcers formed on the foreskin. Doctors measured the penis regularly and reassured the parents that no shrinkage was occurring. Of course the risk here is that the parents might conclude superstitiously that their home-made treatment was actually working.[9]

Although koro is a characteristically Eastern disease, an increasing number of non-Asian (non-Chinese, non-Indonesian) cases have been reported.[10] According to the case descriptions, in the majority of these cases, koro-like symptoms seemed to be a 'covering top layer' of a primary psychiatric disorder, such as depression or schizophrenia, while in other cases different sociocultural and psychological stressors precipitated the appearance of these symptoms. There have also been cases in which organic alterations (e.g. somatic diseases induced by alcohol, brain tumours, stroke, epilepsy) were proven to be the cause of koro-like symptoms.[11]

Other authors have published reports about the development of koro after hallucinogens, amphetamines, heroin and cannabis had been taken by the patient. Given this wide set of possible causes, koro can be considered a universal behavioural expression, the basis of which is an intensive attention paid to the sexual organs. This attention fixation can have several reasons (like psychosexual conflicts, psychiatric and organic diseases, interpersonal effects), and it means vulnerability to the appearance of koro-like symptoms.[12]

Psychiatrist Dr Eliezer Witztum and colleagues from the Beer-Sheva Mental Center, in Beer-Sheva, Israel, recently reported a koro-like syndrome in a Bedouin man living in the Negev desert in Israel.[13] The Bedouin are an Arab nomadic tribe spread throughout Asia and Africa. The patient's disturbance is accompanied by voyeurism and the onset appears to be related to his sexual practices.

The man whose penis was disappearing

The patient is a single, unemployed, illiterate male, aged 34, the oldest in a family of seven children. He was admitted to hospital after being apprehended by police in response to complaints that he was looking into women's bathrooms. In the emergency room he was verbally aggressive and threatened the attending physician. At admission he was fully aware, had dishevelled appearance, was uncooperative, agitated and was yelling. His ability to concentrate was markedly deteriorated and he was angry and hostile. His thought process was tangential and he believed the police and physicians were persecuting him. He denied thoughts of suicide and was diagnosed with psychosis, voyeurism and mixed personality disorder with paranoid and antisocial traits.

The patient was born in Israel and had four years of formal education. He was the victim of severe abuse as a child. As a punishment for truancy, he reported, his father restrained him with an iron chain. During the last few years he worked sporadically as a gardener in the centre of Israel away from his tribe. He describes himself 'outgoing' and as 'having many friends'.

The patient traced his condition back five or six years to a time when he went to a prostitute, after which he became impotent. Thereafter he began to feel his penis shrink and began to fear that it would recede into his abdomen. He began pulling his penis and clutching it, but this did not diminish his fears. He reported that for days he felt a general weakness, headaches and fever throughout his body. He tried a number of times to have sexual intercourse but was unable to because he had no erection. He was examined by several physicians but no biological basis for his impotence was found.

He thought he might have some kind of infection so underwent many tests, which ruled out HIV and syphilis.

He first sought outpatient psychiatric treatment in 1988 complaining of impotence. He returned to the clinic in 1993 again complaining of impotence, and of feelings of hostility on the part of his family. He also felt that the Bedouin community was against him because of his encounters with prostitutes. He was treated with a small dose of antipsychotic medication, which had a minimal effect. During the two years prior to his hospital admission he had broken off all treatment contact.

During his first day in hospital he was agitated and spoke about the need to 'defend himself', and tried to harm himself. He claimed that he had been hospitalized for no reason. His condition improved, he began to eat and drink and his persecutory delusions appeared to diminish. However, he was still worried by his sexual problems and had 'strange' thoughts regarding his sex organ. He noted that 'five and six years ago I felt someone pulling my penis into my belly. I then began feeling pressure all over my body, but I have a root in my stomach and when I squeeze it I feel better.'

Towards the end of his hospital stay he began to co-operate, the delusions disappeared, he gave up thoughts of suicide and was no longer violent. He refused medication and was discharged against medical advice after five days. He did not show up for outpatient follow-up and owing to his Bedouin lifestyle it was very difficult to locate him for the purposes of outreach.

Those who subscribe to the culturally specific view of koro term symptoms that develop in non-Chinese 'partial' or 'koro-like syndrome'. It has been asserted that true koro syndrome appears under very stressful situations among individuals who are otherwise mentally healthy. Partial koro appears among persons with underlying major psychiatric disturbances.

The case described here was koro-like. Although the patient was afraid that his penis was shrinking and would recede into his stomach, he did not feel that he was going to die. Yet he was preoccupied with hypochondriacal thoughts, a kind of partial death. The fear was first manifested after he developed impotence following a sexual encounter with a prostitute. During treatment his strange thoughts of his penis shrinking were understood to be part of a psychotic process. This interpretation may be due to the fact that his therapist, like many others, was not familiar with the diagnosis and treatment of koro syndrome.

While in many cultures masturbation is forbidden and thus may be a precipitant of the disorder, in this case it is probably not, since Islamic culture is tolerant of masturbation. However, this man's visit to a prostitute and his voyeurism conflicted with Bedouin values. Bedouins are very concerned with female modesty, and an attack on this is considered very serious. It is possible that his time spent working away from the tribe may have been as a result of banishment. This would help to explain his strained relations with his family and the Bedouin community.[14]

This appears to be the first description of koro syndrome and voyeurism. This case, together with other pure cases in Britain, Nepal and Israel, and koro-like cases in patients with other psychiatric disorders and organic brain syndromes, strengthens the possibility that koro may be connected with various mental disorders.[15] In the presence of Chinese cultural beliefs the koro syndrome takes on its 'classical' form and can be a cultural idiom of distress; at times it has even reached epidemic proportions. In different cultures the symptoms may take on different meanings relating to conflicts about body image, sexuality and shame.[16]

Most of the Western psychological theorizing about koro is derived from the Freudian psychoanalytic perspective. As is so often the case, from this point of view the problem of koro is ultimately due to the fear of castration. In Freud's theory the male child fears that his powerful father will retaliate against him for his unconscious sexual desires for his own mother. That retaliation is assumed to take the form of castration, a fate the male child fears (falsely) has already befallen females.[17]

In China, the original cultural punishment for incest was not castration alone, but death, either alone or with castration. This association accounts for the prominence of the fear of death in this disorder, which is even greater than the fear of castration. The patient believes he can prevent death by preventing the disappearance of his penis.[18]

From a more obvious psychological standpoint there is also a connection between anxiety concerning the disappearing penis and anxiety about masturbation. In essence, if a boy masturbates he is to be punished by castration and death. The symptom also has a characteristic double meaning for by preventing and punishing masturbation on the one hand, it also leads to the very masturbatory act of holding the penis.[19]

Some psychiatrists, in attempting to explain the much rarer

female form of koro, point out the 'great similarity' of the nipple of the breast or glans clitoris with the glans penis. Women with koro symptoms fear shrinkage and eventual disappearance of their breasts or labia. The psychoanalytic view is that in the female the loss of the breast gives her an opportunity to rid herself of her obvious female identity and to satisfy her unconscious wish to be a man. In other words the female form of koro is actually a version of the Freudian 'penis envy' which all women are supposed to suffer from.[20]

There is a much more straightforward behavioural theory. The behavioural school of psychology sees human problems as having arisen from learned behaviour, and not from unconscious conflicts. This view is that an anxious man may have doubts about his sexual adequacy and may continually check his organ for health and size. Since the penis does shrink temporarily in conditions of cold or fright, it may indeed become smaller. During self-examination, the man notices this and becomes even more fearful, and the penis consequently becomes smaller. He learns by association that his anxieties are connected to his shrinking penis. He assumes it is the shrinking penis that is causing his distress when in fact it is the other way round.[21]

Psychiatrists Dr Attila Kovács and Dr Péter Osváth of the University Medical School, Pécs, Hungary, recently reported the following case of koro in a young Korean female patient found in Hungary.[22] This case is remarkable, because as far as is known, cases of koro in women have only been described in epidemic contexts, and there are no reports of cases of Korean patients.

The woman who needed sex to stay alive

A 29-year-old woman was brought to the clinic by the police because she had been running naked along a highway at night. The patient arrived wrapped in a blanket and although she was aware of the examination situation, she was distracted and tried to control her anxiety by doing exercises when left alone. She started to communicate in German (which she spoke very poorly), and she expressed her wish to learn Hungarian. Later, when she was given a sheet of paper with written questions in English, she gave answers in English, and slowly seemed to become more and more familiar with the language.

She had been living in Hungary with her husband and two children for two years, and she had been studying music at college.

193

She had had a love affair with one of her teachers, but recently they had split up. She said that she had previously been in Pécs with her lover but this time she came by herself, hoping that she might meet him spiritually. Walking on the street she became tense, she stopped feeling her legs, and experienced itching and tingling in her thighs. This numbness spread upwards and she felt she was becoming less and less a woman: her breasts were shrinking and she was gradually transforming into a man. This imagined sexual metamorphosis became increasingly threatening to her, because she believed that by becoming a man she would lose all her energy and finally die. She thought she heard her lover's voice trying to tell her what to do. She took off all her clothes, because it eased her mind and made her 'feel something' in her legs. She was convinced that she would be able to remain a woman only if she had sexual intercourse: by doing so she would receive 'penis and energy'.

Her fear of physical transformation and her sexual impulses gradually took possession of her and she begged the male members of staff to have sexual intercourse with her to save her life. The admission examination revealed no symptoms of internal neurological disorders or trauma-causing external injury. As far as the patient's psychic state was concerned, she was quite lucid. However, she was depressed and her behaviour was characterized by overwhelming anxiety (sometimes as strong as panic), fear of impending death and restlessness. She was losing her sense of reality and thought herself to be seriously ill.

She could be calmed verbally only with limited success, so she was given small doses of antipsychotic medication. By the following morning her behaviour had become composed, co-ordinated and her anxiety had disappeared.

She explained that she had never been under psychiatric or neurological treatment and that she did not take any medicine, drugs or alcohol on a regular basis. She mentioned some conflicts in her marriage. According to the husband, the patient had difficulties with social integration into the Hungarian environment, did not socialize and spent all her time at home. Her studies were a further burden to her. She became impatient with her children and felt that she was not a good mother. Just before this incident her behaviour changed and she became suspicious: she often talked about being watched by the police, and dreaded that they would assault her children. The husband admitted that they had become alienated from each other lately, and the patient had often accused him of not loving her any more. She feared that he wanted to divorce her.

A state of depersonalization, or feeling that she was unreal, was observed in the patient, accompanied by acute anxiety and fear of death induced by the misperception of the shape of her body, shrinkage of her breasts and loss of her sexual identity. Her beliefs were so firm that they appeared to be delusions. Her experience of breast hyperinvolution and her anxiety suggest the koro syndrome.

Numerous authors emphasize the significance of cultural stressors (e.g. emigration) and interpersonal factors (e.g. marital conflicts) in the genesis of koro. Recent events in this patient's life (difficulties with studies, isolation) led to this disorder, although the basis of the syndrome was probably a primary psychiatric disorder. The need for integration into Hungarian culture – which is very different from Korean – created pressure on the patient ('cultural shock'), which was heightened by the marital crisis and by her unstable maternal identity.[23]

Korean culture is similar to Chinese culture in many respects. Traditional Chinese medicophilosophical concepts and folklore (e.g. the role of yin–yang and balance theory in understanding sexual physiology) are widely known in Korea. The patient believed that the shrinkage of her breasts and her whole sexual metamorphosis were the result of having become spiritually and sexually unbalanced. She believed that she needed male (yang) energy transmitted through sexual intercourse to regain her balance.[24]

This case demonstrates that koro represents an intersection of medicinal, psychological, anthropological and ethnographical concepts. The koro syndrome is of interest for many reasons, not least because it introduces the concept of 'cultural relativism': the idea that an individual's pattern of behaviour or complaint may be seen as abnormal or sick in one culture, but not necessarily in another. In fact the very same behaviour may even be prized in the second culture. Conversely, the concept of cultural invariance suggests that some behaviours are so strange or unusual that they are considered abnormal in all cultures.[25]

Koro goes to the heart of the debate at the very foundation of psychiatry as to whether mental illnesses really exist or are constructions – ways of classifying phenomena that are imposed on the world by our perspective. If a heart attack is viewed as an illness or at the very least an undesirable state in every culture world-wide then there is some sense in which perspective-taking is not a major issue here. However, as there is no blood test in psychiatry to establish biological abnormality this raises questions about whether psychiatric illnesses arise from the context in which they exist.[26]

Koro may be appearing more in the West simply because doctors are becoming more acquainted with it through the medical literature and use it to categorize a common anxiety in Western males – concern about penis size.[27]

The results of the largest scientific survey of penis size ever conducted in the world were recently published. The penis proportions of 5,122 men were collected over 25 years at the Kinsey Institute of Sex Research at Indiana University and analysed by US psychologists Dr Anthony Bogaert and Dr Scott Hershberger.[28]

They found that homosexual men have larger penises on all measures of size, from flaccid to erect, circumference and length, than do heterosexual men. For example the average heterosexual man's penis was smaller when erect by over one cubic inch in volume than that of the average homosexual. The finding is all the more remarkable as on average the homosexual men had slightly smaller bodies in terms of weight and height than the heterosexuals, and very generally the bigger a man's body, the larger his penis.

One possible explanation for the difference in penis size is that homosexual men tend to start puberty earlier than heterosexuals, and puberty marks the start of a surge of testosterone secretion in the male body which only begins to decline from the mid-thirties onwards. As testosterone is one of the hormones that determines penis proportion, the longer exposure to higher testosterone levels could explain why gay men end up with larger penises.

This testosterone theory has other implications for male body shape. The group of genes which determine finger and toe size are the same ones involved in fixing penis proportions. Dr John Manning, a biologist at Liverpool University, has reported that the longer a man's fourth finger (counted with the thumb as one) relative to his second, the higher his testosterone levels and the more sperm he produces. Since testosterone partly determines penis size, this also suggests that the longer a man's fourth finger compared to his second, the larger his penis may be. The link with toes may partly explain the origin of the folk story that penis size is linked with foot length.[29]

Now there is added evidence for this common idea, we can expect men to become obsessed with their shoe and glove size, as surveys repeatedly find most men think that their own penises are smaller than average. Yet surveys of penis size have found a remarkable lack of variation between men. In 1999 Bogaert and Hershberger found that two-thirds of men fall within an inch smaller or longer than 6.14 inches at erect length.

But if the size of the penis when erect is so similar, why are men so anxious and obsessed by this? Part of the answer may derive from previous research into penis size which found that flaccid length is not a good predictor of erect length. Smaller flaccid penises tend to 'catch up' with larger flaccid ones when they become erect. It could be that in shower and locker rooms men only see other male flaccid penises and make the mistake of assuming that any variability is reflected on erection, when this is not the case. So you can put that ruler down now.

Another part of the body which is often the focus for disordered thinking is the bowels.

Bowel obsessions have long been recognized in clinical settings and usually present as an overwhelming fear of losing bowel control in public. Disagreement exists as to their proper classification along the spectrum of anxiety disorders but bowel obsession has been conceptualized both as a variant of obsessive-compulsive disorder and as a symptom of social phobia, panic disorder and agoraphobia.

Preoccupation with bowel and bladder control as a psychological issue has been a part of clinical literature as far back as the French psychiatrist Janet's influential 1903 book Les Obsessions et la Psychoasthénie. Researchers assume that the variant involving bowel function is more common than that involving the bladder. The primary symptom in bowel obsessions is an irrational fear of faecal incontinence. Associated anxieties range from possible public humiliation to perceived unavailability of bathrooms outside the home. These give rise to a fairly standard repertoire of behaviours aimed at maintaining bodily control, including spending inordinate amounts of time on the toilet and restricting food intake.[30]

The fear of having an 'accident' often discourages sufferers from leaving home or interacting socially. Neither incidence nor prevalence estimates are documented, but there is reason to believe this problem is much more frequent than is commonly thought. Given society's reticence about speaking openly about bodily functions, it is not surprising that people with this problem should be reluctant to discuss it, even with medical or mental health professionals.[31]

Little has been written about specific treatment techniques for this disorder except for cases in which antidepressants were used to achieve nearly total resolution of symptoms. Despite the tendency to downplay the role of psychological therapy in the treatment, cases which reported the best outcome over time are those in which behavioural therapy is used as an adjunctive treatment.

The following two cases were recently reported by Dr Marjorie Hatch of the Southern Methodist University in Dallas, Texas, because although similar in some ways the treatment of Mr A. was straightforward and short term, while the treatment of Mr B. was complicated by a number of factors, both medical and psychological.[32]

The man afraid of his own body

Mr A., a 25-year-old dental student, dated the onset of his increasing preoccupation with accidental defecation as coinciding with the beginning of professional school four years previously. Situations which causes the most intense distress were those in which an available bathroom was unlikely: driving on the freeway, going to popular dance clubs and travelling by public transport. He reported spending several hours a day worrying about various aspects of this problem. Mr A. said these fears did not prevent him from travelling to and from school, but added that he sometimes carried spare clothes and baby wipes in his briefcase.

Mr A. reported two periods of obsessive-compulsive symptoms in his past. For a year at the age of nine, and again from 12–15, he was very concerned about his family's safety and engaged in checking rituals (gas, electric outlets). These thoughts and urges stopped when he finally convinced himself that 'they were silly', and he never sought treatment. Mr A. stated that he had been diagnosed with a spastic colon in connection with abdominal pains that had begun at the same time as his bowel obsessions. He reported that his father had been under psychiatric care for many years for panic disorder, major depression and bowel obsessions.

The man who experienced one of the worse humiliations possible

Mr B. is a 69-year-old Jewish retired purchasing agent. Four years prior to seeking treatment, he had lost control of his bowels while visiting a cemetery with his wife, soiling himself and the ground around him. This humiliating experience was made worse because it was a religious holiday and the cemetery was crowded: 'I felt like I was in the middle of a stadium with 50,000 people watching.' Immediately afterwards, Mr B. began to experience 'knots' in his stomach and nausea before leaving the house and, feeling as though he needed to void, would spend long periods in the bathroom. He became increasingly fearful of leaving the house. In addition, he reported changes in his eating habits: he would not eat for several days at a time and avoided spicy foods. His ruminations revolved around fears that he had a serious medical problem and that he would not remain continent in public.

Mr B. denied any previous psychiatric history, but said that his mother was 'always very nervous and rarely left the house'. Following the loss of bowel control, he was diagnosed as having irritable bowel syndrome. Mr B. also reported suffering from angina and a hernia, both controlled with medication, as well as from a heel spur that reduced his mobility. Eventually he sought psychiatric help and was prescribed an antidepressant, which he reported gave him excruciating headaches and did not reduce his preoccupation with his bowels. At this point he was referred for psychological treatment.

In addition to similar presenting symptoms, both clients first sought help from a gastroenterologist and were diagnosed with a functional bowel disorder, and both appeared to share some family history of anxiety problems. Nevertheless, several prognostic differences bear mentioning. First, Mr B.'s onset of symptoms was unusual in that it followed a loss of bowel control. In the overwhelming majority of these cases, there is never actual faecal incontinence. This factor made challenging certain of Mr B.'s misconceptions (e.g. lack of confidence in future bowel control) more difficult.

In addition, Mr B. (a much older man) had a number of health problems, which although unrelated to his bowel obsessions would impact on his treatment. For example, his reduced mobility and history of cardiac problems had to be considered in developing exposure exercises. A third difference was the nature and extent of family history of anxiety. Mr A.'s father had suffered from untreated bowel obsessions of many years' standing. This similarity of symptoms became an important motivating factor, in that Mr A. could 'see his future' if he did not successfully complete treatment.

TREATMENT

Case 1: Mr A. was seen for 18 sessions, twice a week. Although medication was considered, it was not used. An early focus was Mr A.'s distorted thoughts about self-control and the need for perfection. For example, by keeping a detailed record of his 'unpredictable' bowel habits, he discovered he was in fact quite regular. Mr A. learned to tell himself to accept the imperfection of delay (in relieving himself) and to focus on 'stepwise' progress – gradual, small goals as opposed to control or 'zero level anxiety'.

Case 2: Mr B. was seen for twice-weekly sessions for approximately six months, after which sessions were gradually tapered to once a month. Total treatment time was 18 months, due to two periods of partial relapse, when Mr B. felt 'devastated and hopeless' and very sceptical of the potential benefits of psychotherapy. Simple and concrete methods were used to help him gain confidence in both himself and the treatment – daily activity records and an exposure hierarchy consisting of steps he was likely to master easily.

Real-life exposure exercises included using public transport, travelling to unknown sites and eating spicy foods (both in-session and as homework). Slowly, Mr B.'s confidence steadily increased and his depression decreased. He was encouraged to allow his wife and closest friends in on his 'secret', a strategy that reduced his overall anxiety level in their presence. Part of his treatment involved taking a trip with the therapist to the cemetery where he had lost control of his bowels. At the cemetery, Mr B. described the original incident in detail and performed an 'atonement ritual' for those whose graves he felt he had desecrated. He later reported this as the single most helpful intervention.

Two periods of relapse occurred. The first was linked to the onset of panic attacks during a vacation about six months into treatment, the only major trip Mr B. had taken in four years. The second relapse occurred about 12 months into treatment, at the time of the death of Mr B.'s aged mother. These crises put temporary halts to the original treatment plan, as Mr B. and his therapist engaged in more traditional insight-oriented therapy to deal with these and other issues. At one point, Mr B.'s depression became severe and he was temporarily placed on antidepressant medication.

Although the vast majority of psychological outcome research for OCD has used exposure and response prevention (which involves exposing oneself to a situation one would normally avoid), there is evidence suggesting that cognitive techniques are effective as a complement to existing treatment methods. Cognitive techniques, a form of therapy based on direct disputation with the patient about the validity of their beliefs, proved to be helpful in the treatment of Mr A. For Mr A., addressing his unrealistic fears and expectations served to prepare him to start the exposure component of the treatment. Similar discussions with Mr B., on the other hand, had little beneficial effect. It seems that Mr A.'s previous success at overcoming obsessive thinking on his own and his high degree of psychological sophistication were central to the success of cognitive techniques. In addition, the sudden, traumatic, and emotionally charged onset of Mr A.'s bowel obsessions may have favoured the early introduction of behavioural techniques.[33]

At the termination of treatment, both men were rated by their therapist as 'much improved'. Mr A. had a decrease in total obsessive-compulsive test scores of 54 per cent, and Mr B. a 57 per cent decrease. At 12-month follow-up, Mr A.'s obsessional scores were unchanged. He mentioned occasional urges but reported success at overcoming them despite new stressors, including his recent marriage and starting advanced training in his field. At both 12- and 24-month follow-up sessions, Mr A. reported being '90 per cent better', stating that although he had occasional obsessive thoughts, he was able to stop them within moments. Both Mr B.'s 12- and 24-month ratings showed a 71 per cent decrease from pretreatment levels. He reported that despite occasional anxious moments, he was regularly accompanying his wife on local outings, and had been on vacation several times. Both men said they were no longer troubled by gastrointestinal distress.[33]

Although bowel obsessions do not fit neatly into the classic subtypes (e.g. cleaning, checking, ordering, hoarding), they seem best conceptualized as a variant of OCD.[34]

Probably the strongest argument for a link with OCD is the shared symptom profile: obsessive thinking which drives up the client's anxiety level and the compulsive rituals aimed at lessening these uncomfortable feelings. The findings of most researchers that the two disorders respond well to similar pharmacological and psychological interventions provide further, although certainly not conclusive, evidence for their relatedness. A third commonality is a family history of OCD and OCD-like behaviour.[35]

Another form of obsessive-compulsive disorder taken in terms of body preoccupation is body dysmorphic disorder (BDD), though this can be so severe as to be indistinguishable from a psychotic illness at times.[36]

Body dysmorphic disorder (also known as dysmorphophobia) is an illness characterized by 'a preoccupation with a defect in appearance' that is 'either imagined, or, if a slight physical anomaly is present, markedly excessive'. It is a socially debilitating disorder that is strongly associated with depression and risk of suicide. Although any part of the body may act as a focus for concern, the dermatologist is most likely to encounter a dysmorphophobic patient with perceived facial flaws such as wrinkles, hirsutism, hair loss or acne. These patients experience profound and persistent feelings of revulsion at their appearance, frequently resulting in marked social, occupational and sexual dysfunction.[37]

Since the first published case of dysmorphophobia by Enrique Morselli in 1891, colourful descriptions of the syndrome have appeared sporadically in the European literature. A famous patient of Sigmund Freud, known as the 'Wolf Man', was said to have 'neglected his daily life and work because he was engrossed, to the exclusion of all else, in the state of his nose'. Such historical examples illustrate the tendency for sufferers to become isolated as they develop the conviction that others find them repulsive.[38]

The understanding of dysmorphophobia is based on a limited number of case reports and study of the condition is hampered by the tendency for sufferers to remain secretive and to avoid medical consultation because of intense embarrassment. Recognized cases may therefore represent the tip of a clinical iceberg. Nevertheless, certain patient characteristics have been identified. The onset of BDD usually occurs during adolescence, when individuals are at their most sensitive about their appearance and may be teased or bullied. However, most patients take up to 10–15 years or so before they seek help from a mental health professional and even then may present with symptoms of depression or social phobia. It shows slight female predominance and nearly all of its sufferers are single or divorced.

Several authors have identified pre-morbid personality traits that may predispose to dysmorphophobia, including extreme sensitivity, shyness, insecurity and perfectionism.[39]

It has also been suggested that the condition may be triggered by emotional stress and introspection, for example following rejection by a sexual partner, or that it may develop during adolescence in response to comments about appearance. An association with in-

202

harmonious family background has also been invoked, as has the presence of extreme dependence on a parent for whom physical beauty is of great importance.[40]

Psychiatrists Dr E. Sobanski and Dr M. H. Schmidt of the Department of Child and Adolescent Psychiatry, Central Institute of Mental Health, Mannheim, Germany, recently reported the case and treatment of a 16-year-old female patient who suffered from the belief that she had a dislocated pubic bone, and had BDD associated rituals and social avoidance.[41]

The girl who thought everybody was looking at her pubic bone

The 16-year-old girl had been suffering for about six months from the belief that her pubic bone was becoming increasingly dislocated and prominent, and that everyone was staring at and talking about it. She could not remember a particular occurrence which had brought on the symptom but was totally convinced that she could only be helped by surgery. In an attempt to achieve a smaller hip girth and also to influence the pubic bone she slimmed down from 48 kg to 44 kg, with a height of 1.68 metres, which corresponds to a body mass index (BMI) of 15.8 kg/m (the normal variation is 20–25, so this is worryingly low). This weight reduction led to her periods stopping.

One month before admission she was admitted to a paediatric clinic where anorexia nervosa was diagnosed. She was fed with high-caloric nutrient solution and gained 2 kilos. Two weeks later the girl had become totally housebound because she was extremely ashamed of her looks. She spent almost the entire day in her bedroom, wearing excessively large pyjamas. On admission her mood was depressed and her drive reduced. She cried often and said she felt hopeless and apathetic. She denied contemplating suicide. Up to 10 times a day she lowered herself to the ground and measured, with her fingers, the position of her pubic bone. She was constantly preoccupied with thoughts about it.

The girl was the eldest daughter of a couple with university education, and had a five-year-old sister. No particular problems in family interaction could be identified and there was no family history of psychiatric disorders. Described by her parents as being ambitious at school and a little reserved and shy with her peers, the girl had no long-term close friendships. She had dated a boy of her age for a month but had discontinued the relationship because she felt too occupied by it. She had no sexual experience.

The patient was treated for 10 weeks. From the second week onwards she received antidepressant medication and therapy with exposure and response prevention. This means exposing yourself to the situation you normally avoid and then not engaging in rituals you would normally perform.

At first she was extremely upset by the programme and had thoughts such as: 'I am an outsider. Everybody looks at my pubic bone. If it was normal, everything would be fine. I need surgical correction.' Gradually it became easier for her to face formerly avoided situations. At the end of treatment, the girl's BDD symptoms were distinctly improved. Although she was still certain about the dislocation of her pubic bone, the belief was less distressing for her and no longer impaired her daily life. She had stopped camouflaging and checking her pubic bone. She dated her peers and attended school regularly; the depressive symptoms completely vanished and when she was seen after six months for a follow-up session with her psychiatrist the therapeutic results had remained stable.

According to the scientific literature, depression is the psychiatric disorder most frequently related to BDD: between 60 and 94 per cent of patients have a lifetime diagnosis of depression. Most individuals with BDD perform ritualistic behaviours related to their dysmorphophobic beliefs that resemble obsessive-compulsive disorder compulsions. Between 6 and 30 per cent fulfil the diagnostic criteria for concurrent OCD. Virtually always, BDD results in social impairment, in particular avoidance of social interactions. Available studies show that between 10 per cent and 43 per cent of BDD patients have social phobia. In a series of 100 patients, 32 had been completely housebound for at least one year.[42]

As we have seen, dysmorphophobic symptoms are treated successfully with exposure and response prevention although there is growing evidence that BDD symptoms and associated depression respond well to antidepressants.

This case report highlighted here shows that it is possible to obtain a satisfying outcome if BDD is diagnosed early and treated appropriately. Severe complications such as being housebound, or suicide attempts, which occur in up to 25 per cent of cases, can thereby be avoided.

But it is not just body shape that can become the focus of preoccupation. Olfactory reference syndrome, a disorder characterized by persistent preoccupation with body odour accompanied by shame and embarrassment, appears also to be an OCD spectrum disorder and is linked to BDD.

Dr Dan J. Stein and colleagues from the Departments of Psychiatry and Nuclear Medicine, University of Stellenbosch, Tygerberg, South Africa, recently reported two cases of olfactory reference syndrome, in which a number of features were at least partially reminiscent of OCD. In particular, despite having poor insight, both patients demonstrated significant improvement upon treatment with an antidepressant.[43]

Olfactory symptoms can be seen in a number of disorders, including schizophrenia, depression and certain medical conditions. An early case series in the Western literature used the term 'olfactory paranoid syndrome'. Japanese patients with similar symptoms have, however, been characterized as having an anxiety condition known as *taijin kyofusho* or 'anthropophobia', a term that emphasizes the avoidance of social situations typically seen in such patients.[44]

The term 'olfactory reference syndrome' (ORS) has recently been introduced to differentiate the olfactory symptoms found in this entity from those of schizophrenia, depression and temporal lobe epilepsy. Patients with ORS hold themselves responsible for the odour, and therefore experience a 'contrite reaction', characterized by shame and embarrassment. Such patients tend to wash themselves excessively, to change their clothes with more than usual frequency, to hide themselves away and to restrict their social and domestic excursions.[45]

The young man who believed he smelt of urine

Mr A. was a 17-year-old male who described a persistent pre-occupation, which had begun about six months previously, with the idea that he smelt of urine. Each time he urinated, for example, he worried that he had wet his underwear. He stated that these thoughts occupied most of his waking time. As a result he would repeatedly check his underwear for urine stains, would change his clothing excessively often and would use more deodorant than usual. Shame and embarrassment gradually led him to avoid social interactions, and he even began to miss days at school. He became increasingly demoralized and exhibited a number of symptoms of depression. On close questioning, the patient said that he was 95 per cent certain that he did in fact smell of urine, although on occasion he recognized that his preoccupation with odour was excessive and unreasonable. He had no history of classic obsessions or compulsions, of definite hallucinations or delusions or of substance abuse, and no underlying general medical disorder.

Following his treatment with an antidepressant, he began to show a gradual reduction in his preoccupation with odours.

The woman who believed she had terrible body odour

A 54-year-old woman presented with a persistent preoccupation that she had a foul body odour. The smell emanated from her armpits, breasts, feet and anal region and was reminiscent of rotting fruit. This symptom had begun about 30 years earlier. A more recent concern was that drains from her house emitted a similar foul smell. Although the patient was able to admit that these concerns were perhaps unrealistic, she was often concerned about embarrassing herself, and this had led to excessive hand-washing, frequent changes of clothing and repeated cleansing of drains. Furthermore, at times these concerns resulted in marked depressive symptoms. The patient also suffered at times from checking (of lights, stove, taps) and counting rituals.

At first the woman was treated with an antidepressant, which improved her mood but did not diminish the olfactory symptoms. When she discontinued medication after 12 weeks her depressive symptoms worsened, and she submitted to a course of electroconvulsive therapy. This again improved mood but not olfactory symptoms. A 12-week course of another antidepressant had no further effect. Antipsychotic medication was similarly unsuccessful although an increased dose of the antidepressant gradually showed some improvement.

The symptoms in the two patients are reminiscent of OCD in a number of respects. Although all symptoms were related to body odour, these met the criteria for obsessions (intrusive thoughts about body odour) and compulsions (repetitive cleansing behaviours). Although symptoms were often not unreasonable or excessive, they were accompanied by significant shame and distress. Both patients experienced onset of the disorder in adolescence, as well as secondary depressive symptoms, features that are common in OCD.

Another delusion linked to the body is delusional parasitosis (DP). Though uncommon, it is a cause of severe distress for affected patients and frequently a cause of frustration for their physicians.

Patients are primarily middle-aged or older women who have the unshakeable delusional belief that they are infested with parasites – tiny animals like mites, bugs or lice. Although the vast majority of cases involve skin manifestations, some patients may have delusions of intestinal infection.[46]

'Delusional parasitosis' was first described by the French dermatologist Georges Thibierge in 1894. Before 1946 the condition was known by a variety of names, including acarophobia, dermatophobia and parasitophobia.[47]

Patients with delusional parasitosis characteristically come to the physician complaining of itching, biting and crawling sensations. They may point to 'tracks' on their skin and describe the 'life-cycle' of the parasite. Frequently they have had multiple encounters with physicians and may describe the hostility and ineptitude of past physicians in recognizing or curing the disease. The patients may report extensive use of pesticides at home, and even get rid of family pets who they believe are hosts for the parasites. They frequently bring 'samples' of the parasites wrapped in tissue, enclosed in small containers (the 'matchbox sign'), or sealed in envelopes. Careful examination of these specimens is imperative as it assures the patient that they are being taken seriously. However, in cases of delusional parasitosis, these specimens generally turn out to be bits of dirt, mucus or skin debris.[48]

The patients spend much time trying to get rid of this 'infection' and patients prefer to go to dermatologists, general practitioners and public health physicians because most do not accept that there is any underlying psychiatric disorder that could account for their complaints. This is one reason why psychiatrists are not very familiar with this syndrome.[49]

An area of interest has been the finding that patients can not only feel but also often see the 'parasite', even drawing it, despite a 'shakeable' belief in the infestation. What do they see? What shall we label the experience? 'Illusion' might best explain the phenomenon, as these patients actually are viewing the 'parasitic' materials they bring with them in their plastic bags and matchboxes. The transformation of the material into 'six-legged arthropods' is probably a phenomenon consistent with hysteria.[50]

One of the particular aspects of this syndrome is its 'power' to induce shared psychotic (delusional) disorder (SPD), that is to transfer the delusional contents (and probably in a first step the tactile sensations) to another person (*folie à deux*). In most of these cases, there is a close and often long-standing relationship between the 'inducer' (primary case) and the 'induced' person (secondary case) who shares the delusional beliefs wholly or in part.[51]

Dr Marc L. Bourgeois, a professor of psychiatry, and colleagues at the University of Bordeaux in France reported the case of a woman suffering from delusional parasitosis who tried to kill her general practitioner.[52] Her husband shared in her beliefs but lost all delusional conviction after she was compulsorily admitted to a special hospital. The case illustrates the intractable nature and potential dangerousness of some of these cases, and their affinity to paranoia.

A *case of delusional parasitosis*: folie à deux *and attempted murder of a family doctor*

A 58-year-old woman was compulsorily admitted to hospital after twice shooting (and missing) her family doctor with a hunting gun. Following the attempts, she proceeded to inflict minor injuries to his head with a stick. The doctor did not press charges against her. For a number of years she had been suffering from delusions of infestation, believing that small animals swarmed under her scalp and crawled under her skin. She could also hear the insects and see them while combing her hair and would present her doctor with 'specimens' in a matchbox. She also believed that she had caught scabies from her cat, and that other villagers were also infested. She sought help from the police and the town mayor, and harassed her family doctor for almost two years. Eventually, she developed the delusion that he had engineered a plot against her, and was responsible for her symptoms. Her husband, who was an alcoholic, shared this belief and threatened the doctor after his wife was compulsorily admitted. However, his conviction then gradually melted away.

Born in Brittany, France, the patient was of humble origins and received a poor education (she could hardly read). Her alcoholic mother had died at the age of 68 from 'dementia', and her father hanged himself in his fifties. Her husband had spent from 1940 to 1945 as a prisoner of war in Germany, and she had had difficulties in rearing two daughters. She had become progressively irritable, developed sleep problems and shown abnormal behaviour. Before attacking her doctor, she had been sleepless for a week.

One of the most worrying features of delusional parasitosis is the great potential it has for leading to dramatic self-harm as the patient persistently attempts to scratch or deal with the imagined infection.

Because the infection lies in the patient's imagination no physical methods for dealing with the diseased skin appear to work. This leads to the use of ever more drastic methods. Doctors appear to be at particular risk of aggression in some cases. The fear of infestation, coupled with the medical profession's reluctance to take this fear seriously, may result in panic and violent assault. In the next chapter we examine in more detail how similar problems produce dramatic cases of self-harm.

7

DANGER TO SELF

No matter how you slice it, self-mutilation is a grisly topic.
Dr Armando Favazza, University of Missouri

Self-mutilation has certainly been around for a long time: in Book VI of the *History*, Herodotus (5th century BC) describes the actions of a deranged, probably psychotic Spartan leader: 'As soon as the knife was in his hands, Cleomenes began to mutilate himself, beginning on his shins. He sliced his flesh into strips, working upwards to his thighs, hips and sides until he reached his belly, which he chopped into mincemeat.'

The Gospel of Mark (5: 5) describes a repetitive self-mutilator, a man who 'night and day would cry aloud among the tombs and on the hillsides and cut himself with stones'. However it is only relatively recently that self-mutilation and self-harm have become the subject of detailed psychiatric study.[1]

Psychiatrists Dr Susan Scheftel and colleagues from the North Central Bronx Hospital in New York describe a modern case of self-mutilation unprecedented in the literature to date.[2] The patient, a 20-year-old male diagnosed as schizophrenic, removed virtually his entire face while in a psychotic state. What is particularly disturbing about this case is the patient's persistent refusal to admit that he had mutilated himself.

The man who removed his own face

The following report is composed of information from several sources, including the patient, his father and previous hospital records. Because the patient has been guarded in speaking of the incident, aspects of this history necessarily remain obscure.

The patient, Mr H., was 20 years old and the eldest of five children. Early one morning several years ago, he was found by his father and a brother lying on the floor of their apartment in a pool of blood, his face totally mutilated. He was promptly brought to the hospital by the emergency medical service and claimed that two of the family dogs had caused the injuries. (The family owned three adult Belgian Shepherds and a new litter.)

At first this explanation coincided with the opinion of the doctors, but soon the 'dog story' was called into question. The wounds were clean and without the jagged edges that would be consistent with dog bites; the family members who were asleep in the small apartment had heard neither growling nor screams; there were no defensive wounds on the patient's hands or on the rest of his body. The father reports that a broken mirror with blood on it was found beside the patient. In addition, the patient claimed that the mother dog had swallowed the severed body parts. The contents of her stomach were examined and they showed intact facial features with straight edges and no teeth marks.

Unfortunately, and despite the growing awareness of how the injuries occurred, at least two of the animals were destroyed. The patient has never admitted that he caused the injuries and has clung to his story about the dogs.

The patient appeared to have been psychotic for at least two weeks. He reported that during this period he had fasted and had not used alcohol or drugs. He was withdrawn but agitated and felt that people were laughing at him and calling him 'a bum'. His family observed that he was preoccupied with the Bible and God. At that time, the patient's father was planning to move his family – without Mr H. – to another state; this development was probably one of the main precipitants of the self-mutilation.

Several crucial events occurred on the day before admission, although their sequence and relation to each other are unclear. We know that, although often uncomfortable about his attractiveness to women, Mr H. was seduced that day by an older woman, the girl-friend of his male friend. During the sexual act, the friend walked in.

Mr H. later confronted his friend, demanded that this man cut his own penis off, and expressed omnipotent certainty that this order would be carried out. He felt close to God and to Jesus, believing that he was 'Ruler of the Heavens' and that no-one could or would stop him from doing whatever he wanted. Perhaps related to this sense of omnipotence, Mr H. stated that he also believed himself to be 'Master of the Beasts' and was beating his dogs for reasons he cannot specify. On at least one occasion Mr H. described eating animals' faeces as a test of repentance mandated by God.

On the same day Mr H. was also involved in a verbal and physical altercation (perhaps related to the seduction) in which his lip was bloodied. He returned home to have the dogs lick the blood off his face, claiming he wanted to 'mother the pups and be mothered by them'. Mr H. also said that when he was handling the puppies he had the feeling that the mother dog might 'tear his face off'. About the mutilation itself, Mr H. has only stated that he 'let the dogs do it'.

Several days before the mutilation, Mr H. went to the locked ward of another hospital where he had been a patient and requested admission. He was walking with a cane and, according to the psychiatrist who saw him, 'looked like an orphan'. Although the exact reason for his request was unclear, the doctor took Mr H. to the emergency room, but Mr H. apparently left without even registering.

Concerned about his son, Mr H.'s father took him to another clinic the day before the self-mutilation. Mr H. was seen briefly and noted to be having auditory hallucinations – voices talking to each other. He denied having either suicidal or homicidal feelings, and an appointment, which he never kept, was set up for the following day. That the patient was not well was clear, but neither the intensity of the delusional system nor the belief that he would act on it was apparent.

By age 20, Mr H. has already had five psychiatric hospitaliz-ations. Although this number of hospitalizations could be attributed to his schizophrenia, his traumatic family life cannot be excluded as a major contributing factor. Mr H. lost his mother suddenly when he was seven years old and was placed in the care of his maternal grandmother, but she too died about a year later. Mr H.'s father, despite remarriage, was not able to cope with the demands of a large family, particularly his eldest son, who manifested behaviour problems from an early age. A further traumatic event in Mr H.'s early life was the destruction of his home by fire, supposedly started by a younger brother.

At the age of 15, Mr H. had his first psychiatric hospitalization, after he put his hands through a glass window with the intention of severing them; however, he sustained only superficial lacerations. The reason for this act was his extreme sexual guilt over the fantasized or actual sexual molestation of two of his step-siblings. Relevant to Mr H.'s sexual guilt was some early history given by his father at this time. While bathing her son from infancy until he was four years old, Mr H.'s mother consistently performed fellatio on him. At first the father thought this action somewhat unusual, but later chose to see it as an 'act of love'.

Mr H.'s first hospitalization was a prototype for the subsequent admissions. He was flagrantly psychotic. His behaviour was dominated by sexual and aggressive acting out, and his thinking was influenced by religious delusions. He remained a diagnostic puzzle throughout this hospitalization.

During Mr H.'s next three hospitalizations, despite depressive symptoms, the prevailing diagnosis seemed to be paranoid schizophrenia. Hallucinations, delusions and acting out dominated the clinical picture although his family remained seemingly indifferent to him and to the hospital staff.

Dr Susan Scheftel reported that when she first encountered Mr H. she found a grotesquely mutilated man, unrecognizable as a living being, yet in no apparent physical pain. Despite the obvious presence of a thought disorder, perhaps the most glaring indicator of Mr H.'s psychopathology was his seeming indifference to his situation. He was friendly and cordial, denying direct responsibility for his injuries.

Certain aspects of Mr H.'s mental status changed as he improved with high doses of antipsychotic medication and frequent therapeutic contacts. His thoughts became organized and coherent, and he spoke quite movingly about his past and present situations, so much so that it was almost possible to forget that he had been a psychotic young man.

He is now painfully aware of his blindness (he is unable to see out of his partially remaining eye and it is unlikely his vision will return), is aware of his disfigurement and is distressed by the impact his appearance has on others. As he has come to comprehend his situation, he has understandably become more depressed. However, due to his treatment he is not only able to express his depressive states, but he also has the capacity to be humorous and high-spirited.

A predominant reliance on projection and denial and the continued credence given to earlier delusions are the remaining manifestations of this patient's pre-existing psychopathology. At times he angrily attributes his own feelings to others, particularly when discussing abandonment and disappointments. Perhaps more significant is his continued refusal to admit that he caused the injuries to himself. Even in the face of direct confrontation, he continues to insist that 'the dogs did it'. Notably, it is before and during stressful periods (e.g. surgery) that such defences become more evident. One should keep in mind that Mr H. has endured nine painful reconstructive procedures, procedures that would tax even the defences of a 'healthy' individual.

Over time his sensitivity to pain has increased and he has talked emotionally of the excruciating physical pain he is suffering. Similarly, although at first he completely denied his blindness, Mr H. now painfully acknowledges his loss of sight. Nonetheless, he has compensated remarkably for this and has become cognizant of virtually everything that is being done to and for him, recognizes staff members by their voices and footsteps and is well oriented to time, despite the lack of visual cues.

In summary, this young man is no longer acutely psychotic. Since admission six months previously, he has changed markedly; there have been dramatic improvements in his thinking, capacity for insight, contact with reality, and relatedness. He remains a 'model patient' quite able to be maintained on the intensive care unit. His days are spent anticipating, or recuperating from, surgical procedures.

As with many cases of radical self-mutilation, this patient's self-mutilation occurred in a context of psychosis, delusional religiosity, sexual guilt, a 'tyrannical conscience' and recent abandonment superimposed on a history of early loss.

There are other features, however, that make this case unique. A strikingly different element is this patient's sustained refusal to admit that he mutilated himself. Even as his thinking has become clearer, even as his reality-testing has improved, and even as he has gained trust in the staff members working with him, our patient continues to assert that his dogs mutilated him. This type of outright disavowal is uncharacteristic of patients for whom the mutilative act is delusionally justified. Other patients have been described as lying or concealing before the act, so that their psychotic intentions will not be thwarted; once the act is complete, however, their delusional thinking seems to obviate the need for concealment or denial. Not so with this patient.

While the mutilation was probably performed to expiate guilt, it has, in a sense, become its own source of guilt. For one thing, a direct consequence of Mr H.'s act was the extermination of two of his dogs. Though no-one knows a great deal about Mr H.'s relationship to his dogs, one speculation is that they may have been more constant and reliable objects than any family members.

Mr H.'s family was never particularly supportive of him, and by moving to a different state they were making themselves even less available. The fact that they have visited him little while he has been in hospital Mr H. may ascribe to the nature of his act. He may feel that not only did he drive the family away, but his grotesque appearance keeps them away. If he denies his role in the injuries, Mr H. may feel that he stands a better chance of regaining the affection of his family.

In a sense, this unwillingness to admit that he mutilated himself means Mr H. understands that his injuries are more acceptable if dogs caused them. It also bespeaks of Mr H.'s wish to conform to social expectations and to be liked. From the start, it seems, he has been enough 'outside' his delusional beliefs to see the unacceptability of their consequences.

The symbolic equivalence of radical self-mutilation and castration is certainly relevant in this case. The same day as Mr H. mutilated his face, he commanded another man to remove his penis. Perhaps being caught *in flagrante delicto* with this man's girlfriend stirred up powerful sexual and Oedipal guilt. Mr H. probably already had a reservoir of such guilt, considering his early incestuous experiences with his mother (which happened under the watchful eye of his father).

Although this history may explain some of the guilt that drove this patient to punish himself so massively, it does not explain why it was his face he chose to punish. He was ambivalent about being attractive to women so was he attempting to destroy an aspect of himself that he knew women were drawn to? Another more specific conjecture that would link this patient's present and past sexual guilt is the possibility that his face actually 'became' a sexual organ. It does not seem far-fetched to suggest that the patient may not only have been caught having sex with another man's girlfriend, but may also have been performing cunnilingus. If so, it would have been a reversal of the original incestuous situation in which the patient's mother performed fellatio on him.

These preliminary speculations suggest that Mr H.'s choice of the face for self-mutilation may have been doubly determined, obtaining symbolic 'fuel' from both the affective and sexual domains of his life.

A multitude of different specialists (general surgery, plastic surgery, ophthalmology, nursing, physical and occupational therapy, anaesthesiology) have been involved in the care and treatment of Mr H. and psychiatric staff members have undertaken the complex task of attempting to co-ordinate these different services. Related to this complexity, it is not accidental that much of the work – therapeutic, consultative, didactic, organizational – has been shared, with two or more psychiatrists involved in these activities.

This collaborative approach arose initially out of the overwhelming visual repulsiveness of the patient and the need for 'moral support'. It is of obvious benefit to have more than one staff member co-ordinating the many disciplines involved with Mr H. However, perhaps the greatest benefit has been in the therapeutic work itself. After the initial contacts with Mr H. in which several doctors visited him simultaneously, two have remained as his co-therapists.

Not only have they been able to share the effort of 'translating' Mr H.'s inarticulate (but intelligible) speech, they have also been able to offer each other feedback. Examination of their own responses to the patient has led them to become more actively aware of the overall phenomenon of staff reaction to him.

Mr H. would inevitably have a profound effect on all those working with him. Previously psychiatrists working in this area have pointed out that there is sometimes a sense in which self-mutilation has a more devastating effect on staff members than even suicide. In facing the patient who has self-mutilated, one is simultaneously confronted with both physical and psychological disfigurement. Others in the field also remark that staff members may experience self-mutilation as both a 'disgusting and titillating experience'.

This double-edged response is a complicated one. Staff members are confronted not only by their own revulsion but also by the curiosity and excitement that the self-mutilating act arouses. The sadomasochism inherent in the act of self-mutilation is evoked in parallel form in the reactions of the staff members. This phenomenon is the same one that sells tabloid newspapers, yet when such responses occur in those identified as 'helping professionals' it is a shock. Inappropriate displays of curiosity, distortion and avoidance seem to be the major modes of 'countertransference' elicited in staff.

Within several days of his admission, Mr H. was known to virtually the entire hospital. The housekeeping staff, security guards and even patients on other floors had heard of him. Some of the curious ones came to the intensive care unit and attempted to enter Mr H.'s room to get a look at him. Although the professional staff tended to view this 'morbid curiosity' critically, few were really immune to it. They found themselves talking constantly about the patient and their visits to him became the most 'interesting', if disquieting, events of their day. After working hours, they even began to inflict descriptions of Mr H. on family and friends who did not share this eagerness to speak graphically about this severe case of self-mutilation.

Perhaps the other side of this particular coin is avoidance. Certain staff members requested not to work with the patient. One anaesthesiologist, during one of Mr H.'s reconstructive surgeries, treated him with a sheet over his face. Although the patient has been ambulatory for some time, few staff members encouraged him to leave his room, a response that seems related to a need to avoid seeing the patient 'in action'. Somehow, if he was lying in a hospital bed, his disfigurement could be more easily tolerated as it would seem to be purely medical. The more ill Mr H. looked, perhaps the less we were reminded that these injuries did not just 'happen'.

Descriptions of bizarre self-mutilation involving the removal of a body part, while not common, are scattered throughout psychiatric and medicinal literature. Case reports have been written about patients driven to amputate, eviscerate and castrate themselves, and enucleate their eyes. These acts are the most drastic form of self-mutilation conceivable; they comprise a unique sub-type which has been labelled 'severing' and almost all those who commit such acts are psychotic at the time. Individuals who dramatically mutilate themselves seem to act with powerful single-mindedness, often in spite of precautions and restraints imposed on them.

Almost all authors who have written on the subject assert or imply that psychosis is a necessary concomitant. Delusions and hallucinations seem to provide the impetus for self-mutilation, particularly when the content is religious or mystical. A preoccupation with the Bible, especially with those passages urging self-mutilation for the purpose of purification, seems to precede many psychotic self-mutilations. Before the act, patients often believe themselves to have a special relationship to God or Jesus: at times this may be a psychotic identification, at other times a belief in being God's functionary. These patients often view the self-mutilative act as having a divine significance. Some experts make an analogy between those who injure themselves in response to psychopathological religiosity and the subjects in psychologist Stanley Milgram's famous experiment on obedience to authority. In both cases, the individuals so revere the authority who is 'endorsing' an absurd and destructive act that they do not stop to question it. The more a person trusts or values his delusions or hallucinations, the greater the likelihood that these psychotic experiences will lead to action.

A remarkable observation contained in practically every case report of psychotic self-mutilation is that these individuals rarely experience pain. To date little is known about how such analgesia can occur. It may be an extreme version of the blunting of emotional range typically found in schizophrenia. Perhaps for an individual to perform the kind of self-mutilation being described, he must have a disorder of body image, a perception that a change of an alarming nature is occurring.[3]

This experience of transformation, 'in the presence of ideas of reference, delusion, and hallucinatory experience, provides the "rationale" for an act such as self-enucleation'. With such a disturbance in body image, the typical thresholds and sensitivities associated with an intact body image may be absent. Rather than pain, these patients seem to experience a sense of relief and a reduction of tension after their acts. The urgency and agitation described when they are prevented from harming themselves bespeak the intensity of the psychotic need.[4]

Minimization and denial of injury also seem to characterize those who psychotically self-mutilate. In 1979 a patient was described who blinded himself and then denied that he could not see, while two years earlier another psychiatrist remarked on a patient who enucleated both her eyes and who had an 'almost monotonous indifference to her blindness'.[5]

There has been discussion as to whether the self-mutilative act is, as termed, a 'focal suicide'. Is the person destroying a part of the self as an alternative to total destruction? Though there are reports of self-mutilating patients who have subsequently committed suicide, most are not overtly suicidal at the time of their actions, nor do they consciously view their act as a suicidal gesture.[6]

Sexual issues (involving either homosexual panic or heterosexual conflict) and Oedipal concerns are frequently implicated in the over-powering sense of guilt that can lead to self-injury. Sometimes these patients imagine that they have done something reprehensible; self-orchidectomy (removal of the testicles) was the solution one patient found for masturbation. In other cases, an actual crime of rape or murder preceded the self-mutilation. While there are instances when the self-mutilator was the offender in a sexual assault, as we have seen there are also cases where self-mutilation occurred after victimization, including incest.[7]

Certain body parts seem more subject to radical self-mutilation than others. Because of their actual or symbolic significance, the genitals and the eyes seem to take precedence. There are fewer reports of hands and digits being amputated and only rare cases of self-inflicted glossectomy (removal of the tongue). There is one report of a patient who anaesthetized himself and removed his adrenal glands.[8]

Even when the organ or appendage removed is not explicitly sexual, the sexual symbolism of these acts seems to be taken for granted by some authors. There are other views, however, as to the significance of the body part removed. One speculation is that the enucleated eye is a 'symbolic condensation of the self, the being guilty of the horrendous act'. In 1973 a patient who had been afflicted with a childhood speech impediment cut out his tongue. A patient in the 1980s who had epilepsy, and so had predominantly left-sided movements, believed his left eye was the locus of his seizures and for this reason removed it. Some psychiatrists suggest that those who self-enucleate may be attempting to stem visual hallucinations or graphic LSD flashbacks. At this level, the self-mutilation seems to serve as a cure rather than a punishment, and indeed some patients refer to their acts as having just such a curative function.[9]

But if self-mutilation has been defined as 'painful, destructive and injurious acts upon the body without the apparent intent to commit suicide' then one of the central puzzles about self-harm remains: what drives this peculiar behaviour?[10]

While most psychiatrists agree that self-mutilation is distinct from suicide in intent, lethality, phenomenology and associated features, some believe it is a compromise between the life and death drives. It is an attempt to avoid complete destruction by channelling the destructive impulses more specifically. Some incidents of self-mutilation serve as 'microsuicides', embracing the self-destructive feelings and creating an 'illusion of mastery over death'. Thus, the anti-suicide model focuses on the behaviour as an active coping mechanism used to avoid suicide in direct contrast to seeing self-mutilation as an actual suicide attempt.[11]

But what adds to the enigma of self-harm is when the form is itself of a particularly bizarre type. For example introduction of foreign bodies into one's own body is one of the uncommon types of self-mutilation. Published clinical reports on this are meagre but Dr Srikala Bharath and colleagues from the Department of Psychiatry at the National Institute of Mental Health and Neurosciences in Bangalore, India, recently reported the following astonishing case of self-mutilating behaviour involving needles.[12]

The man who tried to become the Hollywood movie character, 'The Terminator'

P., a 53-year-old single male, was referred with a possible diagnosis of substance abuse due to the presence of multiple puncture marks on his arms. Detailed evaluation of P. revealed that he had been suffering from paranoid schizophrenia for the previous five years. He was a staunch Christian who hoped to become a pastor. His father was an atheist. P. was closer to his mother, a firm believer. P. had had very rigid and negative views on sex and marriage since adolescence.

His first episode of psychosis occurred at the age of 17 years, and he was treated and remitted. At the time of the current admission P. had delusions of persecution related to Freemasons who he felt were planning to attack and kill him. He also had auditory hallucinations involving his dead mother and had been introducing stainless-steel needles into his limbs to strengthen himself, as in the 1984 film *The Terminator*. This is a movie in which both villain and hero (played by Arnold Schwarzenegger) change into steel robots and have immense power against their enemies. P. had seen the movie 10 times and believed that the steel in his body would make him equally powerful. He did not report pain due to his self-mutilation although X-rays revealed more than 40–50 needles of various types (injection needles, sewing needles, paper pins with the ends broken) in his body.

P. was admitted and treated with antipsychotic medication but surgical removal of the needles turned out to be impossible, as there were so many. During his six-month and one-year follow-up sessions there was no further reported introduction of needles by P. His auditory hallucinations had stopped, but his delusions had not totally disappeared.

Sexual confusion and sexual guilt are identified as the basis for this type of self-mutilation. As noted earlier, the act is seen as a 'sacrifice of a part' to protect the whole self and prevent 'annihilation'.

When an attempt was made to understand the unusual SM of patient P., certain similarities to other reported cases of cutting/maiming were noted even though his actions were very different. In a way, P.'s self-mutilation was an act of preserving himself from nemesis and unlike other reported cases, it was significantly influenced by the media.

This suggests that deliberate self-harm behaviour should not be understood independently of the larger context in which it appears. Culture and religion are some of the determinants recognized by this perspective. In the 20th century the media became very influential so it is not surprising (if unusual) that a popular movie should influence the SM behaviour of a person with psychosis.

Psychosis is characterized by the presence of delusional ideation, defined as a fixed misbelief that is not shared by others in the patient's subculture. The point of this definition is that we are all prone to err in our beliefs, but the deluded hold to gross errors of logic and thinking that most others around them would not commit.

The case of P.'s self-harm was an example of self-mutilation occurring as a result of psychotic delusional beliefs and although his case was considered remarkable, such self-destructive behaviour is not uncommon. However, self-mutilation is much more commonly associated in clinical psychiatry practice with self-hatred, than seen as a result of psychosis.

Dr Robert Cavanaugh Jr of the Department of Pediatrics from the State University of New York, for example, recently reported the case of a 14-year-old girl who appeared to be trying to cut away the skin on her body where her sexual abuser had held her, in an attempt to cleanse herself.[13]

Those in clinical practice often see young women who cut themselves with no intention of committing suicide. The precise motivation for self-induced cutting and carving of the forearms with scarification remains largely mysterious, but is a common manifestation of sexual abuse in young women in particular. One theory is that those who have been sexually abused when younger suffer low self-esteem: they may feel they are responsible for their own abuse in some way or that they could have prevented it. Their attackers are likely to have made them feel terrible about themselves. In the case of incest, children can blame themselves for the abuse, as a way of protecting their need to feel that their parent is a good person.[14]

So there appear to be strong links between low self-esteem and childhood sexual abuse and it may be that self-cutting or mutilation is a physical way of demonstrating the low opinion you have of yourself.[15]

Numerous skin abnormalities have also been described in adolescent girls who have been sexually abused, including bruising, bite marks, cuts, scratches, abrasions or other evidence of struggle. Victims frequently shower or bathe excessively in an effort to cleanse their skin following a sexual abuse encounter.[16]

Dr Cavanaugh's patient was seen in an adolescent medicine consultation setting for evaluation of an anxiety disorder. During the interview the girl related that she had been under considerable stress and that she was having difficulty sleeping. She also had a worsening of facial tics (spasms of the muscle of the face) that had previously been noted in association with obsessive-compulsive behaviours. She had been receiving psychotherapy and was being treated with Prozac, but the symptoms were becoming more severe. On examination she appeared very anxious and demonstrated numerous involuntary, repetitive facial grimaces. Similar twitching movements of the neck were also noted. In addition, she had several well healed scars over both forearms.

Upon further questioning the patient was asked directly about what had caused these marks. At that point she broke down and cried, saying she had been sexually assaulted several months earlier. She stated that she carved out tattoos on her arms to get rid of the skin that the perpetrator had touched when he forcibly held her down and raped her. She believed that the scars were 'clean' as they were covered with newly regenerated skin. Further psychiatric intervention was then obtained as it became very apparent that the patient had numerous unresolved emotional conflicts stemming from the attack.

A key point is that in almost all the cases we have discussed so far the patient was the direct cause of their own mutilation. Most would acknowledge this to themselves at least – in other words they were conscious of their own actions, although the direct causes might remain mysterious to them and their doctors. However, there are cases where self-inflicted injury is suspected by physicians yet they cannot be absolutely certain how the problem is being caused and the patient does not seem to be directly aware they might be causing the problems themselves.[17]

For example psychogenic purpura was first described in four women in 1955 as the occurrence and spontaneous recurrence of painful patches of bleeding into and under the skin after minor trauma. Purpura is the medical term for the patches of red and purple caused by bleeding into the skin. This phenomenon was initially thought to result from immune sensitization of patients against their own blood cells after they had left the blood vessels and entered the rest of the body. The syndrome was first called Gardner-Diamond syndrome, after the two doctors who first reported it, but was renamed after it was postulated that there was a psychogenic basis for the disorder; however, the exact mechanism of this syndrome is still unknown.[18]

The primary clinical feature is recurring patches of bleeding into the skin, accompanied by varying symptoms, including episodic abdominal pain, nausea, vomiting, painful joints, headache and other bleeding episodes such as nosebleeds, stomach bleeding and bleeding from the ear canals. Although bleeding from the eyes is very rare, especially in the West, seven cases have been reported in Turkey.[19]

Some of the patients with psychogenic purpura also had psychological symptoms, suggesting that their physical symptoms were in fact manifestations of emotional distress. In a case recently reported by Dr Baak Yücel and colleagues at Istanbul Medical School a patient with multiple personality disorder (now known as dissociative identity disorder) presented with psychogenic purpura in the form of bleeding from the eyes and various body surfaces.[20]

The woman who cried blood

Ms A., a 22-year-old widow, was referred for psychiatric evaluation of the following complaints: spontaneous and unexplained bleeding from the eyes, nose, ears and mouth as well as several bruises, especially in the extremities.

Ms A. was involved in a car crash with her family two years previously and had been admitted to the hospital with multiple fractures. One month later and after her discharge from the hospital she began to have flashbacks of the accident and developed startle responses upon hearing the sound of any car during daytime. During that year she had recurrent bleeding lesions in her arms: sometimes these were as small as a coin and sometimes they covered her entire arm. Six months before her referral she was seen by a haematologist because of these lesions and her complaint about bleeding from her ears.

Extensive haematological examinations and laboratory check-up revealed no abnormalities. During that time, Ms A. also described bleeding from other parts of her body, such as her eyes, nose and mouth, and irregular menstrual bleeding. These bleedings occurred in staff's presence and were seen by examiners and interviewers; thus, when the patient cried her tears were filled with blood.

When questioned, she said there was a man's voice inside her head that started to give her advice. This began a short time after the bleeding began. She had heard this voice since the age of 17, and called it 'my friend'. This voice was different from her own voice and belonged to an older man who was not a friend or a relative and had a name of his own. When questioned in greater detail about other psychological symptoms, she said she had no memory of any events between the ages of 8–9 and 17–19.

She also complained of not being able to remember what she had been doing during most of the day and at times she felt like a stranger in familiar places and to familiar people. Her family indicated that she sometimes behaved childishly and played with toys or with the children of visiting friends. During psychiatric interviewing, when questioned about depression, she mentioned a two-month period of depressed mood, diminished interest and pleasure in many activities, difficulty in concentrating, feelings of hopelessness, insomnia and recurrent thoughts of death that ended in her attempt to commit suicide by swallowing a large number of pills.

Ms A. is the eldest of five siblings. Her mother, a polio victim, used crutches to walk; her father, an alcoholic and a cannabis abuser, had beaten Ms A. almost every day during her childhood. He would not let her continue her education after primary school, and she had to start working in a factory at the age of 12. When she was 13, her uncle, who was 19 at the time, stayed in their house, and he abused her sexually. When she complained about this to her family, nobody believed her and the sexual abuse went on for about two years. At the age of 15, Ms A. married a young man who worked at the same factory. Although both families at first objected to the marriage, she moved to her husband's house to live with his family. Ms A. gave birth to a baby girl, but two months later her husband and his mother forced her to leave their house. Her daughter was taken away when she was six months old and Ms A. has not been able to see her again. Before returning to her parents' home she travelled to different cities and lived in one city for two years. However, she had little memory of this and after returning home, her uncle, who was still living in the house, resumed his sexual abuse, this time including intercourse.

Apart from Ms A.'s sexual abuse and history of amnesia, she has feared being in social situations and performing in front of others since she was 12. She also reported recurrent obsessional thoughts and repetitive behaviour related to cleaning. For 10 years she has spent 1–2 hours each day washing the dishes.

During haematological examinations, Ms A. was observed shedding tears filled with blood. She did not have any premonition of the bleeding. The tears were analysed with a light microscope, and were found to be full of blood cells of the same blood type as the blood obtained by venipuncture.

Laboratory investigations yielded no abnormalities.

This patient was diagnosed not only with dissociative identity disorder, but also with major depression, chronic post-traumatic stress disorder, obsessive-compulsive disorder, social phobia and an avoidant personality disorder. Here the multiple diagnosis and the sexual and physical trauma during childhood seem to be consistent with the diagnosis of multiple personality disorder. There have been many comprehensive studies of MPD in recent years, and in the 1900s prevalence was estimated to be 0.4 per cent in Turkey. Another survey suggests that MPD patients have an average of 9.3 other diagnoses as well.[21]

It has been reported that new lesions can be induced by hypnotic suggestion in psychogenic purpura. Because those suffering from multiple personality disorder are also characterized by high hypnotizability, there might be a relationship between these two clinical pictures.[22]

French psychiatrists have identified some patients with bleeding from mouth, nose, uterus and skin as a result of the rupturing of superficial blood vessels. This kind of bleeding is reported to resemble the stigmata of Christian saints. However, it is quite improbable that this religious factor could have played a part in symptom formation for this Muslim patient. In Turkish culture, 'shedding bloody tears' is a very common idiom, and it is used in daily language and in literature to express extreme sorrow and emotional suffering. But Dr Yücel and his colleagues who reported the Turkish case have not been able to find any references to a psychogenic purpura case with bleeding from the eyes in Western medical literature.[23]

Psychogenic purpura is a rare syndrome that may occur in association with dissociative type disorders like multiple personality disorder and traumatic events in childhood, and it may also have cultural links.

The incidence of self-mutilation in the psychiatric population is much higher than in the general population, ranging from 4.3 per cent to 20 per cent of all psychiatric patients. If the population evaluated is limited to adolescent inpatients, the incidence rate rises dramatically, approaching 40 per cent in one study and 61 per cent in another. A survey of outpatient therapists indicated that 47 per cent had seen at least one self-mutilating adolescent.

There is a surprising amount of agreement in the accounts of self-mutilation. The precipitating event is most commonly the perception of an interpersonal loss, such as an argument or a therapist's vacation. The individual generally reports feeling extremely tense, anxious, angry or fearful prior to self-mutilating. Often, but not always, the individual reacts to the overwhelming emotion by experiencing dissociation. Isolation from others almost always precedes the actual act of self-mutilation. Self-mutilating is usually quite controlled and, by definition, there is a lack of suicidal intent. Razor blades are the favoured implement and wrists and forearms are the most common targets.[24]

Further statistics show that the majority of self-mutilators are single, female and usually seen and studied as adolescents or young adults. The age at the first episode is usually in middle to late adolescence. Self-mutilators are often underemployed, with a lower vocational achievement than controls in spite of equivalent education. They are more likely to come from families characterized by divorce, neglect or parental deprivation. But while suicidal patients tend to have childhood experiences of complete parental deprivation due to death or divorce, self-mutilators more often experience partial loss through emotional distancing and inconsistent parental warmth.[25]

The attention and concern of others can be powerful reinforcers of behaviour. Self-mutilating patients include the gaining of attention and social status among peers (as a result of being able to endure pain) as two reasons for their behaviour. Some authors have emphasized the secondary gain of control over others and see one of the primary goals of self-mutilation as mobilizing others to react. Some researchers even describe competitions among patients for the most severe or the greatest number of cuts.[26]

The sexual model proposes that self-mutilation offers sexual gratification, punishes, or attempts to avoid, sexual feelings or actions, or aims to control sexuality or sexual maturation. The connection between self-mutilation and sexuality or sexual development is suggested by the absence of self-mutilation behaviour prior to puberty but is linked to sexuality in both positive and negative ways. It serves as a way to obtain sexual gratification while simultaneously punishing oneself for the sexual drive and expressing an unconscious wish to destroy the genitals as the root of this drive. Increased sexual fantasies and the accompanying aggressive impulses may be experienced by self mutilating adolescents as overwhelming. Self-mutilators may feel 'forced' by their bodies to have these fantasies. So it is an attempt to destroy or purify the body, which is seen as separate from the self.[27]

Self-mutilation is also viewed as an attempt to turn passive into active, taking control of penetration and sexual impulses.[28]

Self-mutilation has also been linked to negative reactions to menarche or menstruation. Several connections exist: (a) self-mutilation had not occurred before menses in most subjects; (b) 60 per cent of the self-mutilation episodes investigated occurred during menses; and (c) 65 per cent of patients reported a negative reaction to menarche. Self-mutilation may be a 'means of dealing with genital trauma and conflict centering around menstruation' where the conflict is displaced from the genitals and the bleeding is exposed and controlled. This may also explain why females self-mutilate more than males.[29]

Some conceptualize self-mutilation as the need to feel real physical pain as opposed to just emotional pain. While this is not congruent with the consistent reports of the lack of pain upon self-mutilation, it may be that self-mutilators need to have physical evidence of their emotional injury in order to feel that their emotions are real, justified or bearable. Self-mutilation may translate the feeling into an external injury that validates and expresses the emotion. One self-mutilating subject expressed this function when she said: 'I can look at these marks and say, "This is how badly I felt and it was real." '[30]

Finally, self-mutilation – or the wound or scar it causes – may also serve actually to produce an identity as well as confirm boundaries. It creates or helps to maintain a separate and unique sense of self because 'bleeding became real, tangible evidence that "I do exist somewhere in this world"'. This reflects the fact that these adolescents are often viewed by others in terms of their self-mutilation behaviour: they are known as 'cutters' and defined by this symptom.[31]

As anger, low self-esteem, reaction to abandonment and lack of ability to self-soothe are generally agreed to be issues for individuals who self-mutilate, treatment would do well to focus on these as well as on the specific meaning of the behaviour.[32]

Dr Howard L. Field and Shimon Waldfogel of the Wills Eye Hospital and Thomas Jefferson University Hospital, Jefferson Medical College, Philadelphia, Pennsylvania, reported several cases of severe self-injury to the eye.[33] Severe ocular self-mutilation, an extreme and horrifying act, has long been with us in both legend and clinical practice. The myth of Oedipus who tore out his eyes to atone for patricide and incestuous sex was important to the classical world. The Norse Odin plucked out one eye to exchange for supreme wisdom. Self-enucleation is represented in Christian hagiography by St Lucia. This saint, pursued by a man excited by her beautiful eyes, avoided sexual temptation by cutting them out and sending them to her over-zealous suitor. Myths of eye mutilation are found in many other cultures, though the act itself appears to be confined to Christian cultural areas.[34]

As discussed, severe intentional eye self-injury is an uncommon but not rare condition. Although medical interest began in the middle of the nineteenth century, progress in understanding this symptom has been slow. Of nine recently reported cases of severe intentional self-mutilation of the eye two-thirds of the group were young psychotic individuals suffering from severe sexual and religious delusions, command hallucinations and the propensity to act on delusions. One-third were older and had either dementia or severe mental retardation. That self-mutilation may occur more frequently in confined patients calls for active vigilance on the part of caretakers.[35]

Self-mutilation is best understood as serving a variety of functions. Research suggests that the behaviour is correlated with certain familial experiences and other symptom clusters, and that it may be possible to differentiate self-mutilators from the general psychiatric population on this basis. But we are just beginning to comprehend the underlying dynamics. We lack not only descriptive information about self-mutilators in general but, especially, descriptive information about self-mutilators who are not in-patients. The vast majority of the research is on an inpatient population, but estimates of the prevalence of this behaviour suggest that there is a population of self-mutilators who are not seen in hospitals.[36]

Understanding the function and meaning of self-mutilation and using this understanding to plan and deliver treatment will help us better address the needs of these patients. However, the problem is compounded by the fact that self-harm is often effectively hidden from others. For example in the following case a self-harm be-haviour is disguised as a volunteering act of charity. It also illustrates how far the drive to diet will take people. This disturbing case report comes from Dr A. Missagh Ghadirian, based in Montreal, Canada.[37]

The woman who gave blood as a ritual

Ms A. was a 32-year-old woman whose eating disorder, which began as anorexia at the age of 13, developed a year later into bulimic behaviour that included bingeing, laxative abuse and peri-odic vomiting. For 10 years she had attended a blood donor clinic to donate 'the filthy blood' and to generate 'fresh and clean' blood. She believed that bingeing caused 'internal pollution'. Purging through laxative and blood donation was her way of 'internal purifi-cation'. Ten years earlier, her older sister, also bulimic, had frequently attended the same clinic to donate blood and told Ms A. that it helped her to control weight so that she could eat sweets with peace of mind.

Ms A. had also experienced depression with obsessive symptoms and blood donation became a cleansing ritual that she practised on average once every three months despite her fragility. She would skilfully conceal from the clinic the truth about her bulimia, mal-nutrition and medication. She would observe with fascination the blood flowing from her. She had the fantasy of watching her blood being drained to the last drop so that she would be purged and purified. She also wondered if she could evaporate and disappear in the process and felt relieved and even mildly elated each time that she donated blood.

This appears to be the first case report of blood donation as an obsessional form of purging and 'cleansing' in a bulimic patient. Previous reports have shown bloodletting in bulimic patients to be a sign of severity of bulimic illness.

Indeed, the lingering doubt remains as to whether self-harming acts such as this and other equally disturbing case histories are little more than forms of suicidal behaviour.

This case raises the disturbing possibility that a vast amount of self-harming behaviour is probably successfully hidden from clinicians, friends and family.

It would seem possible that much apparently innocent or even altruistic behaviour is undertaken for a mixture of masochistic, hysterical, depressive or suicidal reasons. However, what isn't in dispute is the extreme danger to themselves the deluded can pose.

8

You Are What You Eat:
The Delusion of Nourishment

Rebecca only liked to eat the damp earth of the courtyard . . . It was obvious that her parents, or whoever raised her, had scolded her for that habit because she did it secretively and with a feeling of guilt, trying to put away supplies so that she could eat when no one was looking . . .

Gabriel García Marquez, *One Hundred Years of Solitude*[1]

Dr Goldman and colleagues from the Department of Paediatric Surgery at C. Sheba Medical Center in Tel-Hashomer in Israel recently reported the following strange case.[2]

The girl who wouldn't eat food

A 16-year-old girl was referred to the emergency room because of lower abdominal pain, nausea and vomiting for two days. Physical examination revealed an apparently healthy well-nourished girl in distress. Mild tenderness and a mass the size of a tennis ball were detected in her right lower abdomen. Ultrasound examination confirmed the presence of a solid mass but there was no sign of any inflammation in the appendix. An X-ray indicated that an obstruction had occurred in her bowels and a large mass of 7 centimetres diameter and numerous other foreign bodies were seen in her right colon on CAT scanning.

At this stage when questioned the girl admitted to having swallowed large amounts of toilet paper. As her clinical condition was stable and there were no symptoms or signs of her bowels being in significant danger, no surgical treatment was undertaken and enemas were used instead. Her stools were monitored for excretion of paper balls and five days after admission she was discharged in satisfactory condition.

It appears that the girl felt that eating something which would make her feel full, but not provide any calories, might be an effective form of dieting. This is possibly the first time such a bizarre foreign body has been reported as a consequence of dieting, or even of eating-disordered behaviour, particularly in a young person.[3]

The medical term for a concretion of foreign material in the gastrointestinal tract is bezoar. This presents a serious medical problem causing intestinal obstruction with complaints of abdominal pain, nausea and vomiting. In about half the cases a mass can actually be felt when palpating the abdominal wall. In children the commonest types of bezoar are referred to as trichobezoars: hairballs swallowed usually by children suffering from learning difficulties. But other items reported include pins, glue, coins, buttons and plastic, wooden or metal particles.[4]

The key point about this case is the extremes to which those obsessed with dieting will go – including eating large quantities of toilet paper.

'Pica' is a medical term unknown to many of the public because it describes a behaviour most would never believe could exist, yet there is some controversy within the medical profession that this condition could be more common than realized. Pica is defined by doctors as 'a perverted appetite for substances not fit as food or of no nutritional value'. Please, for reasons which will shortly become apparent, don't read this chapter if you are about to eat or have just finished a meal.[5]

The symptoms of pica include the compulsion to eat one or more of a number of foreign bodies ranging from dirt and plastic to faeces. Complications and treatment of pica are the best understood features of this condition (the causes certainly aren't). Pica has been found to cause anaemia, iron deficiency, heavy metal poisoning, parasitic infection, bowel obstruction, altered bowel routine, inflammation of the abdominal cavity and obesity.

Objects that can be eaten include cigarettes,[6] as documented in a case study of an autistic 17-year-old male.[7] The chronic ingestion of tobacco has serious medical consequences, including oral cancer, gingival recession, periodontal disease and elevation of blood pressure.[8] These occur with chronic exposure. Other behavioural effects include irritability on tobacco withdrawal.

Bizarre though it might be, pica has actually been reported on all continents.[9] The first description of such behaviour was made by the Greek physician Galen in the second century. The term 'pica' was first applied in the sixteenth century by a French physician, Paré, using the Latin word for magpie, a bird thought to have odd feeding habits and renowned for eating anything. Medical dictionaries of the seventeenth century frequently mentioned the observed association of pica with pregnancy and 'chlorosis' (an iron-deficiency anaemia in young girls sometimes characterized by a greenish skin colour).[10]

A number of terms have evolved to specify pica of a particular substance: geophagia is the ingestion of clay; coprophagia the ingestion of faeces; pagophagia refers to the ingestion of ice; and amylophagia the ingestion of starch. Pica has been observed in three main contexts: in childhood, in certain communities as a culturally sanctioned behaviour, and idiosyncratically.[11]

Culturally sanctioned pica is observed in particular with the eating of clay, and socially acceptable geophagia has been described in several societies. These include African communities and African-American communities. There the practice is most prevalent amongst women, but can occur in both sexes, in children and in adults. In a 1975 study in which 56 women in a Mississippi county were interviewed, ten were regular consumers of clay and 22 consumed it occasionally.[12]

In adults with normal intellect, pica has been observed in a variety of situations. Examples include pica in elderly people with dementia, in those with eating disorders, and in adults with mineral deficiencies. A fundamental conundrum is: does the eating of strange things lead to deficiencies or do the deficiencies prompt people to start a strange diet in some biologically driven unconscious attempt to compensate for a deficiency?[13]

After obesity, pica is probably the most common eating dysfunction among institutionalized people with intellectual disability. But is this because an institutional diet predisposes to boredom or results in mineral deficiencies? Or does the pica arise from the mental problems that led to institutionalization?[14]

Some interesting trends have been observed: it has been found for example that the incidence of pica increases with the severity of the intellectual disability, and that it decreases with age, with a further rise seen after the age of 70 years.[15]

In the eighteenth and nineteenth centuries throughout Europe medical authorities linked pica with either chlorine poisoning or pregnancy. Other nineteenth-century references are to an increased incidence in black slave populations in the southern United States, where it sometimes reached 'epidemic proportions'. Particularly relevant to a case reported later on in this chapter is the report of extensive dirt-eating noted in populations of the West Indies.[16]

In the nineteenth century, mental hospital records frequently noted that 'epileptic, paretic, senile and maniacal cases' could be subject to 'an active perversion of the appetite for food which leads the patient to devour even the most disgusting substances'.

The early part of the last century saw increasing concern about pica in paediatric populations, especially as knowledge of the medical complications of certain forms of pica became clear (e.g. lead poisoning from eating lead-based paint chips). But case reports lie at both ends of the age spectrum. For example, Dr Nicholas Beecroft and colleagues from the Maudsley Hospital in London recently reported the following intriguing case of a 75-year-old woman.[17]

The woman who eats money

A.B. is an elderly unmarried woman who lives in residential care. After she was admitted to A&E with acute abdominal pain, an abdominal X-ray showed a number of metallic objects in her stomach and small intestine. At exploratory surgery of her gut, she was found to have a perforated gastric ulcer and £175.32 in coins in her stomach.

She had been diagnosed as schizophrenic for over 40 years, although without positive symptoms for at least 20 years. From adolescence she had been a 'nervous, isolated person' who was on the fringe of a group of eccentric writers and performers in the 1960s.

The first clue to possible pica-related symptoms emerged when she was 43. By the age of 57 it was noted during an admission to hospital that she 'was taking too many vitamin tablets'. Then, as now, she was quick to deny the consumption and eloquently described the compulsion to eat vitamin C to relieve anxiety. 'I'm not addicted to them, but it's very important that I have them with me in case – I never know when the moment of need will be . . . It's like people who need a cigarette at a certain moment; they can't define when, but something is needed to help one go on to the next thing . . . the need often occurs when there's a new demand coming up – some change of atmosphere . . . Vitamin C is the only thing that helps the devastation of the self due to anxiety.'

Her compulsion to ingest objects to provide relief from anxiety has been maintained since. At different times she has eaten tablets, coins, wire, plastic, 'purple hearts', Bob Martin's dog conditioning powder and dried flowers. There is much comment throughout her medical notes detailing vigorous negotiations about the colour, size, number, timing and supply of medication, including a large batch of handwritten letters to her doctor. She was admitted for assessment to a psychiatric unit where she presented herself as a cleanly dressed lady with loud speech and tangential replies. Her mood was generally warm and friendly but she was easily irritated if not understood or if a demand was not quickly met.

Her thought was vague and she was invariably evasive about coins, which stemmed from a combination of embarrassment and the desire to avoid medical intervention. She said, 'I haven't wanted to do that for two and a half years.' There was no evidence that she had delusions or abnormal perceptions.

Since in the past she had shown a poor response to antipsychotics, a cognitive-behavioural approach was taken with a view to trying to replace the use of coins as a compulsive anxiolytic with the vitamin C tablets which she had used previously. The use of vitamin C tablets for this purpose was regularly reinforced with encouragement, persuasion and a constant supply. In addition, the home staff aimed to provide a stress- and confrontation-free environment.

After the start of this programme, two abdominal X-rays three months apart showed that wire and steel nuts found in the stomach had passed and that there had been an increase in the number of coins from approximately seven to 20. The patient had used vitamin C with good effect, although she had also made considerable effort to gain access to coins.

There were indications of a deterioration in cognitive functioning, but physical examination proved normal, as were all laboratory tests except zinc level, which was low. The programme was judged partially successful.

This is the second case reported to have included the ingestion of coins. A case was reported in 1995 of copper intoxication due to the swallowing of coins, associated with liver fibrosis and hepatic deposits of copper which proved fatal. Although A.B. had a well-documented lifelong history of schizophrenia, there was little symptomatic overlap with the pica. The pica seems to be a compulsion-driven behaviour not related to disturbance of emotion or thought.[18]

The nature and circumstances of pica are far too diverse to expect a single cause or consequence and pica itself probably does not represent a disease entity; it is a symptom which occurs in a number of varied physical and psychological conditions.[19]

Dr Martin Goldstein of the Department of Psychiatry at the Cornell Medical Center in New York recently reported a strange case of pica who discharged herself before her doctors could get to the bottom of what was going on.[20]

The woman who enjoyed the taste of dirt

The patient was a 33-year-old African–American woman with no previous psychiatric problems who had suffered from medical problems in the past, including diabetes, a form of epilepsy and recurrent headaches. She had a complicated obstetric history, including two spontaneous abortions and an ectopic pregnancy. She complained of vague abdominal pains, increasing abdominal girth, weight gain and episodic nausea and vomiting. Substance abuse history included alcohol and the occasional use of cocaine. There was no evidence that psychiatric problems ran in her family.

The patient was born in the West Indies; she had one twin – possibly identical – sister, and one older brother. The patient emigrated with her family to the United States at the age of two, graduated from high school and later attended college. She had been steadily employed as a cosmetics technician.

The patient had had seven pregnancies but of these, only three resulted in live births. Never married, she was living with the father of her two younger children at the time of her admission. She had had many heterosexual partners (each of her pregnancies, except the last two, was conceived with a different sexual partner), as well as an ongoing lesbian relationship (the only homosexual relationship she had ever had).

However, it was doubtful that she had a genuinely bisexual orientation: her sexual fantasies were solely of men and she described her lesbian relationship as consisting more of 'holding and hugging' than actual sexual interaction. The patient was at her most guarded when discussing this relationship, indicating the taboos about homosexuality existing in the culture in which she was raised. She kept this relationship secret, believing that her family (especially her parents) would condemn her for doing something 'dirty' (her word).

The patient was neatly but extravagantly dressed and made-up, with false eyelashes, two-tone nail polish on extremely long, artificial fingernails, and she wore multiple, large gold rings, necklaces and earrings. Her attitude was reluctantly co-operative although initially she was quite guarded. There was occasional contextually inappropriate smirking and intermittent giggling (e.g., when discussing pica). She said she thought she had been depressed. She was very suspicious and almost paranoid about her medical and psychiatric evaluation (e.g., 'You don't have a tape recorder in that briefcase, do you?').

The patient recalled first eating dirt as a child, but she had soon stopped, careful to keep the behaviour hidden from her parents for fear of their punishing her. At the age of 19, she experienced her first miscarriage. After the burial service, the patient described taking a handful of dirt from the grave and ingesting it. There were brief recurrences of pica following the burial of the next stillborn child as well as during subsequent pregnancies. Except for these episodes, pica behaviour was quiescent until about nine months prior to admission, when the patient began instructing her nine-year-old son and 11-year-old daughter to collect dirt from a neighbour's flower garden. Although her children knew why they were collecting it, the patient was careful not to ingest the dirt in front of them.

The patient gave a sensorially detailed account of her experience of eating dirt: she would grab a handful from the plastic toy pail in which her children had collected it, hold it for a moment, look at it, smell it, and feel it with her fingers. She would then thrust the entire handful into her mouth before swallowing it and enjoying the 'gritty feeling' in the back of her throat.

The patient denied ever experiencing any significant immediate adverse effects from eating dirt, and she did not associate her current abdominal complaints with her pica. Her only reference to her current symptoms was, 'I think there's something going on here', pointing to her lower abdomen, and nodding her head when asked if she meant her uterus. She was unable to attribute either the recurrence of her pica behaviour nine months prior to admission or its continuation ('a few times a week') since then to any specific cause. However, she did say that her 'boyfriend' (her word for the man with whom she lived and the father of two of her children) had 'stopped paying attention' to her sexually. This was followed by an intensification of the patient's lesbian relationship.

Two questions psychiatrists ask when confronted with a new symptom presentation are 'why this?' and 'why now?' Let us consider the cultural, psychological and physiologic aspects of this case in turn, to try to answer these questions for this patient.

Depressed individuals have been found to overeat, particularly carbohydrate and sweet foods, and cases are reported of pica diagnosed with depression and treated with antidepressants.

This patient's early experimentation with dirt-eating as a child may be considered, at least partially, to be culturally based: as described earlier, the West Indies is among the places where pica has been observed with some regularity.

The dynamic issues in this case are striking. Two themes were strongly suggested in the way this patient related her potential history: shame and loss. She was ashamed to tell her parents about eating dirt as a child lest they think that she was being 'dirty'. Later, the patient concealed her lesbian relationship, again because she feared her family (especially her parents) would believe her to be 'doing something dirty' and consequently reject her. But more than any other feeling, the patient related a terrible sense of loss when discussing her miscarriages.

The context of the initial adult appearance of the patient's pica and her explanation of it are telling: she took a handful of dirt from the grave of her foetus and ate it, feeling 'like maybe I could put some of it back in me'. The notion of replacement of a lost object (a kind of concrete introjection) is compelling.

So why was this patient presenting with pica? She was neither pregnant nor iron-deficient. Nor was she anaemic. As in most cases, the patient came to the hospital reporting vague abdominal complaints. About a year and a half prior to admission, her boyfriend had stopped paying sexual attention to her and a few months later, the patient reactivated her relationship with a former lesbian partner. Then about nine months prior to admission, the patient started eating dirt again. A few months prior to admission, the patient told her parents for the first time about this habit, but she concealed from them her habit of sleeping with a woman, which, again, she believed they would consider 'dirty'. The sequence of psychological events accounting for this patient's presentation of pica might therefore have been as follows: loss of love object (boyfriend), prompting resumption and intensification of the homosexual relationship, a primarily nurturing relationship but one nevertheless engendering feelings of shame so that the patient feared the loss of her boyfriend, and parental condemnation – a presumably intolerable combination of shame and potential loss in the context of heightened need.

Pica is her solution: regression to a prior behaviour that was less culturally condemned and which was a behaviour she could share with her family that was 'dirty', a sort of 'sin' to confess to her parents that did not carry the higher risk of rejection associated with homosexuality. But 'why now?' Pica was something this patient had long associated with pregnancy, a condition she had experienced with almost every romantic partner. That the patient was presenting nine months following the resumption of pica, with complaints of increasing abdominal girth (unsubstantiated on examination), weight gain (also unsubstantiated), vague abdominal complaints associated with episodic nausea and vomiting, and with her sole attribution being 'something going on in my uterus', strongly suggests that the idea of pregnancy was on her mind.

Although several clinical features have long been associated with pica, no clear causal mechanism has been found to explain any specific form of pica, nor has any single theory been formulated to link varying manifestations.

Psychological accounts have focused on an inadequate parent–child relationship. Comparative studies document a high frequency of parental emotional deprivation among children with pica.[21]

Evidence suggesting a possible hereditary component includes an increased incidence of pica in first-degree relatives. There is also an increased incidence of obesity and drug addiction among parents of pica patients and a childhood history of pica is frequently but not always found in adults with pica.[22]

As we have seen, a major obstacle to both diagnosis and documentation of accurate prevalence rates is that patients rarely complain of pica, and often guard against revealing it at all. Complications of pica, like diarrhoea or weight loss, are what usually prompt patients to seek medical attention. Findings at initial evaluation can include anaemia, iron deficiency, hypertension, high blood potassium levels and disturbed liver-function tests.[23, 24]

The traditional psychological view regards pica as a learned behaviour, perhaps caused by people with intellectual disability being unable to discriminate between edible and non-edible items. Yet other researchers report that an individual can be quite aggressive and focused in their pursuit of a particular item to ingest. Other psychological theories regard it as a form of aggression.[25]

Some propose that it is automatically maintained by the oral stimulation it produces. Others find that pica is greater in an environment with reduced social interaction. The view that pica is a learned behaviour is the basis of the most popular type of intervention, which is to get the client to learn other behaviours instead.[26]

However, can this weight of theory on which treatment is based cope with the most bizarre manifestation of pica – coprophagia?[27]

Eating of one's own faeces has been observed in psychiatric hospitals among adult patients with diffuse brain disease and in individuals with sub-average intelligence. Little is known about its aetiology partly because coprophagia remains uncommon in humans and so has not received any significant attention in the adult academic psychiatry literature. It has, however, received a lot of attention in veterinary literature. For example, it is a relatively common condition in dogs, and several possible causes have been suggested, including thiamine deficits and pancreatic and intestinal enzyme deficiencies. Most cases, however, seem to be psychological in origin. It has been proposed that this behaviour is acquired through boredom or to avoid punishment for defecation in the house.[28]

Dr Sharon Zeitlin, a psychologist at the University of Toronto, describes a case of coprophagia in an adult with normal cognitive functioning, which is extremely unusual, as a lot of pica is associated with those suffering from learning difficulties. The case is also important, not least because an individual can experience avoidance by staff and other residents as a result of pica, particularly coprophagia, and may find it difficult to get the kind of therapeutic attention needed.[29]

The man who ate his own faeces

D. is a 20-year-old white male from a middle-class family. He is an only child and when he was eight, his mother was diagnosed as having bone cancer. During the course of her illness, D.'s father began to drink heavily and about six months after her diagnosis, his

240

father came home inebriated and found D. playing on the floor in his mother's bedroom while she slept. D. alleges that his father became outraged, stating that he had previously told him not to disturb his mother, then took D. to his bedroom where he sexually assaulted him. When D. began to cry his father told him that 'he was bad and had to be punished' and beat him with a leather belt. That night, D. was incontinent and his father forced him to eat his faeces as punishment. D. reported that this pattern of events occurred approximately once every six months between the ages of 8 and 10.

When D. was 10, his mother died and he was placed in a foster home. He was told by a social worker that this was a temporary arrangement to give his father time to adjust to his mother's death, but D. reported that his father said he was 'being sent away from home because he was bad'. D. never saw his father again; he committed suicide two years later and D. blamed himself for his father's death.

D.'s relationship with his foster parents was good; he denied any abuse. When he was 13, his foster mother died of a heart attack. The previous day, D. had argued with her regarding his curfew and reported that his foster father said the cause of her death was 'too much stress'. D. felt responsible for this and was quite anxious. On the day of her death, he experienced recurrent, intrusive thoughts of 'being bad' and felt an irresistible urge (i.e. compulsion) to eat faeces. That evening he ate his faeces and although he tried to resist this urge, he was unable to do so. His anxiety then decreased. The next incident of coprophagic behaviour did not occur for several years.

When he was 17 years old, D. was involved in a minor motor vehicle accident. His foster father told D. that he had 'let him down' and D. became obsessed with the thought that he had disappointed his foster father. In response to recurrent obsessions about being 'bad', he again experienced an irresistible urge to eat his faeces. Again, after doing so, his anxiety diminished. When D. was 19, his girlfriend became pregnant and had an abortion. D.'s foster father told D. that he was 'irresponsible and let him down'. Once again, D. engaged in coprophagic behaviour to reduce his anxiety.

Initially, D.'s obsessions with being 'bad', with letting others down, and being responsible for his parents' deaths occurred in response to infrequent events and he engaged in coprophagic behaviour in response to such thoughts. But in the six months prior to evaluation, the frequency of his coprophagic behaviour had

241

increased and it no longer merely occurred after highly stressful events: for example he ate his faeces on the anniversary of his biological mother's death and his father's suicide. During the three months prior to treatment, thoughts of past events, triggered by family pictures, mention of his parents and learning from the media about people dying, awoke his obsession with letting others down and being responsible for his parents' deaths. The act of elimination also began to trigger these unwanted thoughts and anxieties, which subsided when he ate his faeces.

D. put away all pictures of his family and no longer watched television or read a newspaper. He reduced his food intake and avoided specific foods, such as bran, to decrease the likelihood of a bowel movement. For the month prior to evaluation, D. engaged in coprophagic behaviour approximately once a week, although he had daily urges to do so. He reported that the feeling of anxiety was intolerable and feared that if he did not eat his faeces he would suffer from unending misery. He was aware of the senselessness of this compulsion.

D. said he had no history of psychological or medical problems. He reported, however, that his mother had told him that when he was a child he would 'eat anything he could get his hands on, including rocks and dirt'. He denied currently engaging in any form of pica. At the time of evaluation, D. was a fourth-year university student with an A average. He was in the process of applying to graduate school, and suggested that the stress associated with that may have caused the increase in his coprophagic behaviour. He worked part-time as a waiter and lived with his foster father. He had had a girlfriend for two years, as well as male and female friends with whom he regularly socialized, although contact with his friends had decreased during the past six months.

D. said that he first learned about coprophagia in a psychology course. He had not realized other people engaged in this behaviour and he had been too embarrassed to tell anyone about it before. He reported that he sought treatment because of the increased frequency and felt out of control. His embarrassment and distress were clearly evident during the evaluation.

D. was given various psychiatric and psychological tests and it was found that he met diagnostic criteria for obsessive-compulsive disorder (OCD) and pica. In light of this diagnosis and in the absence of any significant cognitive impairment or organic basis for his behaviour, he began a behavioural treatment programme comprising exposure and response prevention. Several studies suggest that approximately 65–75 per cent of OCD patients who undergo this procedure improve.

Briefly, exposure and response prevention treatment involves repeatedly exposing patients for prolonged periods (45 minutes – 2 hours) to circumstances that provoke anxiety and urges to ritualize. Typically, exposure is graded so that moderately disturbing events precede more upsetting ones. Patients are requested to refrain from ritualizing throughout the treatment programme regardless of their urges to do so.

The principles of exposure and response prevention were explained to D. The exposure component required him to think about events and come into contact with stimuli that triggered anxiety and urges to engage in coprophagia. The response prevention component required D. to resist the urges to eat his faeces.

Based on D.'s detailed accounts of his intrusive thoughts, five different scenes were prepared. During each session, D. was exposed to descriptions of the situations and thoughts that provoked anxiety and discomfort.

He was told to imagine the scene as vividly as possible, and to permit himself to feel he was actually there. Every ten minutes D. was asked to briefly describe what was happening and was also asked to elaborate on (and modify, if necessary) what the therapist was describing. The exposure was continued until D. appeared visibly more at ease and reported a substantial reduction in anxiety (typically 30–40 per cent). This usually occurred within one hour.

Anxiety was also generated by external cues which D. had been avoiding. He was confronted with a graded sequence of items and situations that provoked discomfort, such as looking at pictures of his family, reading newspaper and magazine clippings pertaining to death and suicide, eating bran cereal, and handling a jar in which he had eliminated his faeces. His subjective level of anxiety was monitored every 10 minutes and exposure continued until a reduction in anxiety was achieved.

D. was assigned daily homework which involved listening for two hours a day to a tape made during the imaginal exposure session. He also ate regular meals, including bran cereal, placed pictures of his parents throughout his house, went to his parents' graves and cut out newspaper and magazine clippings pertaining to death and suicide. D. was also instructed to refrain from engaging in coprophagic behaviour regardless of his urges to do so.

Despite the extreme anxiety D. experienced, he was fully compliant with treatment and reliably carried out his homework assignments. Clinical improvements became apparent over time and by the end of three weeks he consistently reported lower anxiety levels. Although no-one supervised his home practice or ensured that he refrained from coprophagic behaviour, his psychiatrist was confident that he was compliant. The evidence is that supervision does not seem to impact strongly on outcome, perhaps because motivated patients comply with treatment instructions without supervision, whereas unmotivated patients will circumvent them.

Following this three-week intensive treatment, D. was seen once a week for a month to ensure maintenance of gains and to address other issues of concern to him, including going away to graduate school and moving away from his foster father and his girlfriend.

In this case treatment was highly successful. At the conclusion of the programme, D. was free of intrusive thoughts and had no urges to engage in coprophagia. Indeed, coprophagic behaviour had not occurred since treatment was initiated. There was also a significant decrease in his level of depression and anxiety. Follow-ups conducted three and six months after the termination of treatment and telephone contact one year later indicated continued remission of obsessive-compulsive and pica symptoms.

Although D.'s behaviour was responsive to a behavioural programme comprising exposure and response prevention, whether such treatment would be effective with individuals with sub-average intelligence is unclear. In contrast to individuals with these disorders. D. recognized the abnormality of his behaviour and was highly motivated to overcome it. Additionally, he was fully compliant with the treatment.

Although coprophagia has traditionally been classified as pica, it appears, at least in this case, that coprophagia can be a manifestation of OCD. A case report of a woman who suffered from an irresistible urge to eat pebbles and rocks also suggests pica may represent a form of OCD in some patients. It is necessary to determine whether anxiety underlies coprophagia in the psychotic patients and individuals with sub-average intelligence in whom it is more usually observed.

It is important to stress that coprophagia in humans is rare. Although described in schizophrenia early this century, little is known about its detailed phenomenology. There is no reference to it in commonly used texts, and mentions in basic postgraduate textbooks are confined to coprophagia as a form of sexual deviance. Faeces ingestion is also a feature of the culture-bound syndrome piblokto which is found in Eskimo communities.

But disturbances of brain and mind can also produce a change in eating patterns, where taste becomes more refined rather than degraded. Such altered eating habits (as a consequence of a brain injury that cannot be classified among known disorders) is best characterized by the name 'gourmand syndrome'. The French word *gourmand* describes someone who is heartily interested in fine food and drink or is simply a food-lover; the term 'gourmet' is reserved for a food connoisseur. Although commonly not considered pathologic, gourmand eating may occasionally indicate brain damage. In particular, passionate eating is significant when it occurs in previously 'normal' eaters and is associated with other behavioural alterations.[30] French doctors Marianne Regard and Theodor Landis describe two patients who drew attention to this condition.[31]

The man whose brain damage improved his taste

This 48-year-old man, who had high blood pressure, non-insulin-dependent diabetes mellitus and chronic smoker's bronchitis, was admitted because of a sudden paralysis to the left side of his body following a brain injury.

The patient had been an average eater. Not especially concerned with food, he ate what his wife brought to the table. He occasionally went to restaurants and had no particular food preferences. His main preoccupation was his profession as a well-known local political journalist. He did not follow any diet, and was slightly overweight. When asked what bothered him most, he instantly replied that he found the hospital food awful, that he felt perfectly healthy, and that he had nothing else on his mind but good, tasty, food served in a nice restaurant. During hospitalization, he wrote in his diary '. . . sex I start to really miss, and it is time for a real hearty dinner, like a good sausage with hash browns or some spaghetti Bolognese, or risotto and a breaded cutlet, nicely decorated, or a scallop of game in cream sauce with "Spatzle" [a Swiss and southern German speciality]. Always just eat and drink! What a connoisseur I am, and now I am dried up here, just like in the desert. Where is the next oasis? With date trees and lamb-roast or couscous and mint tea, the Moroccan way, real fresh . . .'

He recovered partially from his brain injury and after four months was able to take up part-time work. He left his job as a news journalist and chose to write columns on eating, which he subsequently did successfully. He also wrote about food in relation to his experience as a patient. His family was struck by his outgoing and eating-oriented behaviour, which they initially attributed to his new job. However, they noted that the only conversations that aroused him were about food, and his desire and requests for meals prepared at home became more precise and exotic. Indeed, he often left home to dine out and in one year, his weight increased by three kilograms.

The man whose brain damage caused food fantasies

This 55-year-old man was admitted because of severe headache and a sudden weakness of the left arm and face. Tests revealed a haemorrhage in the right side of the brain consistent with having suffered a stroke. Within a few days, he recovered, but his behaviour was altered. He made sexual advances to the nurses and ate 'goodies' even during examinations.

Previously, he was a very active businessman and sportsman, concerned about his looks, but not especially with fine eating. He had no real food preferences, and preferred a tennis match to a fine dinner. He did not follow any diet but did pay attention to his weight. He was a tall, athletic man who did not subsequently gain weight, as measured at a follow-up examination one year later, despite his acquired 'eating passion'.

Five weeks after the stroke, he was asked to write down his experiences as a patient. Astonishingly his writing almost exclusively contained reflections about fine eating: 'After I could stand on my feet again, I dreamt about going downtown and sitting down in this well known restaurant. There I would get a beer, sausage and potatoes. Slowly, my diet improved again and so did the quality of life. The day after discharge, my first trip brought me to this restaurant, and here I was ordering potatoes, salad, sausage and a beer. I felt wonderful. My spouse anxiously registers everything I eat and nibble. It irritates me. A few steps down the street, we entered a coffeehouse. My hand reached for a pastry, but my wife's hand intervened. Through the window I see my bank, damn, if I chose to, I could buy all the pastry I wanted, including the whole store. The creamy pastry slipped from the foil, like a mermaid, I took a bit. From now on, it will be more difficult to put me under stress.' When he returned home, after five weeks in the hospital, the family was struck by his 'eating passion'. His conversation centred around food fantasies, and he grasped every occasion to dine out, being concerned more about quality than quantity of food. Although he resumed his previous business and sports activities, he seemed less engaged with them.

Most patients with Gourmand syndrome appear to suffer from a right-side brain lesion. The eating behaviour does not correspond to any previously known eating disorder, though the closest link would be with 'hyperphagia', or the tendency to eat voraciously, but the distinction and odd thing about Gourmand syndrome is the predilection for *fine* food.

What these cases remind us is that taste is much more biological and brain-based than we might realize. For example, have you ever wondered why food loses its flavour when you have a cold? It's not your taste buds' fault. Blame your stuffed-up nose. Seventy to seventy-five per cent of what we perceive as taste actually comes from our sense of smell. Taste buds allow us to perceive only bitter, salty, sweet and sour flavours. It is the odour molecules from food that give us most of our taste sensations.

When you put food in your mouth, odour molecules from that food travel through the passage between your nose and mouth to olfactory receptor cells at the top of your nasal cavity, just beneath the brain and behind the bridge of the nose. If mucus in your nasal passages becomes too thick, air and odour molecules cannot reach your olfactory receptor cells. Your brain therefore receives no signal identifying the odour and everything you eat tastes much the same. The odour molecules remain trapped in your mouth; the pathway has been blocked off to those powerful perceivers of smell – the olfactory bulbs.

Of all our senses, smell is our most primal. Animals need the sense of smell to survive; although a blind rat may survive, a rat without its sense of smell cannot mate or find food and death becomes inevitable.

Yet, although our sense of smell is our most primal sense, it is also very complex. To identify the smell of a rose, for example, the brain analyses over 300 odour molecules. The average person can discriminate between 4,000 and 10,000 different odour molecules.[32] Much remains unknown about exactly how we detect and discriminate between various odours, but researchers have discovered that an odour can only be detected in liquid form. We breathe in airborne molecules that travel to and combine with receptors in nasal cells. The cilia, the hairlike receptors that extend from cells inside the nose, are covered with a thin, clear mucus that dissolves odour molecules not already in vapour form. When the mucus becomes too thick, it can no longer dissolve the molecules.

Recently, a team led by Charles Zuker and Nicholas Ryba, scientists at the University of California, San Diego, and their colleagues at the National Institute of Dental and Craniofacial Research (NIDCR) reported the discovery of two genes, TIR1 and TIR2, which encode proteins that function as bitter taste receptors.[33]

This new work helps explain, on a molecular level, the 'logic' behind the taste system and how it differs from the olfactory system. The olfactory system is designed to recognize a wide range of odours and to discriminate one odour from another – an essential ability when it comes to avoiding such inappropriate responses as mistaking a mate for a snack. The organization of the olfactory system reflects this need, with each olfactory neuron expressing only one of the 1,000 or so olfactory receptor genes.[34]

Taste is a different matter, especially where bitter compounds are concerned. Virtually every naturally occurring toxin tastes bitter, so bitterness clearly evolved with the sole purpose of warning you against the ingestion of toxic substances. The important thing is to recognize and reject anything bitter, not to get hung up on distinctions among different compounds. Indeed, experimental evidence indicates that humans are unable to discriminate one bitter substance from another.[35]

This imposes an interesting contrast with the olfactory system. Every cell that expresses genes in the T2R family expresses nearly all the genes in that family. So, rather than having one receptor per cell, as in olfaction, you have many. This dramatically increases the repertoire of bitter things you can taste, but since the receptors are all in the same cell, and the cell simply fires when activated, you do not discriminate.[36]

This new advance in understanding the biology of our taste system begins to explain why disturbances in our brain and mind are more likely to lead to the tendency to eat unpalatable items, in contrast to those with Gourmand syndrome, where the tendency is to become more refined in taste. It would seem that the system for detecting the unpalatable is more simple and, therefore, more prone to disturbance than the mechanics of odour, which are involved in more discriminatory taste decisions.[37]

It is possible that these advances in our understanding of basic biology are assisting us in unravelling the mysteries of Pica and Gourmand syndromes.

9

A Load of Old Rubbish:
Diogenes Syndrome

Our hoard is little, but our hearts are great.
Alfred Lord Tennyson, *The Marriage of Geraint*, 352

Most of us admit to hoarding stuff from time to time.[1] We have stacks of reports in our office which we think we should examine at some point; piles of magazines at home we delude ourselves into thinking might be useful. But at what point could this become a problem?[2]

No-one knows how many people fill their homes with what we would regard as junk, but it's sufficiently common for many health and social care professionals to be familiar with the phenomenon. The behaviour even has a name, Diogenes syndrome, though some prefer to view it as an obsessive-compulsive behaviour, and others refer to it as syllogomania.[3]

The syndrome is characterized by extreme self-neglect, domestic squalor, social withdrawal and apathy, but also by a tendency to hoard rubbish. Patients gradually develop a rejection of the community, resenting outside interference and abandoning accepted standards of behaviour. This may represent a reaction to stress in an elderly person, or a disorganized lifestyle becoming exaggerated by ageing and physical infirmity.[4]

Some authors have considered that the social deterioration in many cases is an expression of an attitude of withdrawal from the community by individuals with a tendency to isolation and self-sufficiency: that is, it is a positive reaction rather than a passive deterioration.[5]

In 1966, the first proper research was conducted on this syndrome and it was described as a 'senile breakdown in personal and environmental cleanliness'. This was identified in a study of 72 people living in squalor who had been referred to a specially established psychiatric unit over a three-year period. Almost all were over 60 years old but notably only 53 per cent had a formal mental disorder. The researchers concluded that personality, alcoholism and bereavement were implicated in this behaviour.[6]

Although first recognized in the nineteenth century, it wasn't until 1975 that the term 'Diogenes syndrome' was coined in a description of 30 geriatric patients admitted to hospital in a state of severe self-neglect and who were living in gross domestic filth.[7] The patients' lack of concern for their appearance and living conditions prompted the reference to Diogenes of Sinope (c. 410–c. 320 BC) a co-founder of the ascetic Athenian Cynic (meaning dog-like) sect, who became known for his disregard of domestic comforts, social niceties and material possessions.[8]

A freed slave, Diogenes was an advocate of self-sufficiency, freedom from social restraints and rejection of all luxury. He regarded happiness as lying within oneself and unrelated to personal wealth. Colourful stories of his life abound; he was reputed to live in a barrel and to spend much of his time vainly searching for 'an honest man'. He lived as he preached, sleeping rough in public places and begging for food.[9]

Some doctors have questioned whether 'Diogenes' is a suitable name for this syndrome, on the grounds that patients are 'far from happy or self-sufficient', but many of these people do appear to be at least content with their situation, if not actually happy, and they certainly often survive without external support. The rejection of normal standards of behaviour is common to Diogenes patients.[10]

Perhaps more typical examples in literature are Miss Havisham in Dickens's *Great Expectations* and Plushkin, a Russian aristocrat, in Gogol's novel *Dead Souls*.

Modern sufferers of Diogenes syndrome tend to have a filthy personal appearance unaccompanied by shame. A prominent role is played by syllogomania (hoarding rubbish). They usually live alone and their state is not the result of poverty or poor housing standards. Most are known to social services; often they refuse assistance and have multiple physical problems, including nutritional deficiencies.[11]

Investigators suggest that the syndrome might be a reaction of a certain kind of personality type to stress in later life. Psychiatrists maintain that it is different from the general neglect that they encounter among older people, in particular, those who are suffering from some form of dementia. Not only is the condition not restricted to older people, but those who do collect and hoard are extraordinarily resistant to the efforts of professionals who encourage them to stop doing it. And when the situation affects neighbours and environmental health officers are called in to clear houses or flats, the event is always tremendously traumatic for the sufferer.[12]

That this is more than simple untidiness is revealed by the extraordinarily high mortality rate (46 per cent), especially for females, and the cause of death is often linked to gross self-neglect. There is a good response among survivors, although psychiatric disorder is absent in half the cases. Perhaps this needs to be challenged as the possibility of serious personality dysfunction has been hinted at by most authors. They also have higher than average intelligence, successful professional and business lives, 'good' family backgrounds and upbringing and personalities characterized by aloofness, suspiciousness, emotional volatility, aggressiveness and reality distortion.[13]

Most reviews and original material describe the Diogenes phenomenon as a 'senile breakdown syndrome' but, as previously mentioned, the disorder is not confined to the elderly. Nor is it limited to the intelligent professional. Whilst many sufferers do live alone, others live with a spouse or other carer. 'Diogenes by proxy' has been identified, where neglectful spouses or relatives force someone to live in squalor. Sometimes both cohabitees are afflicted and various attempts have been made to explain this concordance on theoretical grounds, e.g. 'Diogenes à deux'.[14]

The question of intervention in cases of Diogenes syndrome has been hotly debated. One author strongly rejects intervention on the basis of the individual's right to self-determination, but many cannot agree that one must always respect the wishes of a person to neglect him/herself even unto death. (Scottish law provides for social intervention with recourse to mental health legislation.) Others stress the fire risk posed by hoarding.[15]

When a reclusive Polish war veteran was featured in the recent

BBC television fly-on-the-wall series *A Life of Grime*, it was shown that he had spent 35 years building a network of rat-infested tunnels of rubbish to dissuade people calling on him at home.

Some people who collect and hoard in this way are by no means neglectful of their personal hygiene and appearance. Among several examples cited by mental health professionals there is a successful architect, a high-flyer in the City and a musicologist.[16]

Some have suggested that among older people the condition may hark back to the privations and rationing experienced during the Second World War; insecurities in later life may also trigger serious hoarding as an attempt to regain a sense of security.[17]

Should professionals do anything about someone with Diogenes syndrome if the behaviour does not affect other people or put the sufferer's own health at risk? Even then, provided that people are aware of the risks they're taking, what rights do professionals have to intervene?[18]

The problematic nature of the notion of responsibility for choosing to lead a self-neglecting lifestyle is further illustrated in patients who have moderate-severe dementia and have been diagnosed as being self-neglecting. Dementia sufferers may have little control over their actions so it is difficult to see how self-neglect can be described as intentional in such instances. It is questionable whether these individuals have the intellectual capacity to make an intentional choice to self-neglect.

However, in a number of documented cases severe self-neglecters state that their so-called 'self-neglecting' lifestyle is one of choice. It is often assumed that such individuals have an underlying mental health problem or personality disorder which limits choice – a view which is held even when they claim that this is the way they wish to lead their lives. This is a rather tautological argument which does little to clarify the nature and extent of choice in self-neglect.[19]

In one particular case of self-neglect a woman did not seem to give her own care as high a priority as that of her family: she neglected herself so that she could care for them. The paradox is that her capacity to care for others, in what were very trying circumstances, appeared very high. Indeed many sufferers neglect themselves in favour of others.

However, an intriguing community survey of sufferers from Diogenes syndrome, published in the *Lancet* by psychiatrist Dr Graeme Halliday and colleagues from the Institute of Psychiatry, found that 23 individuals (28 per cent) regarded their home as 'clean' or 'very clean'; 14 individuals (17 per cent) did not believe that their home was any less clean than those of other people of their age, 49 (60 per cent) believed it to be equally clean or dirtier, and 18 (22 per cent) were unable to answer the question.[20]

Yet the psychiatrists discovered houses that were often cluttered with bags and boxes of possessions so that it was virtually impossible to move around, with rooms inaccessible or impossible to enter safely. They commonly found all floor space thickly covered with newspapers, cardboard, discarded packaging and other rubbish. Often the occupant had accumulated or hoarded a large number of singular items such as milk bottles (sometimes containing souring milk), newspapers, food containers, carrier bags or fabric. Several homes were dirty and unhygienic due to incontinence or blocked and overflowing toilets. Less striking but not uncommon were rooms and bedsits that were sparsely furnished except for a foul-smelling sofa or mattress, and floors and tables that were thickly covered in dirt, dust and rotting food.

Only 21 individuals (26 per cent) in this study were rated as having a physical health problem such as incontinence, immobility or severe visual impairment which had significantly contributed to the state of their living environment, confirming the psychological nature of the condition.

Hoarding has been observed in several disorders and states of distress, including anorexia nervosa, schizophrenia, biological mental disorders and self-neglect, but there is substantial evidence that it is most closely related to OCD. A cognitive-behavioural model conceptualizes compulsive hoarding as a multifaceted problem, stemming from erroneous beliefs about the nature of saving and possessions.[21]

Psychologists Dr Tamara L. Hartl of the University of Connecticut and Dr Randy O. Frost of Smith College, Northampton, Massachusetts, present this case study of a 53-year-old female suffering from compulsive hoarding.[22]

The woman who gave nothing away

The client, D., lived with her two children, aged 11 and 14, and described her current hoarding behaviour as a 'small problem that mushroomed' many years ago, along with corresponding marital difficulties. D. reported that her father was a hoarder and that she started saving when she was a child. In addition to hoarding, she reported several other obsessive-compulsive symptoms, such as a fear of hurting others due to carelessness, an over-concern with dirt and germs, a need for symmetry and a need to know or remember things. D. also suffered from a handwashing compulsion and engaged in lengthy cleaning rituals of household items.

The volume of cluttered possessions took up approximately 70 per cent of the living space in her house. With the exception of the bathroom, none of the rooms in the house could be easily used for their intended purpose. Both of the doors to the outside were blocked, so entry into the house was through the garage and the kitchen, where the table and chairs were covered with papers, newspapers, bills, books, half-consumed bags of chips and her children's school papers dating back ten years. A few chairs were uncluttered, allowing D. and her family to sit and eat with their plates on their laps. Piles of unopened mail sloped dangerously close to the burners on the stove. In the dining room, heaps of unfolded laundry covered the table. Towers of books, boxes, and brown paper bags stuffed with papers and bills covered the carpet. Very narrow pathways led to the adjacent rooms. What carpet was visible had not been vacuum-cleaned for some time. Everywhere was dingy and dusty. The parlour could not be used for any purpose other than storage. The centre of the floor contained boxes, magazines, books and papers. The two computers in the room were impossible to reach. Again the furniture was covered with clutter so that there was nowhere to sit.

The TV room was the most daunting. Letters, bills, receipts, newspapers and important documents were piled up to three feet high on the couch and streamed over onto the floor, completely burying a coffee table that therapists did not know was there until it was unearthed in a later session. Surrounding the couch were more piles of papers. At one end of the couch was a six-inch-square clutter-free area which D. kept clear in order to sit and sort through 'important papers'. Books were scattered on the floor, toppling out of shelves, and hundreds of videotapes were stacked haphazardly against the wall. Cobwebs stuck to the mantel and covered many of the books and videos piled around the television. In the front hallway were brown paper bags filled with bills and magazines. Books towered three feet high in the corner and the front door was barricaded with towers of paper bags. Upstairs, the hallway was filled with hundreds of gifts that D. had bought with no recipient in mind. Clothes and miscellaneous household items in some places were piled as high as the ceiling. The bedrooms were also cluttered and difficult to walk through.

Clutter severely restricted D.'s life and motivated her to seek treatment. She acknowledged that it was in large part responsible for the demise of her marriage. It also meant her children had no normal house to invite friends to, and exacerbated their dust allergies. Embarrassed by the clutter, D. seldom invited friends over, thereby impeding her social life. She was often unable to find bills she needed to pay, and was frequently harassed by creditors.

Previous treatments, which were largely unsuccessful, included a brief trial of antidepressants that was discontinued due to side-effects, attempts to clean the house and hiring a helper to move clutter from the living space into the attic.

The treatment programme consisted of training in decision-making and categorization, exposure and habituation to discarding, and cognitive restructuring.

D. was entirely responsible for deciding on the placement and status (save/discard) of her possessions. The therapists did not make any decisions for her, nor did they touch any of her possessions unless given explicit permission to do so. Their role was to assist in the development of decision-making skills, to provide feedback regarding normal saving behaviours, and to identify and challenge D.'s erroneous beliefs about possessions.

Treatment strategies were applied first to the kitchen and only progressed to another room once the entire contents of preceding rooms had been sorted and decided upon. D. had to target a specific area in the room, and then decide what type of possession to sort first. Once an area was cleared, boxes of possessions to be saved were moved to a more appropriate destination (e.g. cupboard, garage) or into storage. While it was important to designate a large number of items to the 'discard' category, the crucial aspect in the decision-making was to establish proper categories and proper placement of the possessions (i.e. out of the living area). Early in the treatment the emphasis was mainly on organization. This shifted as D. became more comfortable with discarding.

D. was instructed to designate category types and a comprehensive filing system was developed to provide D. with categorization practice and to make papers more accessible.

The exposure and habituation component forced D. to be exposed to several activities she had avoided, including decision-making, emotional distress at discarding items to which she was

255

attached and putting objects out of sight. For example, D.'s argument that a blank piece of cardboard should be saved for future use was countered by the therapists' question of whether having such a piece of cardboard was more valuable than having an uncluttered house where she could host long-anticipated dinner parties. In essence, D. was encouraged to maintain a more realistic perception of a house filled with unused possessions, versus one that is uncluttered and amenable to daily functioning.

Hoarding symptoms can be successfully treated with a multifaceted cognitive behavioural intervention such as highlighted here. Decreases in clutter in the five rooms targeted for intervention in D.'s home lend initial support for the efficacy of a treatment programme which targeted decision-making skills, exposure and response prevention (ERP) and cognitive restructuring. Furthermore, self-report measures of indecisiveness, hoarding and OCD symptoms all declined after nine months of treatment.[23]

Hoarders are very emotionally attached to their possessions and often describe discarding as equivalent to a part of oneself dying or abandoning a loved one. When D. discarded a 'treasure' book to which she expressed a great deal of attachment, she exclaimed, 'If I could drop dead right now, I would.' D. also reported that she often turned to her possessions for comfort and safety, particularly on days when she felt distressed. Her 'hoarding mood' would sometimes appear in anticipation of the therapists' visit, since she felt anxious about the prospect of throwing away possessions.

In addition to compulsive hoarding, D. suffered from obsessions and compulsions related to cleanliness, which interfered with the programme in several ways. She created duplicate categories, one for 'clean' possessions and one for 'dirty' possessions. Her filing system contained twice as many folders as necessary in order to ensure that 'clean' cuttings and pamphlets did not come into contact with 'contaminated' ones. She was reluctant to sort through 'contaminated' possessions while she was 'clean', and vice versa.

Treatment spanned the course of 17 months. Clearly, the amount of clutter and the complicating features associated with her hoarding require very lengthy treatment. Because of its time-intensive nature, the programme presented here may not be cost-effective. However, attempts to develop and refine this treatment in a more cost-effective format are under way.[24]

In essence, Diogenes syndrome raises the question of whether we must respect the person's right to reject social norms while as a

256

society provide support to help minimize risks both to the person and to neighbours.

However, it is vital to draw a distinction between Diogenes syndrome and severe self-neglect that occurs as a direct result of treatable psychiatric illness. Elke Richartz and Henning Wormstall of the University of Tübingen in Germany recently reported the case of a patient who suffered from irreversible physical handicap as a result of self-neglect.[25]

The woman who wouldn't move

A 67-year-old woman, Mrs A., was referred to the psychiatric clinic from the surgical department of a city hospital, where, for some 12 weeks, she had been under inpatient treatment for extensive gangrenous open bedsores on her buttocks, lower legs and feet. The patient had been in a desolate state at the time of admission. She was weak, her teeth were blackened and full of gaps, and the gums were also black. The open sores were not only infected, but, in some cases, even infested with maggots.

A psychiatrist diagnosed chronic psychosis and prescribed antipsychotic medication. On admission to the psychiatric clinic, Mrs A. appeared animated, despite her obvious suffering, and was friendly and communicative. Her comprehension and concentration were unimpaired, and her memory was undisturbed. Her style of speaking and choice of words indicated intelligence and good education. There were no indications of distorted perception and her basic mood at first seemed well balanced, although she wept frequently. In response to questioning, she admitted to often being unhappy. In the first interview, the patient's concern about her physical complaints predominated. Expressing her fear that she might never again be able to walk unassisted, she complained about severe pains in her legs which, despite powerful painkillers, continued to disturb her sleep at night. Only after several days did she begin to reveal more of her internal life. Gradually, she admitted to a conviction that she was being persecuted as a witch, saying that hers was the only case in which the medieval persecution of witches had persisted into the present.

In contrast to the past, she argued, such persecution is now against the law; thus, the Church, which was certainly involved, pursued its action in secret. She was further convinced that her husband had unwittingly become implicated in her persecution, for example through a kind of espionage. As a young girl, she claimed, she had already had inklings of such persecution. When she visited restaurants or pubs in the evening, she noticed that people seated at nearby tables would whisper about her. She heard children in the neighbourhood calling her a witch and in recent years she said the persecution had intensified. Equipped with special transmitting and receiving equipment, her persecutors were now able to observe her when she was undressed, using what she called 'picture telegraphy'. They could now even touch her. To protect herself, she had ceased to undress. Now she felt secure, even at home, only when sitting in a corner bench or in her chair, which had to stand at a particular place at the table. Her husband regularly served her meals and assisted her in even the most rudimentary activities. Until now, she had feared being observed and molested in a state of undress. Only when the pain in her infected legs had become unbearable did she finally agree to seek medical help.

From her history, it was learned that Mrs A. grew up in Poland as an only child. She recalled her mother as a domineering, emotionally cold woman with strict moral standards. By contrast, she enjoyed a close emotional relationship with her father. He was very sensitive and reserved, well-educated and widely read. She believed that her character strongly resembled his. In her childhood, she was afflicted by a severe case of chronic eczema that was so serious that doctors repeatedly demonstrated her case before medical students. They even wanted to photograph it for use in medical textbooks. Mercifully, her father prevented this.

Following the migration of the family from Poland, the patient completed her secondary school education in West Germany and trained as a children's nurse. Finding working with sick children to be emotionally too draining, she became a telecommunications technician. At the age of 18, the patient became pregnant by her first boyfriend, a classmate at school. On the insistence of the boy's parents, an abortion was performed and the relationship was broken off. At the age of 20 she married her present husband, after once again becoming pregnant. In the course of this pregnancy, she gave up her profession. This son was the couple's only child. He lived with his parents until beginning studies away from home.

Interviews with relatives revealed that, shortly after her marriage, Mrs A. had begun to show mental peculiarities. Although she cared for her child normally, contrary to her previous practice, she refused to leave the house willingly. Very early in her marriage, she withdrew emotionally from her husband. After their son left home, she began to feel persecuted and refused all visitors. For years, she refused medical assistance and her husband was forced to care for her alone, until her suffering became unbearable.

Although she did not give up the idea that she was being persecuted as a witch, after some weeks of treatment she did begin to show a clear reduction in emotional tension. She no longer felt herself to be under the influence of her persecutors: in fact it was they who should feel ashamed. Now her intense pain became the central topic. The sores healed well, and she continued to receive strong painkillers, but her pain continued to dominate the course of further conversations. Slowly she began to show signs of improvement. In the end, she accepted the offer of orthopaedic rehabilitation, continued to take medication and accepted psychiatric treatment.

One year after her release from hospital Mrs A. agreed to move into a nursing home. At the time of writing, she is still on antipsychotic medication and although still convinced of the former persecution, she is able to take part in the daily life of her ward. The delusional experience has receded into the background.

This case reveals the severe consequences that can result from a chronic delusional development. In this patient a systematic delusional structure appeared to go back for decades. While she denied hearing voices and said she had no other psychotic symptoms besides the delusional thinking, the possibility of tactile hallucinations in connection with her delusion of being persecuted, observed and molested could not be excluded with certainty.

The determinant factor in the delusional content appears to be the patient's painful childhood experience of being repeatedly medically examined and of being used as an object of demonstration. Her fear of being photographed as a child is likewise reflected in the later delusion.

The moral rigour of the parents and their high ethical demands, when taken in conjunction with the patient's juvenile pregnancy and subsequent abortion, strongly suggest a guilt problem, which again finds expression in the delusion of persecution. The possibility of Mrs A.'s anxiety about being seen and touched when naked also leads to the consideration of repressed, dissociated sexual needs.

There is a clear temporal connection between the migration from Poland, with its accompanying feelings of insecurity, and the beginning of delusional experience, which the patient described as a 'premonition' coupled with a feeling of something 'uncanny'.

Time and again in the pursuit of detailed analysis and understanding, one encounters the basic 'unintelligibility theorem' enunciated by the psychiatrist Jaspers – which is that what demarcates delusions from other beliefs is the fundamental incomprehensibility of delusions to all others.[26] With most other strange beliefs there will be some 'takers' – people who do not subscribe to your ideas but can see why you might believe them. Here the question remains open: why did Mrs A. fall victim to a delusion rather than to a compulsive neurosis or to depression? In this broad realm, hypotheses about the existence of biological or biochemical factors come to mind, for example the theory of underlying biochemical over-activity.[27]

The patient certainly experienced evident improvement thanks to medication. Although she failed to lose her conviction that she was the subject of a witch hunt, the urgency of this threat and her emotional involvement in the delusion decreased notably.

Remarkably, she continued to suffer from severe pain: despite objective physical improvement, this not only grew more intense, but also dominated her communication for a considerable length of time. This could be interpreted as a defence against problem-laden themes. Another interpretation is that the physical pain is an expression of mental pain. Conceivably, as her outwardly projected suffering, which took the form of the delusion, remitted, Mrs A. became more and more conscious of her real inner suffering. In this connection, the therapist is reminded that the goal of treatment cannot be the mere reduction of symptoms. Bereft of her delusion the patient is all the more in need of a therapeutic human relationship capable of generating trust and opening new possibilities for a healthy orientation in life.[28]

What is odd about Diogenes syndrome is its link with old age and obsessionality, as this is not the age pattern typically found with OCD. Surveys indicate the mean age at onset of idiopathic OCD is between 20 and 25 years, with only 15 per cent of cases present after the age of 35. Onset of OCD after age 50 is relatively unusual. Cases of late-onset OCD may be related to structural cerebral damage and may therefore provide further insight into the neurobiology of this disorder.[29]

Theories regarding the cause of OCD have changed remarkably over the years. The earliest writings focused on repetitive, blasphemous thoughts, which were believed to be the result of demonic possession. Although Jean Etienne Dominique Esquirol, in an 1838 report describing the case of 'Mademoiselle F', was the first psychiatrist to describe the phenomenon, Pierre Janet is often credited with providing the first rational psychological explanation.[30] In his 1903 book *Les Obsessions et la Psychoasténie* he saw psychic fatigue as being responsible for a lack of control over one's thoughts. Within a decade, Freud's case of obsessional neurosis, the 'Rat Man', led to the belief that OCD resulted from unconscious conflicts. Alongside this psychodynamic conceptualization, behaviourists began to apply learning theory to the symptoms of OCD, viewing the obsessions and compulsions as learned responses that lower anxiety.[31]

Psychologists Dr Thomas E. Joiner, Jr, and Natalie Sachs-Ericsson of the Department of Psychology, Florida State University, Tallahassee, report the following excerpt from a therapy session with a patient with obsessive-compulsive disorder to illustrate their theory that there is a fundamental link between anxiety, territoriality and obsessive-compulsive symptoms:[32]

> Therapist: 'How have things been going with obsessions and rituals?'
> Patient [excitedly]: 'Very good. I'm much better – I don't shower and wash all the time; I'm not always cleaning and wiping things down; I can leave my house without checking everything. The only thing I'm still having trouble with is my bedroom. I still check the door about 20 times before I leave.'
> Therapist: 'Why has that been difficult to shake?'
> Patient: 'I think because it's my own special territory. Everything in there is mine and just the way I like it. I feel safe there, and I check the lock to make sure no one violates my own special territory.'

Pathological behaviour may represent exaggerations of behaviour that were adaptive during the course of human evolution. For example, it is possible that the grandiose delusions of manic-depressive disorder represent a maladaptive exaggeration of behaviour and cognition related to leadership and dominance. Depression-related states and behaviours represent evolved forms of a strategy that arose as a way of coping with losses in social competition. Perhaps humans are 'prepared' by natural selection to develop phobias in relation to some but not other stimuli. Panic disorder could be viewed as a maladaptive triggering of an evolved suffocation alarm system.[33]

A similar argument has been made regarding OCD. Perhaps it is an exaggeration of fixed behavioural action patterns related to grooming. But such views do not adequately explain the other symptoms, which encompass a range of phenomena, including hoarding, checking and aggressive ideas.[34]

Human territoriality has been defined as the lasting tendency to express the need for personal and physical space, as well as for security of self and possessions, by reacting aggressively to potential or actual violations of these. Territoriality, in the form of repeatedly checking boundaries, is similar to the lock and door checking commonly seen in OCD patients. Indeed, numerous findings suggest such a link. Functions of territoriality include security and defence (e.g. lock checking) but also reduction in the spread of disease (excessive grooming and washing). Exaggerated territoriality, then, is similar to OCD patients' concerns and behaviours related to defence and contamination.[35]

Human territoriality can also be seen as an ordering of the environment. Here, too, a similarity between territoriality and OC symptoms (counting, partitioning, stacking, etc.) exists.

Third, territory restrictions are clearly associated with a range of OCD-like stereotypes in fish, reptiles, birds and mammals. These stereotypes often include pacing, as well as 'route tracing', following a precise and invariable path within an area (e.g. boundary checking).[36]

To the degree that it is related to territoriality, hoarding also points to a possible link between OCD and territoriality. Approximately 30 per cent of OCD patients report hoarding obsessions and compulsions. Interestingly, drugs that benefit OCD patients have been shown to reduce hoarding in rats, and drugs that activate OC-related brain areas increase hoarding in rats.[37]

A territoriality view may account for many features of OCD that are not well explained by other approaches. For example, the 'grooming' model is not well suited to explain checking and hoarding compulsions. Moreover, the OCD feature best explained by the 'grooming' model – contamination obsessions and washing compulsions – can be incorporated into a territoriality model. That is, extreme territoriality can be viewed as a means to restrict exposure to strangers and to the pathogens they carry.[38]

A territoriality model is better able than one based on grooming to explain the association of OCD and aggression. Although there is controversy as to whether aggression is a fundamental aspect of territoriality, it is clearly involved in establishment and defence of territory among several species of animal. Similarly, OCD patients sometimes experience obsessions regarding an aggressive act they fear they may have committed (virtually always, they have not actually committed the act: e.g. infanticide or running someone over with a car). In one study approximately 27 per cent of OCD patients reported aggressive obsessions. These patients may also be prone to aggressive outbursts, and an association between adult OCD and childhood aggression problems has been found. If OCD phenomena are meaningfully linked to territoriality, as is argued here, an association between OCD and aggression would be expected (and appears to exist).[39]

Dr Thomas E. Joiner, Jr, and Natalie Sachs-Ericsson have tested their theory about the link between territoriality and obsessive-compulsive disorder in several ways but most intriguingly by posing the question: do OCD patients choose to sit farther from therapists?

If OCD is associated with territoriality, this relation may be manifested in the distance OCD patients keep with regard to others, argue Dr Joiner and Sachs-Ericsson. This possibility was assessed in a study where therapists agreed to provide ratings on the distance individual (not group) psychotherapy patients chose to sit from them. Results indicated that patients with OCD chose to sit the farthest from their therapists. Even when compared to non-OCD anxiety-disordered patients (many of whom experienced social phobia), who might be characterized by social avoidance (physical distance), distance ratings for OCD patients were significantly higher.

Does age of onset of OCD in humans mirror the developmental emergence of territoriality in animals? Among men, the average age of onset for OCD is in adolescence, whereas for women it is in early adulthood. Perhaps a similar gap exists regarding animal territoriality, with male animals benefiting from relatively early emergence of territoriality, so that territories can be established and mates attracted. As far as female animals are concerned, pehaps they benefit from a slightly later emergence of territoriality, when offspring are born and are most vulnerable. There does appear to be an association between pregnancy/childbirth and OCD among women.[40]

Is there cultural variation in territoriality, and is it reflected in cultural variation in OCD rates? In a study of territoriality and culture, psychologists Worchel and Lollis placed a bag of litter either in a residence's front yard, on the front pavement, or on the front kerb, in Greece and in the US. These researchers predicted that, because territories are more strictly delimited in Greece than in the US (in Greece, the pavement and kerb are not considered as part of the residence, whereas in the US they are), the litter on the pavement and kerb would be more quickly removed by residents in the US. Regarding litter in the yard, they predicted no difference between Greek and US residences. Results confirmed the prediction. It is interesting to speculate that, in settings where territories are strictly delimited (e.g. urban areas) and territoriality may be higher, OCD prevalence may also be higher.[41]

In other words, obsessive-compulsive disorder could be the product of an age where order is both desired and possible.

10

Obsession

The best things carried to excess are wrong.
Charles Churchill, 1731–64

Obsessions are defined as recurrent and persistent thoughts, impulses or images which may cause anxiety. Common obsessive thoughts include the fear of harm/injury to oneself or to loved ones and fear of contamination by dirt or germs. Compulsions are repetitive and seemingly purposeful types of behaviour that are usually, but not always, performed in response to an obsession, in a stereotyped fashion or in accordance with certain rules. Typical compulsions include excessive cleaning (e.g. repeated handwashing, showering), checking rituals, reordering or arranging habits, repeating rituals, and counting. The obsessive compulsive disorder (OCD) patient often feels driven to perform such behaviour to neutralize distress associated with the obsessions or prevent a certain stressful situation.[1]

The prevalence of OCD in the general population has been estimated at around 1 to 2 per cent, although this may be an underestimation due to a general reluctance to admit to obsessions and compulsions.[2]

The diagnosis of obsessive-compulsive disorder traditionally assumes that the patient at some point recognizes the obsessions or compulsions as excessive or unreasonable. However, patients with OCD exhibit varying degrees of insight into the validity of their beliefs. Psychiatric manuals make some acknowledgement of this, using the term 'poor insight' for individuals who, 'for most of the time' during the current episode, do not recognize that their obsessions or compulsions are excessive or unreasonable.[3]

Psychiatrists Dr Anne-Marie O'Dwyer and Professor Isaac Marks from the Institute of Psychiatry and Maudsley Hospital, London, recently presented these relevant case vignettes and suggest that such cases are best regarded as severe 'atypical' OCD with delusions.[4]

The man who feared the black dot

Z. suddenly developed rituals at the age of 17. While watching television he looked up and saw a man's face at the glass kitchen door and heard a voice say: 'Do the habits and things will go right'. He came to believe in a 'power' that would bring him luck if he could keep it in his possession through ritualizing. He bought an electric guitar which he felt contained the 'power', and would turn the controls ritualistically. Often he saw a 'black dot' the size of a fist leave his body and enter some object near him. When experiencing the loss of the 'black dot' he felt compelled to ritualize to regain the 'power' that he believed it contained. When he was 19 he began to believe that a workman possessed a second 'power' for evil and began a second set of rituals to ward off this evil power while striving to retain the good one. He believed absolutely in the 'power' and feared disastrous consequences for himself and his family should he fail to retain the good and repel the evil power.

Before his admission to hospital, obsessions and compulsions affected every area of his life. Before performing any action he felt compelled to imagine the letter 'L' and repeat the phrase 'X away, power back' for up to 20 minutes. He felt unable to sit on chairs or walk on grass or leaves, and slept with his feet uncovered for fear of the 'power' being transferred to some object (i.e. the bedclothes) from which he might be unable to retrieve it. On leaving home he constantly retraced his steps to place his foot on a crack in the pavement or a leaf that he felt he had trodden on earlier and so lost some of the 'power'. If he saw the black dot leave his body (which he felt occurred about 20 times a day) he had to touch the object it had entered and superimpose the letter 'L' and the phrase 'X away, power back' in his mind until he saw the black dot return.

From the age of 18, Z. also had recurrent depression, feelings of hopelessness and suicidal urges, with deliberate self-harm (overdoses and wrist-slashing) when he was in a depressed mood. He said he harmed himself to appease the power or as a wish to die 'when everything was perfect' after a day of ritualizing.

The man who had the power

Y. developed beliefs about a 'power' at the age of 13. He felt that everyone had a certain 'quality' or 'goodness' which was stored in the brain as a power. He believed that other people drained the power from him and replaced it with their own rubbish (faeces and urine). The exchange of power was triggered by an image in his mind of a face or object. When it happened he felt distressed, 'dirty' and 'horrible'. He could only regain the power by doing complex rituals. He imagined the person's face and that he had detached their head from their body and sucked the power from the major vessels of their neck or from their eyes. He then transferred the power back into himself by banging his palm on a particular spot on his forehead and breathing out repeatedly. This made him feel relieved and 'good', but as the events recurred up to several times a minute the relief was short-lived. He felt compelled at times to get revenge on people who stole his power by drawing with his finger on a wall a deformed and ugly representation. If he touched anything he left a 'power trace' behind and so had to touch it repeatedly to get the power back. Y.'s belief in the experience was absolute. He knew it might seem strange to others but believed that if they experienced it, they would understand.

From the age of 17 he also had recurrent depression, felt hopeless and had suicidal urges that required hospital admission.

The woman who had to count from 0 to 8

At the age of eight, X. had transient counting rituals associated with her fear that harm could come to others. When she was 15, after a relative died, she feared that harm would befall her family and friends unless she completed specific tasks. She thought a supernatural 'power' inserted unpleasant thoughts into her mind, e.g., 'If you read that book a relative will die.' She believed unshakeably that the power was supernatural, but could not explain it. To appease the 'power' and the thoughts, complex counting rituals pervaded her daily activities. She also did ritualistic handwashing and checking. She avoided specific numbers, colours and clothes and counted from 0 to 8 on her fingers and toes throughout the day. She repeated rhymes, avoided multiple numbers she associated with death or harm, and brushed her hair hundreds of times a day. She felt unable to resist the rituals and before she was admitted to hospital the rituals took up all of her time until she fell asleep.

X. had two episodes of moderate depression at the ages of 25 and 34, both associated with worsening of her OCD. She had never harmed herself.

The man who feared being transported to another world

For 20 years W. had a fear of being transported into another world. When he was 17 he worried that reflections in mirrors represented another world, and had complex checking rituals involving mirrors. Gradually this spread to all reflective surfaces. He believed that turning on electrical switches, using the television remote control or hearing car engines could cause him to be 'transported' and constantly checked to make sure this had not happened. He believed that if he ate while in another world he would be forced to stay there, and so either avoided eating, or ate with complex rituals, or induced vomiting. Other rituals involved wearing particular clothes. The 'other' world was tangibly the same as the real one, but felt different – friends and family, although appearing the same, were different and might have been replaced by doubles. The symptoms gradually worsened, occupying all of his time prior to admission to hospital.

When he was 27 he suffered severe depression requiring inpatient care; this happened again at the age of 30. He had no history of self-harm.

All of these subjects had fixed beliefs of 'bizarre' content. Resistance to the compulsive urge and insight were lost. Early writers noted similarities between psychosis and OCD, so how should such cases be classified? For example, patients may logically repudiate their belief while in the safety of the therapist's office, but when in a 'dangerous' situation may be 100 per cent convinced of it.[5]

A key feature in these cases that suggests obsessive-compulsive disorder rather than psychosis is the clear logical link between the thoughts and the rituals. The rituals are all cued by intrusive thoughts concerning a central belief, the patient feels compelled to carry them out to relieve associated distress, and they are all carried out 'ritualistically'. The patients are severely disabled by the illness but are otherwise intact. In particular, none of the subjects had other forms of thought disorder. Case 1 had transient perceptual abnormalities.

Most of the patients took several medications. None had improved significantly with antipsychotic drugs, although several had improved somewhat on antidepressant medication.[6]

The diagnostic issues posed by these patients are not unique to OCD. Anorexia nervosa subjects may believe with 'absolute certainty' that they are fat, despite evidence to the contrary. These beliefs, despite their fixity, are generally called 'overvalued ideas', the distinction from delusions perhaps being that the content of the belief is not 'alien' beyond normal understanding, although some would argue that the disturbance is of 'delusional proportions'. Patients with body dysmorphic disorder also have a range of beliefs from 'obsessional' at one end of the spectrum to 'delusional' at the other.[7] Such cases highlight the artificial nature of current diagnostic boundaries, and the limitations of the dichotomy between neurosis and psychosis in understanding and treating these disorders.[8]

How one labels the psychopathology in these OCD subjects is of more than mere academic interest. A diagnosis of schizophrenia or delusional disorder may lead to a lifetime of antipsychotic medication and a reluctance to consider other, more effective, interventions.[9]

Perhaps, developments in brain-scanning technology will soon allow us to distinguish more reliably between psychosis and neurosis.

Dr H. Tei and colleagues of the Neurological Institute, Tokyo Women's Medical College, describe the case of a computer operator who experienced paroxysmal attacks several times in which she felt a compulsion to handle keys with her right hand, or her right hand actually moved involuntarily in a key-handling rhythm. Brain scanning revealed a tumour: after its removal there were no more paroxysmal attacks. They suggest that voluntary movements controlled by the brain's supplementary motor area were deranged by seizures provoked by the tumour. This case is important in relation to obsessive-compulsive disorder as it suggests a direct location in the brain with which the phenomenon of obsessions could be associated.[10]

The woman with a compulsion to handle keys

The patient was a 35-year-old woman who had been working as a computer operator for several years. She was right-handed and one evening, after overworking for several days (operating a computer for more than 10 hours a day), she was writing a report with a pen at her desk. After she put the pen down on the desk, she felt a powerful compulsion to operate a computer with her right hand. Immediately, she held her right hand with her left hand. This compulsion disappeared within two minutes.

Similar events occurred three times within six months. One afternoon about a year later, she met a friend. They began chatting and when the conversation stopped for a minute, she felt a powerful compulsion to operate a computer with her right hand for a moment, then actually started moving involuntarily in a key-handling rhythm for a few seconds. She held her right hand down immediately and she intended to explain this phenomenon to her friend, but could not speak at all. This involuntary movement and speech arrest resolved within a few minutes without any disturbance of consciousness. In the following week, she experienced another similar attack. This time, instead of speech arrest, continuous vocalization of 'zu, zu, zu, zu, . . .' occurred for a minute.

She visited a hospital and a general physical and neurological examination revealed no abnormal findings. However, cranial CT and MRI brain scanning showed a mass lesion in the left medial frontal lobe. Total removal of the tumour was performed and although she felt slight weakness in the right leg for several days after the operation, the woman was discharged with no residual symptoms. There have been no paroxysmal attacks for two years.

The paroxysmal compulsion to handle keys was probably caused by epilepsy provoked by the mass lesion. The clinical manifestations (the compulsion to handle keys), motor abnormality (key-handling rhythm) and speech arrest correspond with the characteristics of seizures caused by tumours in this part of the brain.[11]

Recent studies have suggested that the supplementary motor area plays a major role in the initiation and control of voluntary movements, especially in complex ones. When electrical stimulation on the supplementary motor area of 13 patients with intractable epilepsy was performed, three types of subjective-sensory response occurred, the third type being a subjective 'urge' to perform a movement or the anticipation that a movement was going to occur.[12]

At some sites where such responses were elicited, stimulation at higher current evoked an overt motor response. These results correspond to those of this patient well, in that at first, she merely felt a compulsion to operate a computer with her right hand, but later, her right hand actually moved in a key-handling rhythm. This suggests that enlargement of the tumour changed the character of the seizure.[13]

The symptoms of the compulsive urge to operate a computer with inner resistance also indicate an association with obsessive-compulsive disorder.[14]

Related to OCD is Tourette's syndrome (TS), a disorder characterized by simple and/or complex motor and vocal tics. Tics are usually defined as repetitive, stereotyped movements or vocalizations that are involuntary, although more recent clinical observation suggests that some of the repetitive behaviours in TS are voluntary in nature. At onset, which is predominantly before 10 years of age, the TS patient typically exhibits one or two simple motor tics, such as eye blinking or neck movements. These symptoms progress over time and usually become more severe and complex. More complex tics include touching objects, squatting, twirling while walking, retracing steps, and hopping. Vocalizations include inarticulate sounds, such as barking, coughing and grunting, as well as the more complex palilalia (repetition of one's own words/phrases), echolalia (the repetition of another's words or phrases) and coprolalia (uttering of obscenities).[15]

A diagnosis of TS occurs in approximately 1 in 1,500 children and studies suggest it is a genetic disorder affecting three times as many males as females.[16] The latter are more likely to exhibit obsessive-compulsive behaviours, with or without tics. Behaviour such as hyperactivity, impulsivity and distractibility are also commonly associated with TS, which has led to speculation regarding possible genetic links between TS and attention deficit hyperactivity disorder (ADHD).

Tourette's syndrome was initially described by Itard[17] in 1825 but became known as Tourette's syndrome after Gilles de la Tourette (1857–1904), a Frenchman who published a review of the disorder after reading about Itard's original patient and following the study of eight of his own patients.[18]

TS follows a similar progression to OCD in that patients usually suffer initially from simple motor tics/obsessions and compulsions but as the disorder progresses these become more complex and severe.[19]

Increasing tension is experienced if the behaviour is inhibited, followed by relief as the act is carried out. The close similarity between OCD and TS symptoms was emphasized in a recent study, which found that in addition to unintentional repetitive behaviour, intentional repetitive behaviour also occurred. The symptoms of both TS and OCD are exacerbated by stressful situations, fatigue and emotional states. Another area of similarity is the appearance of scatologic and obscene material. In OCD, contamination, excretory functions, sexual material and aggressive behaviour are common obsessions, and in TS many of the tics are aggressive or obscene.[20]

Georges Gilles de la Tourette was a young colleague of the great French physician Jean-Martin Charcot. The history of the designation of the syndrome was marked by controversy (which has persisted to the present day), partly because of the unusual nature of the symptoms. These include cursing and obscene gestures that often seem alien to the basic personality structure of the patient and are particularly noticeable in persons of refined manners who suddenly blurt out the most obscene language imaginable.[21]

It is easy to see why one of the early controversies about the origin of this syndrome broke out between the psychoanalysts and the more organically oriented physicians – the first group believing that these behaviours represented the release of repressed sexual and aggressive material from the unconscious, and the second that the gestures were more in the nature of tics. The latter idea gained ground when it was discovered that rheumatic fever was associated with tics, even though these did not have the complex nature of the tics of Gilles de la Tourette syndrome.[22]

George Eliot in *Silas Marner*, published in 1861, precisely describes the clinical features of Tourette's syndrome. A minor character, Mrs Crackenthorp, is described as follows:

Mrs Crackenthorp – a small blinking woman, who fidgeted incessantly with her lace, ribbons, and gold chain, turning her head about and making subdued noises, very much like a guinea-pig that twitches its nose and soliloquizes in all company indiscriminately – now blinked and fidgeted towards the Squire, and said, 'O no – no offence.' . . .

'Did you ever hear the like?' said Mrs Kimble . . . aside to Mrs Crackenthorp, who blinked and nodded, and amiably intended to smile, but the intention lost itself in small twitchings and noises.

Perhaps the first real breakthrough was the trial of haloperidol, an antipsychotic medication, given to patients with TS. It was quickly recognized that relief of tics involved blockade of brain dopamine receptors.[23]

Tic disorders form a continuum from simple transient tics to chronic Tourette's syndrome. Rarely occurring before the age of two, tics have an average onset age of seven years and often begin with repetitive, simple movements of the face (grimaces, mouth movements, twitches) or eyes (blinking, eye widening), or as recurrent utterances (throat clearing, grunting, sniffing, snorting and barking). Often quite subtle, early tic manifestations are frequently dismissed by teachers or parents, who may attribute them to stress or allergies. The sudden, rapid, recurrent and non-rhythmic nature of tics, however, is distinctive, as is the tendency to progress to more complicated and elaborate movements or vocalizations. Simple motor tics can proceed to quite complex acts involving head, neck and torso which appear as gestures, grooming actions, jumping, touching, stamping and smelling. There is an involuntary character to these events and, at least at first, children themselves may be unaware of these acts. The anatomical location, frequency and obviousness of tics can change dramatically over time. Although most individuals with TS/tics have mild, subtle and transient symptoms that may go unnoticed, some experience severe and chronic symptoms that cause personal distress or social rejection, which then prompts professional evaluation.

Tics themselves are often the starting place for intervention. Allowing the student with severe tics to leave the room when the urge becomes unmanageable is suggested for social and humanitarian reasons. Tics are extremely difficult-to-suppress urges and while temporary suppression is possible, long-term inhibition of the urge generally is not. Experience shows that it is almost always vocal tics (humming, grunts, snorts or swearing) that prompts concern.[24]

The histories of patients with TS who presented with utterances of swear words were studied by psychiatrists Dr Jordi Serra-Mestres and colleagues who have tentatively named this behaviour 'palicophrolalia'. The following cases illustrate this condition.[25]

The girl who couldn't stop herself repeatedly swearing

A.B. was a 14-year-old schoolgirl who suffered from TS and also from attention-deficit/hyperactivity disorder and oppositional defiant disorder (ODD). When she was first seen, more than 50 motor tics and up to eight vocalizations were documented. She also had a range of obsessive-compulsive behaviours (OCBs) such as clicking her fingers, forced touching, compulsive counting and other actions. She did not have classic palilalia, but she had palipraxia (repetition of her own acts).

She showed no evidence of coprolalia, but uttered swear words in contextually appropriate situations – followed by the compulsion to repeat the swear word (usually four or five times) in a palilalic fashion. She said that she could not stop repeating herself.

As we have seen, OCD is characterized by intrusive thoughts and irrational urges to carry out ritualized actions, and all current psychiatric diagnostic and classicatory systems concur in seeing OCD as a form of anxiety disorder.[26] Comparisons are frequently drawn between the symptoms of OCD and certain religious practices and it has been suggested that both may stem from the human propensity to produce socially meaningful rituals.[27] However, the following cases demand a wider interpretation than the mere maintenance of social cohesiveness.[28]

Psychiatrist Dr F. J. Jarrett from the Department of Psychiatry, Queen's University, Kingston, Ontario, recently reported the case of a man with an unusual phobia. The term 'locophobia' has been used because the fear is associated with a specific geographical place. This distinguishes it from agoraphobia, in which the fear is usually associated with any of a number of places that fulfil certain criteria – open, crowded, silent, dark, etc.[29]

The man who suffered from locophobia

Mr K. is a 50-year-old married man. He referred himself to the psychiatric department of a general hospital complaining of a lack of energy, poor sleep and a loss of interest in life. These were recent symptoms, but on more careful enquiry, the following story emerged.

He was unable to visit a small town, St Thomas, Ontario, about 200 miles away from where he presently lives, because of the incapacitating anxiety that this would induce. Furthermore, he could not talk to people from the town without experiencing anxiety, and he felt tense when he saw the name in a newspaper.

He had some relatives in St Thomas with whom he occasionally corresponded. When he received letters from them, he adopted a fixed routine. He washed the letters in soap and water, following which he washed his hands thoroughly, then changed his clothes and made sure that those which he discarded were cleaned.

Since moving to the house in which he and his wife currently live, all the mail has been washed. Shortly after moving there, he discovered that a neighbour had at one time lived in St Thomas, and Mr K. suspected that this neighbour must still have contacts there. He presumed that if so, then the neighbour would occasionally receive mail from St Thomas. Because their mail is delivered by the same person, he was afraid that his own mail might be 'contaminated' and so, 'to play safe', he washed it.

On one occasion, he and his wife were visited unexpectedly by some relatives from St Thomas. He refused to let them enter the house, saying that if they had come in he would have to fumigate the house.

Mr K. was born in Brantford, a medium-sized town in Ontario. His parents separated when he was seven and he went to live in Guelph, Ontario, with his father, who worked as a tenant farmer. When the boy was 13, the owner of the house in which they lived began to exhibit aggressive and bizarre behaviour. Within a few days of the onset of this episode, this man killed himself in a most gruesome manner. The lad was so upset that he and his father had to leave the district.

They moved to St Catherine's, Ontario, where his father obtained another job, but this patient began to notice that he experienced distress whenever he had to handle mail from Guelph. This persisted for some years.

In his early twenties he married, and he and his wife opened a store in St Catherine's. One day there was a brutal murder in the town, and Mr K. visited the scene of the crime. A few days later, he began to feel uneasy when touching objects connected with the scene of the murder, or meeting people who had also been to the scene. This uneasiness became so incapacitating that he and his wife sold the business and moved back to Guelph.

When Mr K. was 30, he was running a summer resort franchise in Tillsonburg and was involved in the search for a 16-year-old boy who had drowned in a nearby lake. The day after this episode, he felt acute anxiety when he came across some of the equipment which had been used to drag the lake. This anxiety persisted and became more generalized and, as happened in the previous incident, he and his wife sold their business and moved elsewhere – this time to the town of St Thomas, not far away. Because of the repeated contact with people and objects from Tillsonburg, he had to leave St Thomas, too, and eventually they moved to a a large city where they lived for 15 years. He obtained employment in a major company where his wife also found work.

Mr K.'s work involved him in meeting many people, but whenever he talked to anyone who came from St Thomas, or handled goods or mail from there, he experienced acute anxiety symptoms. No anxiety symptoms were associated with Guelph, St Catherine's or Tillsonburg. Over the period of 15 years, his anxiety connected with St Thomas became progressively more incapacitating, until at last he and his wife moved into a small summer resort area far away from the towns in question. (They still live there today.)

Mr K. and his wife are childless, but he has refused to allow his wife or himself to undergo investigations for this distressing problem. He has long liked the company of children, especially girls, and this interest seems to be frankly sexual in nature. He has never divulged such information, but according to his wife, he has occasionally had illicit physical contact with girls in their early teenage years.

This man is interesting for a number of reasons. A careful study of the available literature on phobias has failed to locate fear of a specific geographical location.

Mr K. did not show a typical agoraphobic behaviour pattern, and was accustomed to travel many miles away from home, often alone.

It is at first sight curious that the phobic object, in this case the town of St Thomas, does not seem to be associated with any traumatic event in the same way that the other places were. In fact, it is a relatively neutral object for our patient. There were well-documented fear situations associated with three other towns, and yet Mr K. could visit and receive mail from these places without experiencing any distress.

It is interesting to speculate on how this situation might have arisen. Recently it has been suggested that a neutral stimulus, when presented to an individual in an approach-avoidance conflict, may become associated with the anxiety produced in such a situation. Perhaps a particular town could be considered the appropriate stimulus or group of stimuli.[30]

There is no doubt that Mr K. exhibited a number of obsessive-compulsive features. Together with the compulsive rituals already described, he was orderly, rigid in manner, 'a worrier', parsimonious and subject to periods of morose brooding.[31]

Some psychiatrists suggest that in human subjects approach-avoidance conflicts 'often centre on sex and aggression'.[32] In the case of Mr K., we might guess that the conflicts would be associated either with situations in which violence was involved, or with his sexual relations with young girls. The conflict over sexual relations with minors must be a continuing one for Mr K., and it might be expected that the present geographical location would become associated with this. He and his wife have recently put their house up for sale, at his suggestion, and wish to move elsewhere. This seems to suggest that their present place of residence, a previously neutral stimulus, is acquiring the properties of a feared object in the same way as the town of St Thomas. It will be interesting to note whether St Thomas reverts to neutral status, and whether the place in which they now live does become a phobic object.[33]

Locophobia is undoubtedly an unusual and rare condition, and so too is Glenophobia, or the fear of dolls, both cases adding to the puzzle of how fears arise and are maintained in the absence of any obvious danger from the feared objects.

Psychiatrist Dr James Briscoe of the Uffculme Clinic, Queensbridge Road, Birmingham, recently reported a case of 'Glenophobia' – only the third time it has been mentioned in the literature.[34]

The woman suffering from Glenophobia

A 19-year-old single secretary was referred by her GP to outpatients complaining of a fear of dolls which she had experienced since the age of four. She recalled having had her photograph taken with a doll at that age, but since then had experienced varying degrees of anxiety in the presence of dolls and had not played with any form of doll as a child.

In the three months before seeking help, she had been experiencing distressing dreams and her lifestyle had been affected. In one dream she described being in a taxi 'with loads of people and my boyfriend. I sat in the front and noticed a rotating type of ashtray which had 12 segments. The taxi driver stopped by my house near a wood and we started playing party tricks. He spun the ashtray and there were cracker presents in each compartment except mine, in which there was a doll. I noticed then that the rest of the compartments were full of dolls. Despite my objections the taxi driver got them out and I ran out of the taxi towards the wood. The taxi driver threw the dolls at me and they stuck on my sweater. I looked down and opened my mouth to scream and they flew in.'

She had become acutely conscious of her fear in the presence of dolls and described how she experienced panic attacks when unexpectedly encountering dolls. She avoided coming into contact with children who carried dolls and would cross the road rather than expose herself to this fear. She also described an image of herself swallowing toy soldiers.

One of the prime reasons for seeking help was her wish to start a family. She was concerned that her fear of dolls might extend to her envisaging the foetus as a doll, leading to possible rejection of it following birth, and indeed she was worried that if she did have children her relationship with them might suffer because of her inability to tolerate dolls.

The patient was born in Birmingham and her early development and education were normal. Her mother had been married three times and she was the only girl, with three brothers and six half-brothers. One brother (aged 27) had learning difficulties and severe epilepsy. She was a sociable and mostly confident person who tended to establish good relationships with people. However, she did exhibit some traits of low self-esteem and low self-worth.

Examination revealed no evidence of depression or other mental illness except for this unusual phobia.

The dolls' eyes were the most feared feature, followed by fingers, arms and legs. Dolls which actually moved or simulated movement generated more fear than those that were motionless. The more fragile the material a doll was made of, the worse the fear, but clothing or sex of the doll made no difference. However, any missing limb was associated with worse fear, especially if the dismembered limb was lying nearby. The worst scenario was of a small, realistic plastic toy soldier with a snapped-off arm beside it, as this engendered acute anxiety and a fear that she would inadvertently swallow it.

The patient was treated with exposure therapy during 12 sessions in the outpatient department, and undertook homework using self-rating anxiety scales and relaxation techniques. The fear hierarchy that had been drawn up was addressed using pictures from magazines and the presentation and eventual handling of a large baby doll. Other dolls included porcelain dolls, Action Man and toy soldiers of varying size. Imagery techniques involved imagining toy soldiers in a battlefield with various limbs missing and walking through a toyshop encountering dolls.

By the end of treatment and at follow-up three months later there was a marked reduction in this patient's phobic symptoms. She was able to pick up any doll or toy soldier, was no longer avoiding dolls and could walk through a toyshop without fear. Her dreams had disappeared and she was confident at the prospect of having a family.

This is the first reported case of doll phobia occurring in a female. Doll phobias occurring in a 38-year-old man and a 14-year-old boy have been previously described. The first underwent four years of psychoanalysis whereas the second patient was treated with 12 weekly sessions of graded exposure and desensitization. The present case was also treated effectively with behavioural techniques but might equally have been treated with a psychoanalytic approach, though this is more consuming of time and resources. In all three reports the eyes (particularly their mobility) caused severe anxiety and in two of the three cases fragility, fear of coming to life and upper limbs were all identified as severely anxiety provoking. This may imply a similar explanation for the genesis of the phobia in both males and females.[35]

Individuals and society generally do not consider doll-like figures as threatening – unlike spiders, dogs or open spaces with no escape – because there is no evolutionary reason for it. The observation that it is the individual aspects of the dolls that cause differing degrees of fear, however, points to the doll being a symbol of, or a vehicle for, the true phobia rather than the fear being that of a doll *per se*. This was indeed true in another case report, in which the fear was associated with touching or breaking the fragile and untouchable ceramic dolls in the patient's childhood home and was allied to his anxiety about touching his penis and indulging in masturbation. Fear associated with touching the penis was displaced to the dolls, setting up the doll phobia and resulting in a penis being portrayed as a doll.[36]

It is difficult to speculate on a psychoanalytic explanation for the second patient's phobia because of lack of information but in the present case the areas of interest are her early childhood in an all-male family, the experience of growing up with a learning-disabled and epileptic brother with whom she had contact from an early age, and her thrice-married mother; this may have raised doubts about her own femininity, thereby devaluing the role of a doll as a symbol of femininity to her.[37]

What is most intriguing about these examples of fears and obsessions is that the patients agree that their fears make no sense. If there is no conscious awareness of why, for example, a doll should be feared, this is good evidence of how Freudian ideas or biological concepts can help to explain these puzzling behaviours.

11

MUNCHAUSEN SYNDROME AND THE
DELUSION OF ILLNESS

There are men and women whom the operating table seems to
fascinate: half-alive people who through vanity, or hypochondria, or
a craving to be the constant objects of anxious attention or what not,
lose such feeble sense as they ever had of the value of their organs and
limbs.

George Bernard Shaw, *The Doctor's Dilemma*, 1906

Dr Marc Feldman and Dr Charles Ford are psychiatrists at the University of Alabama and probably the world's foremost authorities on the strange group of disorders known as factitious.[1]

The term 'factitious' comes from the Latin for 'made by art' – in other words artificial, self-induced or not natural. A factitious dermatitis, for example, is an inflammation of the skin produced by the patient, by picking or scratching the surface.

Feldman and Ford report cases such as that of Billy, who so skilfully simulated the symptoms of a brain tumour that he had been scheduled for surgery before it was discovered that no tumour really existed. They claim that there has been a dramatic tenfold increase in published case reports of factitious disorders like that of Billy (and Jenny, see below) since the 1970s, yet the reasons for this sudden rise remain obscure.

The woman who needed to think she was terminally ill to feel alive

This case report involves a woman named Jenny, who shortly after being left by her boyfriend announced to work colleagues one day that she had terminal breast cancer. With this announcement Jenny became an instant 'somebody', the object of sympathy and attention from people who never noticed her before. Suddenly co-workers became best friends. Everyone rallied to support her. Indeed, people were willing to change their own lifestyles to accommodate Jenny. They offered to include her in car pools to cut down on the amount of travelling she had to do and to share her workload, even though that meant they might have to work overtime without compensation. But Jenny declined their offers, saying that she wanted to carry on as she had before in spite of her illness. Her co-workers were moved by her spirit.

Jenny was rewarded with the nurturance and support she had been craving. She had watched a neighbour suffer from breast cancer and knew how a woman would look as the disease progressed. Gradually, Jenny too lost her hair. She seemed to lose the incentive to wear makeup that would hide her haggard appearance, and her already slight figure reflected drastic weight loss. As her hair disappeared (later to be replaced by a wig), and as her weight dropped 20 pounds, making her look more gaunt and pale each day, Jenny's life was ironically transformed and she became emotionally fulfilled.

Several months after breaking the news about her illness, Jenny enrolled in a weekly hospital support group for women with breast cancer. She became a diligent member, never missing an opportunity to be with the caring group of cancer patients and the social support team from the local cancer centre.

Because Jenny had emphasized the deadly nature of her illness, co-workers naturally talked among themselves about what would happen to her as she got closer to the time when the cancer would claim her life. But when months passed and Jenny's condition didn't seem to get worse, support from co-workers levelled off and even began to wane. At that point Jenny shared another personal tragedy with her colleagues – her beloved grandfather had been seriously injured in a fire. A few people rolled their eyes as if to ask, 'What next?' but most were upset by the thought of the increased emotional burden Jenny would have to bear and they pitied her. One woman spent her lunch break reassuring Jenny and sharing intimacies about how she had dealt with the death of her grandmother. She even offered to accompany Jenny to a 'Death and Dying' counselling group which was sponsored by a local church. But Jenny boldly squared her shoulders and pronounced, 'I'll be all right. I'm learning to deal with these things in my cancer group.'

The student body of her mother's elementary school supported Jenny as well. The children raised money to help Jenny pay for chemotherapy treatment and although Jenny didn't want to take the money, her mother insisted, saying she shouldn't disappoint the students. Feeling guilty about accepting it, Jenny squirrelled it away with the intention of somehow paying them back. A local newspaper even wrote about her courage and strength.

Although some people wondered about her ability to report to work every day, and despite Jenny's failure to file insurance claims (normal practice in the US), there were surprisingly few questions from her co-workers and supervisors. It wasn't until her support group leaders tried to gain more information about her medical status that suspicions arose. 'Jenny, we haven't been able to reach one of the doctors you said has been treating you and the other doctor you referred us to doesn't know you,' a counsellor told her one night. 'Can you help us?' Jenny hesitated momentarily then quickly explained that one of them had retired and moved to Florida, but that the other was her specialist: 'Of course he knows me. Call him again.' Jenny continued to provide the group's leaders with the names of doctors who had treated her but it seemed that she was sending them on one wild goose chase after another. After following Jenny's dead ends, the leaders became convinced that she was lying.

Dr Feldman was consulted and he advised the group leaders to avoid being harsh or judgmental. He also asked them to let Jenny know that she was not in trouble and that psychiatric help was available.

Jenny's initial reaction to the confrontation was the same as that of many sufferers of factitious disorders when they are discovered. She vociferously denied having feigned the cancer. But she did eventually collapse and admitted to having faked everything when she realized that the counsellors wanted to help her, not punish her. By then Jenny had simulated cancer for two years but she responded well to Dr Feldman's treatment of what he believed was an underlying depression.

One theory about why people might go to such lengths to fake an illness like cancer is that underlying emotional pain or disorder is particularly difficult for them to talk about or own up to. Pretending to have a physical illness instead may be a way for them to gain the attention and sympathy they crave without having to admit to psychological disturbance.

The key point about these factitious disorders is that the motive appears obscure to the casual observer and requires an in-depth analysis of the psychological or emotional pay-off that is being gained. This is in marked distinction to the other group of disorders where illness is manufactured by the patient – termed malingering.[2]

How many of you, after a particularly good weekend, have felt disinclined to return to work on Monday morning, or if you have tickets to your favourite sports event that day, you phone in 'sick'? You know you are not unwell, but are pretending to be ill in order to gain an obvious reward: an extra day's holiday. In Britain this behaviour is now so common it has attracted its own slang, and the term for pulling the wool over the eyes of others by pretending to be ill in order to get off work is called 'pulling a sickie'. Or so I am told by my secretary, who seemed disconcertingly aware of these terms![3]

Doctors use the designation 'malingering' in order to distinguish this behaviour from a galaxy of strange syndromes associated with physical symptoms that have been manufactured by patients, when no biological or organic cause can be found for them. As some people will go to incredible extremes to deliberately produce painful or mutilating but verifiable symptoms for doctors, there is an overlap here with the syndromes found in the chapter on self-destructive behaviour.[4]

Malingering then refers to feigned disability, the intentional and fraudulent production of symptoms that do not exist, or the gross exaggeration of ones that do. The essential feature is the deliberate falsification of one's medical condition in order to obtain specific tangible rewards – like a day off work or insurance or compensation money for an injury that was never sustained.[5]

In contrast, the psychiatric term of 'factitious' disorders refers to a more chronic condition whereby the person simulates or creates somatic problems in the absence of clearly identifiable objective rewards. While many of the symptoms appear similar to malingering the motivation underlying factitious illness can be understood only by examining the patient's psychological functioning rather than environmental factors. A diagnosis of factitious disorder implies the presence of psychological problems while malingering does not.[6]

An extreme form of factitious disorder was identified in 1951, when Dr Richard Asher dedicated to Baron von Münchhausen a syndrome in which the patient provides a dramatic, plausible, but wholly false medical history.[7]

Baron Karl von Münchhausen (1720–97) was a German soldier who possibly exaggerated his exploits while supposedly travelling the world, hence the link with Munchausen patients. His tales were first published by Rudolf E. Raspe (1737–94), and more recently were chronicled in a 1989 film, *The Adventures of Baron Münchhausen*.[8]

Munchausen syndrome is a particular type of factitious disorder in which patients create potentially life-threatening physical symptoms for unclear psychological reasons. The disorder is difficult to detect and treat. It is also known as 'hospital hobo syndrome', as patients tend to present to multiple hospitals.[9] This is also known as peregrination. Classic cases of Munchausen syndrome involve itinerancy where the patient is hospitalized many times across a wide geographic area. Commonly associated features are chronic lying and the use of false identities. While cases of factitious disorder often display the classic symptoms of Munchausen syndrome, most of these patients do not wander from town to town, and typically do not develop such an extensive falsified history.[10]

The advantage of travelling to a wide selection of hospitals is that you will be meeting staff who have not seen you before and this increases your chances of duping them. And if you venture to clinics widely separated, medical gossip about you between staff is unlikely to have arrived before you do. Another possible benefit is that you can pretend to have much more dramatic illnesses: if you stay in an environment where people know you well, after a while they will expect some end point to the medical problems – that you should die or be cured.[11]

This, after all, was what in the end exposed Jenny: the fact that she was supposed to be seriously ill yet didn't produce the correct course of the disease over an extended period of time. If she had moved around over large distances and presented to different groups of people she might have been able to carry off the deception for much longer. The very need to travel far in order to facilitate the deception is a marker that the need to pretend to be ill is so strong that it has taken over a person's life to the extent of displacing them from their homes.[12]

Dr Edi-Osagie and Dr J. Patrick of the Department of Obstetrics and Gynaecology of the Royal Oldham Hospital in the UK recently reported the following extraordinary case which they could only explain as an example of Munchausen syndrome.[13]

The woman who inflicted serious pain upon herself

This case involves a 21-year-old single woman with no children who presented to doctors with vaginal pain. Pelvic examination failed because of pain and difficulty inserting the speculum (the instrument doctors use to gain access to the internal vaginal area).

However, X-rays revealed two Stanley-knife blades in the pelvic region. These were removed from the vagina under general anaesthetic, to reveal, astonishingly enough, an intact vagina.

The patient opted for an early discharge, only to return two days later with another pair of Stanley-knife blades in the same location. Removal was again easy. She was transferred to psychiatric care, but discharged herself the following day after she was recognized by a doctor from another hospital where she had been admitted several times with similar complaints, receiving various unnecessary treatments.

Munchausen syndrome was suspected at the first visit, but a sexual accident was also considered. It is not uncommon for strange objects utilized for sexual gratification to become retained. Increased lubrication and ballooning of the upper vagina in the excitement phase of sexual arousal would be conducive to the insertion of two 6 cm blades with pointed ends into the vagina with minimal damage.

This woman's psychiatric evaluation, treatment and follow-up highlight the frustrations encountered with this syndrome. Patients lie about themselves and their illness, making it difficult to conduct a proper evaluation and delaying diagnosis. Treatment in any form is difficult to institute, and optimum therapy remains obscure. When confronted, patients deny knowledge of their illness and rapidly discharge themselves from hospital, and as already mentioned, represent in another unit or hospital.[14]

The health care burden of this condition is enormous. The following extraordinary case was reported by Drs Robin Powell and Neil Boast who were at the time at the Maudsley and Hackney Hospitals in London. The title of their case is 'The Million-Dollar Man', which is the amount in US dollars that the authors of the case report estimated this example of Munchausen syndrome cost the British Health Service.[15]

The million-dollar man

The subject was an unemployed man in his thirties who lived in London. The authors have documentary evidence of 545 treatment episodes in 84 hospitals over a 12-year period. As he provided an inaccurate history, information was obtained from his mother and from social service and probation reports.

His early development was complicated when his mother nearly miscarried when only four months pregnant. He was born after a prolonged difficult labour, and at nine months suffered from measles, requiring hospital admission. He received schooling for educational delay from 7 to 16 years, at which time he had no friends and was often truant. Also, he was untruthful, disobedient and engaged in petty theft. Employment has consisted of brief, unskilled manual work, his main source of income being begging. Although he indicated a heterosexual orientation, there are no substantiated relationships. There have been inappropriate sexual advances to female relatives, patients and staff. He is not dependent on alcohol or drugs but has abused phenobarbitone and phenytoin.

He had convictions as a juvenile hoax telephone caller to the fire brigade and as an adult for handbag theft, and assaulting a nurse. He set fire to a prison cell, from which he received severe burns, and was suspected of causing minor hospital fires. Allegedly he engages in petty thefts and frauds. Psychiatric reports cite him as immature, of low intelligence and psychopathic. Following criminal proceedings he was made subject to a section 60 hospital order, which proved ineffective in altering his behaviour. He responded best to 13 months of youth custody; prison medical reports describe improvements in confidence, self-care, relationships and work record.

The authors contacted 205 hospitals (187 in the four Thames health regions and 18 other selected hospitals), of which 161 (79 per cent) replied. During 12 years, this man spent over six years in institutions, comprising 1,300 days in psychiatric units, 556 days in prisons and 354 days in medical care. He has had 284 casualty attendances and 261 hospital admissions, the length of stay varying from a few hours to 13 months (average 6.3 days). He has often been detained under sections of the Mental Health Act (62 times).

Reasons for hospital admissions have varied but predominantly concerned self-harm (305 instances). These have included overdose (192) with drugs. Drug intake detected on 28 per cent of admissions, although levels were never high enough to require treatment.

Dangerous behaviour (85 instances) has included running in the traffic (56), threatening to jump from heights (17) and walking on railway tracks (12). He has presented with psychiatric disorders (69) including reaction to feigned bereavement (51) and hearing voices (18). Most episodes of physical illness (156) were feigned or self-inflicted, for example epilepsy (50), head injury (28), collapse (21) and asthma (8). However, biological disease of the brain has also been confirmed frequently (28).

Although he is the tenant of a council flat, it is bereft of furniture or personal effects. He spends his time seeking hospital admission, visiting unstructured day centres, travelling, living in reception centres or as a vagrant, and, as mentioned, generates income by begging. His family feel unable to help him and only remain in contact through agencies attempting to establish the patient's identity. He can be polite, co-operative and plausible but may be angry if challenged and has assaulted patients and staff.

This patient's personal history contains gross distortions and fabrications. On occasion there is an ironic concealment of truth, such as giving his place of birth as Leicester, where he received nine months inpatient treatment. Occasionally he complains of hearing voices in the second person which take the form of pseudo-hallucinations. Cognitive examination is consistent with low intelligence and physical examination reveals old injuries and an unhealthy pallor. His standard reply to the question of his motivation for seeking hospital admission is, 'It's a dangerous world out there, doctor.'

The sum of £450,900 represents only part of the costs involved in treating this patient and does not include assessment under sections of the Mental Health Act, police, ambulance, social service and legal costs. Neither has it been possible to estimate the cost of outpatient and primary health care treatment, including pharmaceutical expenses. Also hidden from this figure are costs such as those arising from interference with train services.

Doctors Powell and Boast conclude that this is a case of Munchausen syndrome combined with anti-social personality disorder.

One superficially obvious solution to the problem Munchausen syndrome patients present to health services is the keeping of clinic 'blacklists', or even a centralized register, although, admittedly, patients easily sidestep such obstacles. They use aliases, and most blacklists are hopelessly out of date and rely on staff to refer to them regularly. In a health service with limited resources and an increasingly rapid turnover of staff, Munchausen syndrome becomes ever more difficult to detect.[16]

The circulation of a blacklist outside a particular hospital and the keeping of a national or regional central register might even be considered legally questionable and ethically doubtful as patients are usually considered to be entitled to confidentiality when it comes to their medical records. In the UK a doctor who discloses information without patient consent may have to answer for this to the General Medical Council.[17]

It is also not entirely clear precisely what detection and immediate discharge from a hospital achieves, as this merely enables the patient to wander off and present elsewhere. The situation is further complicated by the fact that Munchausen syndrome patients may also have concurrent real illnesses. Doctors Powell and Boast point out that although this is a spectacular case and the vast majority of hospital admissions were engineered needlessly, their patient did suffer from severe anaemia and fractures that were often missed.[18]

A key dilemma with factitious disorders in general, and Munchausen syndrome specifically, is whether to regard these patients as basically out of control, and so closer to suffering from a kind of psychotic illness rather than straightforward malingering. If doctors go down this route they would seek to admit such patients for long-term psychiatric care in order to attempt a cure of their problem. Obviously this could be seen as a kind of 'victory' for the patient. Isn't this, after all, what they were trying to engineer all along? This approach could be defended clinically; these patients may seek admission to hospital for manufactured physical and psychiatric symptoms, but they would not recognize themselves as needing help for the underlying pathology which drives the behaviour. So an inpatient admission to a clinic for treatment of factitious disorder would not necessarily be to their taste.[19]

Loren Pankratz and James Jackson of the Portland Veterans Affairs Medical Center and the Departments of Psychiatry and Medical Psychology of the Oregon Health Sciences University in Portland, Oregon, conducted perhaps the most extensive study to date of what they termed 'wandering patients'. These are patients most likely to suffer from Munchausen syndrome because they gain admission to one hospital after another. Little is still known about them, their use of hospital resources or the costs of their medical care. To better understand what was going on Drs Pankratz and

Jackson used the extensive computerized records across the United States to analyse the characteristics of wandering patients served by the Department of Veterans Affairs Medical Centers (VAMCs).[20]

For each patient they admit, all 159 hospitals in the Veterans Affairs medical system submit demographic and diagnostic information to a central database at the Data Processing Center in Austin, Texas. Pankratz and Jackson identified patients who were admitted to four or more Veterans Affairs Medical Centers each year from 1988 through to 1992. Patients identified with this frequency in any one year were called 'habitual wanderers'.[21]

Pankratz and Jackson identified 1,013 wanderers in 1988, and in 1991 there were 810 wandering patients who averaged about eight admissions per year and more than 100 days of inpatient care; they accounted for about $26.5 million in costs for inpatient and outpatient care in that year. Only 35 patients (all male) wandered in all five years from 1988 to 1992. The most common discharge diagnoses of these 35 men were related to substance abuse (mostly alcoholism) and mental disorders. Their 2,268 admissions and 7,832 outpatient visits cost an estimated $6.5 million over the five-year period. All 35 would probably be regarded as suffering from Munchausen syndrome.[22]

Homelessness has been proposed as an explanation for some so-called revolving-door patients. However, among the habitual wanderers identified, homelessness is not an adequate explanation for their transient lifestyle. Hospitals may be the preferred living situation for some patients who need structure, support and basic amenities when faced with social problems. Habitual wanderers have complex problems of maladjustment, characterized by impulsivity, substance abuse and character disorders. It is not surprising therefore, that they can cause diagnostic confusion.[23]

An even stronger form of Munchausen syndrome

So far, we have discussed Munchausen syndrome, in which an individual manufactures illness in themselves for various mysterious psychological reasons. There is however a recently identified variant – Munchausen syndrome by proxy (MSBP), a rare condition in which a child is admitted to hospital for medical care with symptoms that are fabricated or produced by a caretaker. The deception often is repeated on numerous occasions, resulting in many hospitalizations, considerable serious complications and sometimes death.[24]

Nearly always committed by the mother (father perpetrators have been recently described), the motives are usually unknown. Overt psychiatric disturbance is infrequently found, and denial by the mother is common, even when confronted with substantial evidence of her duplicity.

Munchausen syndrome by proxy was recognized by Dr Roy Meadow in 1977. It is a serious form of child abuse, often overlooked for several weeks, months or years. Numerous patients have been described with a wide variety of symptoms, including apnea, seizure disorders, intractable vomiting and/or diarrhoea, gastrointestinal bleeding, septicaemia, hypoglycaemia and cystic fibrosis. In all of the cases so far reported the mother or a female caretaker was described as pleasant, co-operative, and appreciative and supportive of good medical care. They were also intelligent and medically knowledgeable.

The recognition of Munchausen syndrome by proxy is a milestone in child protection, and the increasing number of these tragic case reports is a testimony to Dr Meadow's astute observations. Some had suggested that 'Meadow's syndrome' be used not only as a tribute to Dr Meadow's work but also in recognition of the fact that Baron von Münchhausen never harmed a child.

In one case report tracing the death of a child, a mother remembers that as a youngster she fantasized about being sick, avidly watched television medical shows and read medical dictionaries. She also reported that she was raped by a gang of teenage boys when she was 10 years old. 'Shaking' spells experienced a year later persuaded the family physician to prescribe barbiturates. Her mother would arbitrarily increase the barbiturate dosage when she was under stress or when her mother thought she was experiencing puberty-related emotions. Treated and hospitalized numerous times as an adult for depression, she had severe marital problems. She attempted suicide by overdose and on another occasion by deliberately driving her car into a tree.

After episodes of Munchausen syndrome, a pair of cuticle scissors was surgically removed from her bladder, a paper clip from her urethra and drain cleaner crystals from her eyes. She fabricated a kidney infection for which she claimed she needed dialysis, but later allowed her fundamentalist church members to think she had been 'miraculously cured'.

Tragically, this woman's son died after she placed him in a freezer and left him there until he suffocated. At the time, sudden infant death syndrome was diagnosed, and postpartum depression was diagnosed in the mother. Later it was learned that the mother had formerly been married to a physician, had a dental and nursing background, and had a history of factitious medical conditions of her own.

The following warning signs alert paediatricians to the presence of a factitious illness: (1) unexplained, prolonged and extraordinary illness; (2) signs and symptoms that are incongruous or apparent only when the mother is present; (3) ineffective treatments; and (4) a mother who is at ease on the paediatric floor and who forms unusually close relationships with the staff.

In reports on intractable diarrhoea in children due to the surreptitious administration of laxatives, mothers of these children provided continuous care, seldom left the bedside and had a history of suicidal ideation and of psychiatric intervention. A profound symbiotic relationship existed between this kind of parent and her child. Separation anxiety on the part of the child and over-protectiveness on the part of the mother were most evident. This abnormal relationship appeared to serve various purposes.

Another common finding is that of a poor emotional relationship between the mother and father. In some families, the child's illness brings about a closer relationship between parents; in others, it seems a welcome distraction from personal difficulties at home. Thus, the parent's need for help often finds expression in the child's 'illness'.

It is important to mention here that children may engage in self-injury that is intended to alarm their parents and mislead the physician. At an early age, children become aware of the attention they receive as a result of minor bleeding and of the alarm with which adults attend to greater amounts of bleeding or bruising. Physicians who work in correctional settings report that self-inflicted bleeding is extremely common in delinquent youths. Such children are imaginative in obtaining cutting instruments (paper clips, staples, plastic cutlery) and in locating a site for the self-inflicted laceration so as to give the appearance of internal bleeding. But, of course, not all factitious injury in childhood is self-induced, and the possibility of a parent producing the injury in a young child, or colluding with self-injury in a child, must also be considered.

If Munchausen syndrome and Munchausen syndrome by proxy are disorders where the attempt to produce illness is driven by mysterious motives, in malingering the intention to fabricate disease has a more straightforward drive – usually the attempt to gain financially.

Malingering, the feigning of an illness for the purpose of secondary gain, is an act seen with increasing frequency, especially among emergency department patients. Malingering should be distinguished from factitious disorder because factitious disorder may be found in a patient who is in danger of harming himself. In malingering this is much less likely, as direct benefit to the patient is always the fundamental motivation.[25]

Malingerers' portrayal of psychosis will be based on their understanding of it, and they will draw on their experience of contact with mentally disordered individuals in the past. Eager to call attention to their illness, these patients frequently overact their part, over-emphasizing their supposed symptoms in an effort to convince the doubtful clinician. The malingerer is 'determined that his insanity should not lack multiple and obvious signs, piles symptom upon symptom and so outstrips madness itself'.[26]

Malingering is obviously easier to detect when objective verification of whether an illness is present or not is possible, as in the use of X-rays. But what happens in the realm of psychiatric disorder when no objective physical tests exist to make a diagnosis?[27]

The difficulty of detecting malingered psychosis has long been recognized. Rosenhan's 1973 classic study, which is probably the most famous test of simulated psychosis, demonstrated mental health professionals' inability to distinguish normality from mental illness. Eight volunteer 'pseudopatients', comprising one psychology student, three psychologists, a paediatrician, a psychiatrist, a painter and a housewife, were secretly admitted to psychiatric hospitals claiming to hear voices. Such claims were designed to stop immediately following admission, yet once they had been admitted, medical and nursing staff were unable to spot that these 'patients' were now devoid of symptoms. All were still diagnosed as suffering from schizophrenia and their length of stay in hospital varied from 9 to 52 days. Fellow patients, however, did sometimes recognize the 'pseudopatients' as frauds. Rosenhan concluded that 'it is clear we cannot distinguish the sane from the insane in psychiatric hospitals'. In part, such difficulties are due to the fact that psychiatry is far from being an exact science; instead of definitive physical tests diagnosis is reliant on clinical observation and objective interpretation of symptoms.[28]

Paul Chesterman of Three Bridges Regional Secure Unit in Middlesex recently reported a case of a man who was convicted of indecently assaulting a teenage boy, but subsequently presented to forensic services with a variety of psychotic symptoms he was later proved to have feigned.[29]

The man who pretended to be insane

J.S., a 35-year-old single male, was conditionally discharged from a regional secure unit approximately two years ago following an admission under the 1983 Mental Health Act. The second of four male siblings, he was the only one to have been physically abused by his father. His parents separated a number of years ago and there is no family history of mental illness. Prior to the events described below, J.S. had no psychiatric or forensic history of note. His offence was the indecent assault of a 14-year-old boy, for which he was convicted and remanded in prison for reports. He first came to the attention of psychiatric services in the weeks preceding his court appearance. At that time he complained of low mood and suicidal thoughts; indeed he attempted to hang himself.

On assessment he was withdrawn and anxious in manner, and had little memory of many aspects of his personal history, including his date of birth. He described having heard voices over a 12-month period but was unable to describe these in any great detail. He denied the offence with which he was charged and described himself as bisexual with a preference for female partners. Following conviction and remand to prison he continued to describe psychotic symptoms, particularly persecutory beliefs regarding prison officers. He stated that cameras in prison watched him. In light of this, and his vulnerable appearance, he was transferred to the hospital wing where he suffered a broken jaw following an unprovoked attack by a fellow inmate. He was subsequently referred for a further psychiatric assessment and it was then considered that his behaviour was in keeping with a developing psychotic illness. Admission to hospital under the provisions of the Mental Health Act 1983 was therefore recommended.

In hospital he remained guarded about his personal details; he was adamant that he was born in 1971, and gave conflicting accounts of his educational achievements. He was especially reluctant to discuss both the assault he had committed and his sexuality. On admission he stated that he had been treated in prison for both tuberculosis and heroin addiction; however, the prison medical service had no records of this.

Particularly anxious in social situations, he displayed compulsive behaviour in the form of checking and repeated washing. His mood, both objectively and subjectively, remained low, he continued to express persecutory beliefs and described second person auditory hallucinations of a derogatory nature. He also reported vivid, violent fantasies, and claimed that he was William the Conqueror. Although his precise diagnosis remained far from clear, he was commenced on a trial of both antipsychotic and antidepressant medication.

Subsequently he described a wide variety of possible psychotic symptoms, including delusions of being watched and delusions of reference from the television. On one occasion he described a visual hallucination of a black man talking to him in the corridor. When questioned by staff he demonstrated suggestibility in his responses; for example, when asked whether the man was wearing a black hat he replied in the affirmative. However, his behaviour and accounts of such symptoms were often inconsistent.

During his admission J.S. remained in close contact by telephone with his mother but did not inform her of his claimed psychotic experiences. When asked to explain this omission he merely smiled and refused to elaborate. He continued to describe in a convincing manner a number of strange experiences, including what appeared to be a multimodal hallucination, stating that while in hospital he had seen a Victorian gentleman who had spoken to him for several hours. He had not informed staff of this experience at the time as he did not feel that anyone else had witnessed it. Of note is that J.S. revealed this symptom soon after his case was transferred to a new consultant.

Personality assessment demonstrated that he displayed avoidant, dependent, obsessive-compulsive and paranoid traits with an IQ of 80. In an effort to clarify his personal history, and especially his sexual history, information was obtained from his immediate family. His mother reluctantly agreed to be seen on three occasions. She denied any knowledge of her son's psychotic symptoms and strongly expressed her belief that he was only suffering from depression. She added that J.S. was well known in their home town as he had claimed to be the only survivor of both the King's Cross station fire and the Clapham Junction train crash. J.S. was unable to remember the names of the hospitals where he had been admitted following these traumatic events. He reluctantly gave his permission for the medical team to have access to his flat and belongings, having initially prevented this by legal means. These investigations revealed that:

- his date of birth was 11 years prior to that he had previously stated;
- he had used in excess of 20 aliases in the past and was in possession of a false passport;
- he was in possession of a large amount of homosexual, heterosexual and paedophilic pornographic material, videos inter-spliced with children's programmes, numerous children's books and many items of children's sports clothing. He continued, however, to adamantly deny any sexual interest in children and denied the significance of these findings but was unable to provide any explanation as to why he was in possession of such items.

His accounts of his past history remained contradictory; indeed he was unable to provide any details for a five-year period of his adult life. Such findings cast further doubt on J.S.'s diagnosis. Further information obtained from his mother was strongly suggestive that the appropriate diagnosis was one of a pervasive developmental disorder, specifically Asperger's syndrome, a type of autism characterized by limited, obsessive interests and difficulty in relating to people. She revealed that J.S. had shown a marked impairment of social interaction during his childhood with few, if any, peer relationships. He appears to have been a clumsy child with an odd gait and was terrified of balloons. His mother also described a lack of spontaneous seeking to share enjoyment with others, and a pattern of restricted behaviour and interests, including an almost obsessive interest in history.

When the extent of his deception became clear, it was put to J.S. that the situation he had found himself in while in custody had been extremely distressing and had resulted in his describing symptoms that were not true. He reluctantly acknowledged that he had done so in order to obtain a psychiatric diagnosis. He went on to describe the origins of some of those symptoms; for example, his considerable interest in history had given him the idea of claiming to be William the Conqueror. He had described seeing the Victorian gentleman after nursing staff had told him that part of the hospital was built on the site of a Victorian cemetery.

He continues to deny his offence, claiming that his victim led him on. He remains unwilling to admit the extent of his sexual interest in children and since the cessation of treatment over three years ago, there has been no deterioration in his mental state and he has described no further symptoms of a possibly psychotic nature.

The onset of J.S.'s psychotic symptoms can be traced to the weeks preceding his court appearance following the charge of indecent assault. It is unusual for people in custody to develop psychotic illnesses in response to the stresses they experience: the term 'prison psychosis', however, is still occasionally used to describe such reactive episodes.

With the benefit of hindsight, we can see that the fearful prospect of imprisonment served as the stimulus for the creation of J.S.'s fabricated psychotic symptoms, an understandable response given his propensity for fantastic stories.

The importance of distinguishing real from fabricated illness is clear. However, the potential pitfalls of assessing someone as a malingering psychotic must also be appreciated, as classically demonstrated in a study published in the aftermath of the trial of Peter Sutcliffe in which the judge overruled psychiatrists and asserted that Sutcliffe was malingering although he later went on to develop schizophrenia. (Four out of five cases of simulated psychosis subsequently develop schizophrenia.)[30]

A distinction has also been made between *pure malingering*, defined as the feigning of disease when it does not exist at all in a particular patient, and *partial malingering*, the conscious exaggeration of existing symptoms or the fraudulent assertion that previously experienced genuine symptoms are present after their resolution.[31]

The term pseudo-malingering has been used to describe those who fabricate mental illness before becoming unwell.[32] For example, in Leonid Andreyev's novel *The Dilemma* (1902) a doctor commits murder with the premeditated plan of appearing insane; he then begins to experience true hallucinations and realizes that his psychosis is indeed genuine. Such pseudo-malingering is a mechanism to maintain an 'intact self-image', which would be damaged by the realization that certain psychological problems cannot be overcome consciously.[33]

It appears that the incidence of malingered psychosis may have increased in recent years as a consequence of the closure of long-stay psychiatric institutions and the move towards care in the community. Many chronically mentally ill patients, who may have preferred the stable environment of the asylum, are now living in marginal circumstances in the community.[34] Such individuals may therefore consciously exaggerate their symptoms in an effort to obtain shelter in the new generation of psychiatric hospitals. It has also been proposed that there has been a change in coping strategies in society's disenfranchised individuals, who now present with psychological rather than physical symptoms.[35] This shift has been precipitated by the lack of precision in psychiatric diagnoses, the increased availability of mental health services and the decreased stigma attached to mental illness.

12

BORN INTO THE WRONG BODY:
THE DELUSION OF GENDER

He ran back into the yellow house, stood before the mirror as he had stood so often when painting a self-portrait, and hacked off part of his left ear with the razor.

Jean-Francois Barrielle, *The Life and Work of Vincent van Gogh*, 1987

The first case of genital self-mutilation was published in 1882 – a 29-year-old farmer on two occasions accused his neighbours of cutting open his scrotum and removing a testicle.[1] His assailants were imprisoned but then released a year later when the farmer made a deathbed confession that he had inflicted both wounds. Even at that time the thinking in psychiatry was that psychologically disturbed patients mutilate their genitals because they are unable to cope with their own sexual desires. It might also be considered a self-cure for masturbation and to protect against perverse sexual cravings. The term Eshmun complex was coined to describe the psychology of patients who actually or symbolically castrated themselves and is named after Eshmun, a handsome Phoenician deity, who castrated himself to avoid the sexual advances of the mother-goddess Astronae.[2]

Self-castrated priests were common in early Rome, but this form of religion-based castration appears to have been replaced by celibacy in some religions. In recent times there have been religious overtones in the commission of genital self-mutilation.[3]

In relation to spirituality, body modification activities are found in many religions: these are thought to be pleasing to spirits and are seen as capable of helping humans achieve special states of holiness, ecstasy and insight. Priests devoted to the great mother-goddess Cybele castrated themselves to demonstrate their mourning and identification with Attis, who had castrated himself, died and was resurrected. By their wounds, the Old Testament Suffering Servant and the New Testament Jesus brought holiness and salvation to humankind.[4]

Castration is discussed in great detail in psychoanalytic articles during the first half of the twentieth century. Although it is rarely encountered, the fear of castration is thought in psychoanalysis to play a vital role in both normal childhood development and later emotional disturbance.[5]

The genital mutilation of John Bobbitt by his wife Lorena in 1993 was sensationalized in the media and it is easy to understand how a psychologically fragile woman might strike back at an abusive husband. But why did she wait to attack him on that particular night? Why did she confine her attack to his penis? Why did she take the severed organ with her? And why did she pause when fleeing the house to steal their houseguest's Game Boy?

A new analysis of the case published by psychiatrist Dr David Reardon of the Elliot Institute in the USA offers intriguing answers to these questions. According to Dr Reardon, her violence was secondary to psychiatric symptoms of depression and post-traumatic stress disorder (PTSD) and these were precipitated by a coerced abortion three days before their first wedding anniversary. Lorena pleaded to keep her child and gave in to the abortion only because she was pressured into it by John. Like other women before her, Lorena experienced the unwanted abortion as an attack on both her maternity and her sexuality. That is the key to understanding her subsequent attack on John.[6]

Dr Reardon argues that guilt, shame and resentment over the abortion fuelled the rapid rise in violence and sexual abuse in the Bobbitt household. This atmosphere of violence culminated in Lorena's cutting off of John's penis on almost exactly the third anniversary of the abortion. To Dr Reardon the timing of the cutting incident was not coincidental, as between 30 and 40 per cent of women who report post-abortion problems experience more intense symptoms around the anniversary of the abortion. For these women, the anniversary date of an abortion is a connector back to unresolved grief, which can exhibit itself in the guise of psychosomatic illnesses, increased depression, and uncontrollable fits of rage, all of which Lorena experienced.

Lorena's abortion was on 15 June 1990. On 18 June 1993, she went to her doctor complaining of hyperventilation, cramping and anxiety attacks. Reardon says these symptoms are all typical of a post-abortion anniversary reaction. The cutting incident occurred five days later, only minutes after she experienced flashbacks to the abortion, another common post-abortion reaction.

According to Lorena's sworn testimony, she became sexually cold towards John immediately after the abortion. It was then, she claimed, that John began to sexually force himself upon her and that they began to experience frequent and violent altercations.

Lorena's traumatic abortion is implicated in the cutting incident not only by the timing of the attack, but also by the manner in which she attacked John. 'Lorena felt as though her abortion had left her sexually mutilated,' Reardon says, 'and she blamed John for making her have it. That she chose to attack John's sexuality, not his life, indicates that Lorena was subconsciously choosing to retaliate in kind – "an eye for an eye", so to speak.'

The fact that Lorena carried off the severed penis may also be significant. 'Lorena desperately wanted to have a replacement baby. The grief and shame surrounding her "missing child" were at the heart of her psychological problems,' says Reardon. 'In the moments when she fled the house, she was highly upset and disoriented. Subconsciously, the severed penis may have symbolized her missing child; it embodied her desire to have her child.'

Reardon supports this theory by pointing out that when Lorena fled from the house that night she also grabbed their houseguest's Game Boy. He believes this bizarre act had psychological significance. According to his written analysis of the case, 'In her hands she clutched both a phallic symbol and a child's toy, which even by its very name – Game Boy – symbolized the missing "Little Boy" she so desperately wanted. When fleeing the house she was, on some subconscious level, simply trying to take "her baby" with her'.

The biting off of the penis during fellatio has been recorded, as has group ritual genital mutilation, which is a custom carried out by a sect of Australian Aborigines. (This also involves the drinking of

300

the blood by the infirm who believe that it restores health.) Genital self-mutilation (GSM) has also been observed in mice.

But there is a group of psychotic patients, often those suffering from schizophrenia, who have committed autocastration due to religious delusions that are based on a rather literal interpretation of the Bible's comment on celibacy (Matthew 19: AV 12): 'There are some eunuchs which were so born from their mother's womb: and there are some eunuchs, which were made eunuchs of [by] men: and there be eunuchs, which have made themselves eunuchs for the kingdom of heaven's sake.' Another famous biblical passage often quoted by psychotics who have self-mutilated is Matthew 5: 29–30, 'And if thy right eye offend thee, pluck it out and cast it from thee: for it is profitable for thee that one of thy members should perish, and not that thy whole body should be cast into hell. And if thy right hand offend thee, cut it off and cast it from thee: for it is profitable for thee that one of thy members should perish, and not that thy whole body should be cast into hell.'[7]

Because genital self-mutilation is considered to be a severe form of bizarre behaviour, there is a tendency to assume that the victims are psychotic. This view is too simple, however. Three groups of men are thought most at risk: psychotics, personality-disordered individuals including transsexuals, and those under social or cultural influence. The last group includes schizophrenics with religious delusions and men who consider themselves failures in the male role.[8]

Genital self-mutilation is usually carried out in a state of clear consciousness, often after a period of planning, and it may be the first and only manifestation of psychiatric illness. The major psychotic illnesses in these patients are delusions in chronic paranoid schizophrenia and command hallucinations (i.e. those that command the patient to do something). Drug-and alcohol-induced psychosis have been reported, as well as lesser psychiatric illnesses including pathological guilt feelings associated with aberrant sexual conduct and conflicts, and aberrant body image in transsexuals.[9]

The motives for GSM vary; it is estimated that roughly 10 per cent of self-mutilators intend suicide and the recognition or incidence of this motive is increasing. Many people believe that amputation of the penis is fatal and given this widespread belief in China (see 'koro' in Chapter 6) it has been suggested that GSM among the Chinese be considered a suicide attempt.[10]

Other motives are less obscure; an avowed anti-circumcisionist mutilated his penis while trying to reconstruct his previous circumcision. One patient is reported to have carried out bilateral orchidectomy (removal of the testicles) to prevent alopecia, believing that reducing testosterone levels would help his condition.[11] GSM has also been associated with unresolved sexual conflicts. In Canada, a group of transsexuals amputated their genitals in anticipation of a change of policy on sexual reassignment surgery (SRS).[12] Another impatient transsexual sequentially amputated his left testis, right testis and finally his penis over a period of nine months in a vain effort to secure SRS. And a woman malingered abnormal placement of her placenta or placenta praevia in four pregnancies by mutilating her vagina each time, to secure a Caesarean section.[13]

The severest form of GSM recorded is total amputation of the penis, scrotum and testes in the male. This occurs in around 10 per cent of GSM cases, and the term 'lock, stock and barrel' mutilation is used to describe it.[14] The most frequent type of self-mutilation of the genitals is complete transection (slicing through) of the penis. This, along with those who remove both testicles, accounts for 51 per cent of cases.[15]

The extent or severity of mutilation is similar between those considered psychotic and those not. In females, the reported injuries include third-degree perineal tears, gouging of the internal genitalia with fingernails and vaginal mutilation with a hatpin and knitting needle. Other instruments used in GSM include scissors, razor blades, an electric chainsaw, axe (hatchet) on a wooden block, a kitchen knife and saw and a soup can lid.[16]

Most patients show no interest in their amputated parts, although some who have sought help after mutilation take the amputated organs with them. A few patients who did not want the amputated parts to be retrieved and replanted have flushed them away or ritually burned them. In one extreme case, a 51-year-old German repeatedly practised GSM and ate the mutilated parts of his body. On the last occasion, after he had bled to death, his penis was recovered from his colon at autopsy;[17] a similar case of autophagia (eating oneself) has been reported in the USA.[18]

Motive often remains difficult to discern. Doctor Arnold Waugh, formerly a psychiatrist at the Princess Alexandra Hospital in Queensland, Australia, demonstrates this problem in the following case, though here religious delusions appeared to play a major role.[19]

The man who thought the bible was about him

The patient was born in a Queensland provincial town, of elderly parents. He was one of non-identical twins, and the birth was difficult: the patient's mother described him as a 'blue baby'. His father was a retired farmer who taught his sons to castrate bulls, using the technique that the patient later used on himself.

As a child this patient was very quiet and close to his family; he had few friends and his mother described him as her 'pet'. His early school performance was fair, but he struggled in his senior years. He worked for a year in the public service, but left this job, claiming all the men were homosexuals and smoked too much. He denied any homosexual or heterosexual experience. Indeed, his only sexual experience was masturbation, the source of his guilt and anxiety. Although his immediate family were not particularly religious, at the age of 17 he became greatly influenced by an eccentric elderly aunt, who was described by the patient's parents as a religious fanatic. She introduced him to the Bible and he was baptized. Eventually, he spent every spare moment sitting in his room reading the Bible from cover to cover. At the time of admission the patient held a low-key job as a storeman and he lived at home with his parents. He did not drink, smoke or take illicit drugs, and his only interests were the Bible and attending church.

At the age of 31 he incised his scrotum with a razor blade, severed his testicles and flushed them down the toilet. He was brought to hospital in shock which was caused by extreme anaemia as a result of the loss of blood.

When surgically stable he was transferred to the psychiatric unit. The patient stated that he had castrated himself in response to Matthew 19: 12; he felt evil, as he had been masturbating and saw castration as the only way to gain forgiveness. He had considered cutting off his right hand in response to Matthew 18: 8, but considered that 19: 12 was a specific reference to himself. He admitted to occasionally hearing non-hostile voices describing his actions, but these were not prominent in his illness.

The patient had considered castration for at least five years prior to actually committing the act: at times he had consulted surgeons requesting this, and had been referred for a psychiatrist's opinion. After a self-inflicted laceration to his penis had required suturing he was admitted to another psychiatric hospital. A diagnosis of schizophrenia was made and he received outpatient treatment for five years. Eight weeks prior to the present admission he had appeared agitated and refused his medication.

When he had been fully resuscitated he seemed a vague perplexed man. His speech was soft and quiet. He felt a great sense of relief at having finally castrated himself and at no stage did he request analgesia. His thoughts contained many bizarre delusions. No biological or organic cause for his psychosis could be found.

The patient was started on antipsychotic medication and his acute symptoms settled rapidly. He became more sociable and outgoing but continued to be preoccupied with the Bible, and showed no regret for castrating himself. He refused to take replacement testosterone for fear of getting renewed sexual desires. Simple religious arguments were incorporated into a supportive psychotherapy programme.

The patient's parents were bewildered at their son's plight. They were involved in psychotherapy to overcome their horror and disgust and to encourage them to support their son. After six weeks he was discharged home on antipsychotic injections and has remained well.

In the management of self-induced genital injuries surgeons stress the importance of preservation or replacement of testicular androgen activity. This was not possible in the case reported here as the patient became quite anxious at the prospect of replacement testosterone. This is not surprising, considering his delusions and the way in which he disposed of his testicles originally. It has been noted that those individuals adamantly opposed to surgical repair of the severed genitals almost always dispose of the organs at the time of the act; those who are ambivalent about the act may bring their organs with them to hospital.[20]

This patient is one of the small group of psychotic schizophrenics who castrate themselves in response to a biblical passage. Following years of obsessive study they develop a complex delusional system in which they feel the need to castrate themselves to atone for perceived sexual guilt. The autocastration follows careful deliberation: the patient has usually requested surgical castration before taking matters into his own hands. The need to recognize the serious implications of such requests is clear.[21]

Over 110 cases of male genital self-mutilation have been reported in the medical literature since 1901 and the age range is 17–72 with the average age being 36. According to one review only 57 cases were reported between the turn of the century and 1986, so there is evidence of a worrying increase in this disorder in recent years.[22]

There are just four cases on record of GSM by women.[23]

Religious psychotic experiences, often the direct motives for the act, include auditory hallucinations of the voice of Buddha criticizing the patient, sexual lust hallucinations of commands from the Devil, visual hallucination of Jesus, delusions that the patient himself is Buddha as well as the delusions based on a literal interpretation of Bible passages. Religious psychotic experiences have been found in 34 per cent of psychotic self-mutilators, and again these seem to be related to guilt about sexual problems.[24]

Doctor David Ames, a psychiatrist at the Royal Free Hospital in London, has suggested the term Klingsor syndrome for the kind of case reported by Dr Waugh where religious preoccupation and delusions are prominent. Klingsor was a character in Wagner's *Parsifal* who 'unmanned' himself in a vain effort to gain entry to the brotherhood of Grail Knights. The suggested title thus incorporates both the element of autocastration and the religious motivation so often encountered.[25]

The following Klingsor syndrome is reported by Dr Isaac Schweitzer, Senior Lecturer in Psychiatry at the University of Melbourne in Australia.[26]

The man who was convinced he was a sexual sinner

D.W., a 32 year-old divorced Chinese man, was an emergency admission to hospital after he stabbed himself in the chest and abdomen with a carving knife and then severed his penis, leaving a 2 cm stump. The knife had entered the right chest cavity, exposed his heart, lacerated his stomach, bowels and colon. He required emergency surgery and the removal of a large portion of his colon. His penile stump was refashioned and a plastic conduit was inserted into the urethra to allow urine to flow out.

D.W. had been experiencing constant third person auditory hallucinations for four months prior to this self-amputation: he had heard a male voice speaking in Cantonese accusing him of many sins, mainly sexual. According to D.W. he had been told he would become the King of China, a position he felt unworthy to fill because of his excessive masturbation and visits to massage parlours. Consequently he made the 'ultimate sacrifice', intending to end his life.

D.W. was born in Canton, the eldest of three children of a poor peasant family. When he was six his father died suddenly in a farming accident and he went to Hong Kong to live with his grandmother, later migrating to Australia. He worked as a chef in Chinese restaurants. He had an arranged marriage at 19 but this was never consummated, so D.W.'s social activities were mainly drinking tea at Chinese clubs and frequenting massage parlours. He had no steady girlfriends or significant relationships. D.W. denied drug and alcohol abuse and this was confirmed by his sister.

D.W. had had many psychiatric admissions since he turned 20 years of age and had been given several different diagnoses including schizophrenia, other psychotic disorders, depression and manic depressive illness. He had a range of symptoms, including auditory hallucinations, persecutory and grandiose delusions and suicidal ideas. Apparently his recovery between episodes of illness had been good and he had a reasonable employment record until three years previously when he'd made a suicide attempt with a handsaw, cutting his wrist to bleed to death and partially amputating his hand. He was preoccupied with the concern that he had contracted AIDS and had been tormented by persecutory hallucinations telling him to 'get stuffed' and 'to have sex with a girl'. Several months later he completed the amputation with a meat cleaver.

Psychiatrist Dr Laura Roberts and colleagues of the University of New Mexico Health Sciences Center, in Albuquerque, New Mexico, report a case of a man requesting an unusual, but biblical in origin, operation.[27]

The monk with a strange request

A man who introduced himself as Brother David, a monk from Ascension Monastery, was referred by a urologist in private practice for a psychiatric evaluation at the University of New Mexico Health Sciences Center during the summer of 1995. The consultation was prompted by concern about the patient's request for the removal of his testes. The patient could not explain the urgency behind the request, and he denied a recent or specific reason for it. He was willing to comply with the psychiatric evaluation simply because he thought that the urologist would help him if the psychiatrist said it was OK.

After five evaluative sessions the patient stated that he wished to undergo an orchidectomy because his sexual impulses interfered with his spirituality: he described his sexuality as a stumbling block and a barrier between himself and 'the Creator'. He had worked hard for many years to minimize and master his sexual feelings and felt that he had achieved a lot. Nonetheless, he felt that castration was the final answer. His body, he said, was merely a tool of the mind and spirit. He described his testicles as obsolete, useless and harmful to his purpose in life, his genitalia were 'a pest, a fly you swat away that keeps coming back'. He felt guilt, shame and conflict about his sexual impulses. However, he considered his nocturnal erections as normal. He reported that past medication had not been helpful. He had been considering the testicular removal procedure for 10 years and thinking seriously about it for the preceding two years.

In describing the beliefs behind his castration request, Brother David talked about other monks he knew who felt that castration had helped to diminish or eliminate their sexual impulses. Repeatedly he suggested that his hormones might be partially responsible for his rebelliousness with respect to following rules in the monastery.

In explaining his wishes, Brother David referred to the two passages from Matthew mentioned earlier (see p. 303). When asked whether it might in some way be a spiritual failure to need an orchidectomy to deal with his sexuality, he replied, '[God] cares about overcoming, not *how* you overcome. Is it a failure for a cripple to be given crutches?' He expressed chagrin over the difficulties he had experienced in complying with the restrictions of his religious life, but he felt that overall he had gained much more than he had lost by joining the monastery.

Brother David was the second of three children. He described his family upbringing as 'laid back' but punctuated by occasional chaotic emotional responses from his homemaker mother. However, he always felt cared for. During childhood he felt closest emotionally to his grandfather. He denied physical and sexual abuse. He was raised as a Catholic, but during his young adulthood became disillusioned with the Church and abandoned his early thoughts of becoming a priest.

The patient's first sexual interaction occurred at the age of eight and involved another boy of similar age. He found this 'homosexual' experience pleasurable. From early adolescence he realized that he was aroused by males and not by females. He became openly gay during college, and briefly underwent supportive psychotherapy, which he described as very helpful overall. Brother David described his behaviour over the next few years as promiscuous; he reported numerous homosexual partners, daily masturbation and brief experimentation with transvestism and sadomasochistic sexual practices, which he did not like. He received frequent treatment for sexually transmitted infections. In retrospect, he said he had never felt satisfied, experiencing life and sex as if he were 'marking time'.

In his mid-twenties, Brother David felt that he wanted to change in order to 'learn the truth', so he returned to reading the Bible. He found out about a monastery from two monks whom he met one evening at a public gathering and joined the religious community shortly thereafter.

Brother David had been celibate in the ensuing years and had little contact with his family. Nevertheless, his commitment to 'rising to a higher level' was not as strong as he would have liked it to be. He engaged in frequent masturbation and felt considerable remorse. He had left the monastery for a time three years before the psychiatric evaluation, to take up an outside job. However, he soon 'realized that there was nothing in the outside world' for him. He felt that his religious dedication had been intermittently undermined by his rebellious nature but that he belonged within the monastery's spiritual community.

Brother David agreed to ask one of the other monks if he would come in to discuss his positive personal experience of castration. At the fifth meeting, he was accompanied by Brother Thomas, a middle-aged heterosexual man who had been involved with the monastery for more than two decades. Brother Thomas had undergone bilateral testicular removal in 1994 and since that time he had noted a '75 per cent decrease' in sexual interest in women. This change pleased him and he said the procedure had helped with his spirituality.

Brother David stated that other than the counselling he had received in college, he had received no psychiatric treatment. He reported having symptoms of mood disturbance, sleep disturbance, appetite changes, mild suicidal thoughts and feeling that at times he 'didn't belong'. Once during college he had taken a handful of aspirin when feeling confused, depressed and impulsive, but he had not attempted suicide again. His most recent period of significant depressive symptoms had occurred three or four months before the evaluation and was short-lived.

The patient did not appear impulsive and denied the desire to hurt or mutilate himself. His capacity for self-reflection, his insight and his judgement were adequate and in general, his thinking appeared to be flexible yet he was concrete and fixed – even to the point of lacking language – regarding his options for spiritual growth.

The consulting psychiatrist concluded that Brother David's wish for castration was authentic, long-standing, and non-psychotic in nature. Although the request was thought to be unrelated to delusional beliefs, his overvalued ideas regarding the relationship between sexuality and spirituality seemed unusual, rigid and intractable.

The private practice urologist chose not to perform the surgery and the patient was then seen by a second urologist at the university hospital, who conducted his own evaluation. The second urologist also chose not to perform the operation. He did, however, prescribe hormonal treatment, which should have had an anti-testosterone effect. The patient complied with treatment and was pleased by the results. He agreed to follow up with psychiatric care but stated that the monks were going to travel for a while so he could not commit to another appointment.

Brother David and Brother Thomas were two of 39 members of the Heaven's Gate cult who, apparently believing that they would evolve into a supernatural life form, committed suicide in Rancho Santa Fe, California, in March 1997. Eight of the men who died were reportedly found to have been castrated; we do not know whether Brother David was one of them.

The doctors who reported this case were naturally distressed to learn that this patient's life may have ended in such tragic circumstances. It is only after careful study, thought and consultation that they chose to publish this case report because of the many morals of its story.

Brother David joined the cult in young adulthood, when he felt that his sexual behaviour was excessive and would not provide satisfaction or fulfilment. By adopting the lifestyle of the cult and no longer engaging in sexual activity, he reportedly felt less anxious and unhappy. In this sense, the cult's sexual beliefs and expectations apparently helped him to defend himself against his conflict over his sexual identity and behaviour. Like many defences, however, this psychological 'solution' was inflexible and limiting.

In retrospect, phenomena related to destructive cultism may be identified in Brother David's clinical presentation. Milieu control was evident in the fact that Brother David could never be reached directly by letter or telephone.[28] He was typically unable to characterize and articulate his internal emotional state. Demand for purity could be seen in the rule of total celibacy, both mental and physical. The issue of sexuality was probably the one about which Brother David felt the most shame and guilt; this suggests a possible role of cultic confession. Loading of language and doctrine over person were evident in his narrow and concrete reasoning about options other than testicular removal for enhanced spirituality. Impressively, these features existed in an otherwise flexible, likeable and bright person.[29]

Finally, Brother David had become highly dependent on the cult to find meaning in his life. He was unable to tolerate life away from the monastery, and saw those outside the cult as incapable of reaching the higher plane of spirituality. It is uncertain whether he was uncomfortable with his homosexual orientation or his core gender identity. Nevertheless, gender itself was felt not to exist at the 'next level', and Brother David's castration request may have represented a first step towards departing from earth and earthliness. This way of thinking, conceptualized as dispensing with ordinary existence, relates directly to the stated motivation behind the group suicide of Heaven's Gate members.[30]

Concerns about the role of gender in the clinical care of this patient are pertinent because of a question raised by Brother David. He expressed puzzlement that physicians have performed elective oophorectomies (removal of the ovaries) for women's subjective and persistent symptoms. He said that although his own analogous symptoms would be cured by the orchidectomy, the procedure was, he felt, more difficult for him to obtain because he was a man. Another area of controversy relates to the greater acceptance of medical interventions that appear to enhance nature or natural sexuality (e.g. breast or penile implants, in vitro fertilization) than of those that diminish or seem to distort natural sexuality (e.g. orchidectomy, transsexual surgery). While conscientious differences of opinion persist around such topics, this case is valuable in that it makes explicit the values that operate within and throughout ethics-laden clinical decision-making.[31]

A moral of Brother David's story – complete with its lessons, supernatural events and untruths – is the value of recognizing patients' immense need for personal meaning in their lives. Brother David was a very likeable, intelligent man who felt that his search for spirituality through the monastery had helped him. We can see how it may also have destroyed him, and, for this reason, we may be tempted to dismiss the nature and magnitude of his everyday cult experience over two decades. Brother David's life history reminds us that spirituality is an important domain of psychological health that should be respected.

However, while the desire to escape from troubling sexual feelings may drive some to self-mutilation, other attempts at disfiguring the body arise out of the eroticization of disability.

A connection exists between genital self-mutilation and amputee fetishism, though this is extremely rarely reported. Some individuals with long-standing amputee fetishisms have gone to the extreme lengths of even amputating their genitals.[32]

Amputee fetishism is a sexual deviation that has traditionally received very little formal research attention from psychiatrists. The current thinking is that it may be more common than previously thought, since a surprisingly large number of Internet sites offer pornography for such fetishists.[33]

In the nomenclature of the paraphilias there is no term for the syndrome of erotic obsession or fetishism for amputated limbs or digits. However, in accordance with the tradition whereby a philia is assigned its appropriate Greek prefix, this syndrome is known as 'apotemnophilia', literally meaning 'amputation love'. The term was coined by Dr John Money and colleagues from Johns Hopkins Hospital, Baltimore, Maryland, in 1977 and it denotes the desire for amputation to be performed on one's own person, or a preference for a sexual partner who has undergone amputation.[34]

Little is known about apotemnophilia, although the German neurologist and psychiatrist Krafft-Ebing, in his 1890 report 'Lecture on Sexual Perversions', told of a man who had a relationship with a woman whose leg had been amputated. When this relationship broke up the man sought another woman with the same handicap.

Krafft-Ebing gives descriptions of preferences for a number of body handicaps, such as limping or walking with crutches.[35]

One man, as part of his very complicated paraphilia, simulated the amputation of his lower leg. He stuffed hip-boots full of newspapers in such a way that his leg, bent at the knee, fitted in. In this way he simulated an amputated stump and when no-one was around, walked through the house like this. Sometimes he would, in addition, put on one of his mother's skirts.[36]

More recently, Money and colleagues have reported cases of apotemnophilia, a preference for partners with amputations. Most of the patients had fantasized about amputation of their own legs and one of them had made serious but unsuccessful attempts to infect his leg in order to force doctors to amputate the limb. He failed because the wound was continually treated.

The relationship between sexual attraction and amputated limbs is a little-known phenomenon. It was brought to public attention in 1972 with a series of letters published in the forum section of the September and October issues of the magazine *Penthouse*. At first glance, it may have seemed that these letters were pranks. The writers seemed to be erotically obsessed with getting limbs amputated, and some had succeeded.

The two cases show that self-demand amputation is related to eroticization of the stump.[37] The apotemnophiliac obsession represents an *idée fixe* rather than a paranoid delusion. It may be conceptually related to, though it is not identical with, transsexualism, bisexuality, Munchausen syndrome and masochism. Like most paraphilias, it undoubtedly occurs more frequently, if not exclusively, in men.

Dr John Money and colleagues from the Psychohormonal Research Unit (PHRU) of Johns Hopkins Hospital report two cases of men voluntarily applying for amputation of a limb. In the following case apotemnophilia was manifested as an obsessive desire to have one leg surgically amputated above the knee.

The man who was a cryptic transsexual

The patient began his contact with the PHRU by way of a telephone call. He stated that he was a 'cryptic transsexual', and that his problem did not involve his genitals but his leg. His purpose for calling was to obtain a referral to any surgeon who would amputate his left leg. He was informed that this would not be possible, and having been assured of a confidential and non-judgmental consultation, he continued correspondence by way of telephone calls and mail over a period of four years.

He gave the impression that he had been referred by a well-known psychotherapist and a physician who was active in the care of pre-surgical transsexuals. When these professionals were contacted it was found that, although they were acquainted with the patient, they had not actually referred him. For three years prior to his communications with the PHRU he had engaged in group and private sessions with a psychotherapist. The physician's notes confirmed the patient's various problems, especially with regard to his active attempts to self-inflict injury to the left leg.

The patient succinctly expressed his complaint in the following written statement:

Since my 13th year, my conscious life has been absorbed, with varying intensity, in a bizarre and prepotent obsessive wish, need, desire to have my leg amputated above the knee; the image of myself as an amputee has as an erotic fantasy (each one different) accompanied EVERY sexual experience of my life: auto-, homo-, and heterosexual, since, and beginning with, puberty.

He ascribed an erotic component to seeing amputees performing, despite their handicap. He would fantasize on the achievement aspect of a leg amputee walking with crutches more than on the possibility of having that person as a sexual partner. Photographs of semi-nude or fully dressed amputees served as a visual aid during masturbation.

On two separate occasions the patient was able to have homo- and heterosexual experiences with amputees. The first entailed homosexual relations with an older male amputee. Although he would have preferred an adolescent male amputee, he expressed satisfaction with this experience. One specific thing that contributed to his pleasurable experience was the asymmetry of the man's body. Coitus with a female amputee, however, was not as pleasurable, and he proved unable to ejaculate with her. Indeed, he considered his heterosexual experiences generally unsatisfactory. His first marriage, when he was in his mid-twenties, ended in annulment after two years. He married again in his early thirties and this marriage lasted 12 years, during which time he had his first and only child, a daughter. The marriage ended in a legal separation. Retrospectively, he described this marriage as 'turbulent'.

Between marriages, he actively engaged in what he termed 'promiscuous homosexual activity', preferring adolescent males. He had first been sexually attracted to boys younger than himself when he was 14, but he had maintained nothing more than a platonic relationship with them. By this age his self-demand amputation desires were firmly established.

The patient himself perceived a relationship between his gender identity and apotemnophilia:

There are scattered occasions when I 'feel like a woman', viscerally, in terms of body image, and in these situations I loathe myself – it

313

makes me very apprehensive. Somehow this seems linked with the amputation fantasy. I would rather this [amputation] than lose the penis which would mean that I would be like a woman . . . My entire erotic activity now consists of trying to make 'real' the fantasy that I am an amputated homosexual adolescent, for in possessing my stump I can, concurrently, possess my penis.

The patient was serious in his quest to 'make "real" the fantasy'. Once doctors had refused to perform a proper surgical amputation, he began contemplating various accidents which could injure his leg enough to require amputation. He finally settled on inserting a tapered stainless steel stylus into his left tibia, using a hammer to drive it into the porous structure of the bone. Upon removal of the stylus he attempted to infect 'the fistula' with facial acne pus mixed with nasal and anal mucus, hoping to produce serious infection. When his leg showed signs of infection, he reported to a hospital. During his stay nobody challenged his pat story of an occupational accident. Much to his dismay, however, the infection cleared up and he was released.

He continued the attempt to get rid of his leg by placing a tourniquet around his left thigh and numbing the area with ice and injections of an anaesthetic. When the pain eventually became unbearable he stopped. There were other attempts with the stylus, and he informed a physician of his action. The physician provided remedial care to the infected area of his leg and gave him antibiotics. Aware of the patient's psychological status, this physician was reported to be unable to help further.

Reflecting on the seemingly masochistic aspect of his actions, the patient said:

The most disturbing aspect of these acts is that I am inflicting injury on myself – I do not like this. Pain is related to one's appetite for non-pain. The pain involved is trivial, and it is the result of these actions, not the anguish of the process, which is my goal.

He also disclosed his fear of social disapproval and loss of insurance benefits if it was discovered that his amputation was self-induced.

The patient expressed the idea that the cause of his apotemnophilia extended back into his early childhood and familial relationships. Prominent in his recollections was a domestic accident that had occurred when he was two years old. His left leg and foot had been severely burned when he capsized a pot of boiling oatmeal, rendering him unable to walk for almost a year.

He supplied a large amount of information on his early family life. He considered his mother to have been highly overprotective of him throughout his childhood, and he closely identified with her. She, too, had been severely burned by fire in another domestic accident when he was five years old. His father, he said, was overbearing, repressive, remote and above all hypercritical of his close association with the mother:

> Most of my emotional unrest accrues from the fact that I am acting out an overwhelmingly forbidden wish – like to be a girl – savagely forbidden. It is almost as if I will be establishing my male identity by means of the amputation. I could get trapped in a kind of surgical masochism . . . in trying to acquire characteristics more apt to secure my father's love or at least sympathy. Homosexuality is my retreat from overt masculine functioning. One of the anticipated 'pleasures' (for me) of being an amputee is the possibility of a genuine experience of identification.

In addition to apotemnophilia, this man had a rubber fetish, and a homosexual interest in adolescent youth. He disclosed that he had an adult older brother who was a chronic nocturnal neurotic and a divorced younger sister who was a lesbian.

The patient was discharged from the armed forces in his early twenties as 'undesirable', because he requested a release from service to enter psychotherapy. After he graduated from college he was employed for several years as a design engineer in a technical institute but became dissatisfied with his job as he felt he could perform the same work if he were an amputee. His ambition focused on a new career of helping amputees – and himself as a voluntary amputee – to achieve and possibly exceed the capabilities and performance of normal persons. He began the introductory courses at a university which he would need in order to take up prosthetics as an occupation. He expressed satisfaction in having embarked on a new career which would allow him to express his obsession in a more personally and socially acceptable manner.

He said that the non-judgmental approach taken in counselling served to lessen his anxieties regarding his identity and his guilt for inflicting injuries to his leg. In follow-up correspondence he mentioned some attempts to contact other well-known sexologists and psychiatrists for application of, amongst other programmes, LSD therapy. It is not known if he ever entered any such special therapy programmes. In the final follow-up report, he still had his leg and was working. He expressed more depression regarding apotemnophilia as he could resolve it neither by self-amputation nor by psychotherapy.

The apotemnophiliac patient finds no surgical tradition within which he can expect to obtain the service he requests. So if he arranges self-mutilation or amputation and presents himself for follow-up care, he has little choice other than to be secretive about the origin of his injury. In this sense, the apotemnophiliac may have something in common with the patient with Munchausen syndrome. The latter is obsessed with self-inducing symptoms repetitively for the sake of being a patient. By contrast, the apotemnophiliac induces symptoms for the sake of being an amputee, and for the sake of erotic arousal, and usually does not repeat self-injury.

One may think that apotemnophilia is synonymous with masochism. In the above there was no history of the eroticization of pain itself, but only of the healed, amputated stump. Thus, apotemnophilia, because it involves injury and pain, bears only a peripheral relationship to masochism: it is not identical with it.[38]

Less frequently, patients may be obsessed with persuading a partner to be amputated. More commonly, they search for a partner to be amputated or search for a partner among male and female victims of involuntary amputation. Pictures of amputees, revealing the amputated limb, with or without covering, may become their pornography or visual erotica. To involuntary amputees it comes as a surprise that there are some people for whom their deformity makes them a primary erotic choice, instead of a reject.

All of the paraphilias occur either predominantly or exclusively in males although it is also possible that the occurrence of female apotemnophilia has not yet been uncovered. If it does exist, then, as in the case of other paraphilias, it almost certainly occurs less frequently than male apotemnophilia.

In this case the patient cited non-erotic imagery of masculine over-achievement as providing an erotic turn-on in his amputee fantasies. Such imagery primarily consisted of amputees overcoming the adversity caused by a handicap. This reversal fits apotemnophilia into the schema of other paraphilias, as all paraphilias transcend the forbidden. In apotemnophilia the fear of losing one's limb and struggling with a handicap is metamorphosed and eroticized into an impulsion to be amputated and to emerge as superior or super-normal in achievement.

Though the patient mentioned here did not want an alteration of his gender status, he perceived a relationship between amputation and transsexualism in the sense that both involve surgical alteration of the body on demand. Transsexualism has been known to be associated with self-mutilation and self-castration: it is one manifestation of a transposition of gender identity from masculine to feminine, or vice versa. A lesser degree of transposition was evident in this case study, in that bisexualism was a feature; the amputee impulsion could be interpreted as a way of preserving the penis and masculinity.

The Freudian view that there is a link between sexuality, castration fears and apotemnophilia finds some support in the following case.

Psychiatrists Thomas Wise and Ram Chandran Kalyanam from Johns Hopkins University in Baltimore, Maryland, and Inova Fairfax Hospital in Virginia, USA, report the case of a man who amputated his penis following instructions that he had obtained from the Internet.[39]

The man turned on by body parts

Mr A., a 49-year-old accountant, was admitted to the urology service from the emergency room after he severed his penis with a sterilized razor blade. To his horror, he was unable to stop the bleeding and experienced severe pain. The patient called an ambulance and was taken to the hospital, where his penis was reattached through microvascular surgery. This was his second attempt to remove his penis. Six weeks earlier he had bound the base of his penis for 24 hours, using the 'elastrator' that he had purchased on the Internet.

He recalls intense sexual arousal during puberty when he was looking through his physician father's textbooks and found pictures of women with amputated limbs. He found such pictures highly arousing and began to seek out similar pictures in medical libraries. Until the six months prior to his self-mutilation, his preferred masturbatory fantasies involved making love to women with amputated limbs.

At the age of 28, he met and married a woman who had lost her leg during adolescence. He found her amputated stump intensely sexually arousing and when making love to her, he would try to fondle and kiss it. She rarely permitted this and it was at this time that he began to develop a large collection of pornography focused on women with amputations.

His wife discovered these materials and became enraged. The marriage became increasingly difficult and the couple divorced after 8 years. The patient has an 11-year-old son, who has been in psychotherapy for many years because of a developmental disability. Mr A. continued a close relationship with his son and was a leader of his son's Scout troop. He had been living alone for the past six years, with his major interest being the Internet.

Mr A. said that during the year prior to his penile amputation, he had undergone a lot of stress. His elderly mother had become very ill with chronic pulmonary disease and was on a ventilator at the time of his attempted amputation. His former wife had become increasingly difficult regarding child support payments, and Mr A. began to experience both financial difficulties and stress at work due to a new supervisor. It was during this period that the ideas of genital amputation developed, along with symptoms of depression, which included insomnia and diminished motivation.

The patient was an only child. His father, he said, was always distant and rarely at home, and his mother, in the patient's words, 'cared more about herself than me'. He had friends at school, excelled in academic activities and described college as being a happy experience. He entered military service after college and served overseas without difficulties. During that time, he sought out prostitutes with amputations. He denied homosexual activity, cross-dressing or other forms of fetishistic activity.

On the morning after his surgery, the patient was alert and co-operative. He appeared ashamed of his behaviour and was not sure why he had actually done it, but he admitted that it was exciting; he could not honestly assure the staff that he would not try to remove his penis again. He openly admitted that he continued to be inter-ested in amputees although there was no evidence of psychotic thought processes, hallucinations or delusions.

During his three-week hospital stay, Mr A.'s initial conviction that he wished his penis removed diminished, and he began to experience a more depressed mood and was tearful in discussing what he had done to himself. His depression was exacerbated by the fear that he might lose visitation rights to his son. His wife expressed her rage at his fetish, which she felt diminished her self-worth. She did recog-nize, however, the impact of his mother's illness upon his psychological state. In fact, she had been helping to care for her former mother-in-law despite the divorce. Eventually, the couple was able to agree on future visiting arrangements with their son. After discharge, the patient was seen in outpatient psychotherapy, where his depression was treated with antidepressants.

He continued to remain interested in amputee eroticism but denied any renewed interest in mutilating his genitals. Restorative surgery allowed him to urinate without difficulty, but he was unable to obtain an erection. This did not seem to disturb him, since he was able to masturbate with some pleasure, despite a flaccid penis, and described a sensation of ejaculation.

As mentioned, little is known concerning the origin of the desire for amputation but the first conscious fantasies probably originate in prepuberty. In the histories of several cases transvestite and transsexual fantasies and desires also occur. Money and his colleagues point to the possibility that with amputation the fear of castration is averted. (As previously mentioned, one of the men they described said that 'in possessing my stump I can concurrently possess my penis').

Dr Walker Everaerd recently reported a case that is similar in a number of ways. The desire for amputation is the same. The patient's history, however, deviates essentially on a number of points from the men described by Money and colleagues.[40]

The man who had a sexual preference for handicap

Doctor Everaerd first saw Mr B. after he had contacted the doctor by letter. In the course of two and a half years Dr Everaerd regularly spoke to Mr B. about his problems. In the first session Mr B. immediately said that he had not come for psychotherapy. In his letter he had pointed out the similarity between his desire for change and those in cases of transsexualism: 'Just as a transsexual is not happy with his own body but longs to have the body of another sex, in the same way I am not happy with my present body, but long for a peg-leg.'

Mr B. himself had gone to great lengths to find information about apotemnophilia. He located a volume of letters and articles published by a commercial organization (Ampix/IMC Enterprises, California) and from this it became evident that alloapotemnophilia occurred in men and women.

Several of the paraphilias can be classified in reciprocal pairs, as in sadism/masochism, or exhibitionism/voyeurism. The same reciprocity occurs in apotemnophilia, in that it may be both self-directed (autoapotemnophilia) and other-directed (alloapotemnophilia).

Besides a number of contacts with amputees, Mr B. met or corresponded with people who had alloapotemnophilia. In this way he heard from a correspondent friend in the US about two people who had had amputations: one person's leg had been misformed through use of a brace, after which amputation was obtained. The other had his leg amputated by a surgeon with whom he originally had had a paedophilic relation.

For years Mr B. had attempted to contact amputees via advertisements. This course of action wasn't particularly successful although almost all the 'porno' magazines printed his advertisements and a few did result in meetings or correspondence. Mr B. also tried to get his advertisements printed in *Vrij Nederland* (a Dutch weekly), but they were rejected: the advertising editor found the 'choice of words' requesting a partner with an amputation inappropriate. He added as an important personal argument: 'I find that the relation between the affliction of one person and the sexual preference of another oversteps my bounds.'

Mr B. was 65 years old, and was born into the lower middle class in a large city. His parents were very religious and had a strong sense of social status. They forbade him and his siblings to play with other possibly lower-class children in the neighbourhood. The general atmosphere in the home was good, according to Mr B., although physical affection was totally absent.

During his childhood he experienced feelings of loneliness. He was a good student in elementary school, then went on to a Roman Catholic seminary, but had only a mediocre scholastic record. At the age of 18 he went back to live with his parents. He had worked as a clerk in an office and was always active in club and group activities. At the time of writing, he had been unfit for work for several years.

He began to masturbate when he was 14. He was never attracted to girls or women and until his 44th year he had had no sexual partners. It then became increasingly obvious to him that he felt attracted to men. He is very hesitant about entering into relationships, saying he has a need for warmth and tenderness; his sexual needs for a partner are less clear.

Mr B. described in detail his experiences and the desire for amputation:

'When I was eight years old, I became conscious of the fact that I was strongly attracted to people who were missing a leg. It was in

320

the beginning of the 1920s and at that time prosthesis was not paid for by national health insurance. There were, therefore, few people who could afford it. Some amputees walked with crutches, by far the majority had a peg-leg. Amputees were thus more easily recognizable then than they are now. Men and boys were way in majority. I remember only a few cases of women with peg-legs and only one girl. The fashion was also different then; without exception young boys wore short pants until about their 17th year. In the case of one-legged boys, a large piece of the wood was exposed, something which fascinated me enormously. I became extremely aroused by it. Because such boys were not troubled by their mutilation and cheerfully, and with a certain ease, took part in all the street games, including football, I never felt any pity towards them. Naturally they had lost a leg, but I never had the feeling that they really missed it. I was jealous of children who played in the street. They got attention and seemed happy to me, even the boy who struck me the most (attracted me the most) had a wooden leg and he was a so-called unhappy boy. Nevertheless I considered him happier than myself and felt that it was not so awful to be without a leg.

'This opinion steadily became stronger and developed into the idea that it must be nice to have a wooden leg. I, indeed, became more attracted and aroused by it, since the boy was surely happier than me. Unconsciously such a peg-leg became synonymous with happiness and because I also wanted to be happy I longed for a peg-leg. I was about 10 years old when I first became aware of this desire. The desire took hold of me and did not diminish or disappear even when I was old enough to realize intellectually what it actually meant to be mutilated for life. For me the peg-leg remained synonymous with happiness and it still does.

'In the beginning, the desire was kept alive by seeing people (especially boys) with a peg-leg with whom I identified; later the desire sustained itself; I no longer needed to be stimulated by seeing a peg-leg. In fact in the last 15 years there has been hardly any question of that. And yet it has been precisely in these last years that the desire has gotten stronger, so strong that I can no longer control it but am completely controlled by it. The realization of it has become indispensable for my personal happiness and peace of mind. Through this unfulfilled desire my entire existence has been seriously hindered. It controls and limits my thinking. It has hampered my social intercourse because I cannot be, or can hardly be, interested in others. It has paralysed my life so that I can only very irregularly, and then with the greatest of difficulty, force myself into any kind of activity. The only alternative I can see is ending my life.

'What does having a peg-leg mean to me now, and moreover what kind of feelings does it give me? First of all it is still, and undiminished, synonymous with happiness. Besides that, it also satisfies to a large extent my desire to be different from others, also physically. Dissatisfaction with present-day society? Rancour? From that also arises my aversion to prosthesis; I want to be visibly amputated, visibly different from others. Furthermore, the sensory experiences (seeing, feeling, hearing) of my own peg-leg could give me a feeling of physical and mental well-being; to walk in such a way gives me a feeling of intense happiness. I cannot speak from experience but rather from the inner certainty that it is so.

'In the area of sex, the seeing and touching of a leg stump gives me an enormous kick; it does not have to be my own leg stump. I have had experience in this area. This is, however, not the reason I want to be amputated. To be amputated is only important for me insofar as it is the necessary condition for wearing a wooden leg. Without this consequence I do not need to be amputated . . . in the year 1976 the use of a peg-leg is for nearly everyone a completely incomprehensible thing and one which in no possible way can be made attractive. Thus it is merely a personal question based upon an inner conviction that a peg-leg is necessary to my personal happiness and peace of mind and is an absolute condition for my existence. Naturally over the years I have thought of many arguments against amputation, have carefully considered them and rejected them, and not only for emotional reasons. It is not normal. But what is normal and who is normal?

'Naturally I have considered the consequences as far as possible. First of all we are concerned here with a matter that once realized is irreversible and impossible to bring back to its former state. It is a question of "a life sentence". But it is precisely this "life sentence" which is an essential part of my desire. It has nothing to do with walking "one time" on a peg-leg; rather it is the permanent possession of a wooden leg which I deem necessary for my personal happiness. Certainly it is true that one's desires or fantasies are often more beautiful than reality in that a desire once realized can sometimes lead to nothing more than disillusionment. That could also be the case with me, I know. In each case one must consider the possibility of a setback after the first exhilarating moment of realization, a phenomenon that is explainable psychologically and is even to be expected. Only after the working through of the new reality can there be real satisfaction and joy, in a given case happiness being very well possible, albeit on more realistic grounds than previously, because reality has now taken the place of fantasy.

'Moreover, I do not believe in ideal situation. Naturally it is no joke to go through life with one leg. Nevertheless I will be happy when one of my legs is amputated, since this is the condition necessary for me to wear a peg-leg.

'Yet walking on a peg-leg will be decidedly less pleasant than the fantasy which now deludes me. I feel that I must take the chance and bear the consequences. Nothing can be achieved now without taking a risk. And the proposed goal, my personal happiness and peace of mind, is definitely worth the risk. In the case of a disappointment I will continue to live without blaming anyone else or being a nuisance to others with my self-complaining, just as I have done in previous situations (also caused by my own actions and also irreversible).'

Mr B. describes a temporary solution:

'Several years ago I bought a pair of crutches with which I walk through the house. I then imagine that my leg has already been amputated and that gives me a very good feeling. In anticipation, I am already in love with my stump, which I still don't have, and with a wooden leg, which I also don't have yet. It pleases me to be visibly, physically different from others: a man with one leg, a man with a wooden leg. I go through a range of feelings that I, in fact, can't possibly have, because I have not yet experienced them. It's as if I've already walked on a peg-leg before and am now going through the experience again. I find these feelings, real sensory feelings, so pleasant, because they give me happiness.

'I like feeling how my body supports itself on a peg-leg because the stump rests against the side of the stump shaft, fairly high off the ground, while the surface touching the ground is not larger than the 30 cm of the rubber knob. Feeling how I walk on a peg-leg: the jerking up of the shoulder, the swinging out of the stiff, unbendable stick, the shock felt all the way up to the stump of my leg when I set the peg-leg down. Hearing the dull thump each time the rubber knob touches the floor when walking. Seeing the painted black stick and rubber knob that stick out of my pants leg, the realization – with joy – that I have not any leg. In short: the sensory experience of my peg-leg and the knowledge that I have one.

'Having taken into consideration the possible disappointments and a certain amount of setback, one shouldn't make a too hasty decision. The conclusion is that, despite everything, it must nevertheless happen. Besides that I want it to happen (a freely made decision), and I will, without exception, accept all the foreseen consequences. The real difficulty is then not "how do I get rid of this desire?" nor "how can I get a peg-leg?" but "where do I find a surgeon who will amputate a (healthy) leg?" I need and ask for help to answer this question.'

Mr B. became attracted to amputation in his 10th year. An amputated boy is, according to him, happier than he himself. The oppressive situation at home also plays an important role. Being handicapped by missing a leg was apparently an advantage in comparison to his situation.

Mr B. currently realizes that the fulfilment of his desire is impossible. Certainly one of the main reasons for this is the unfamiliarity of health professionals with apotemnophilia. Informing these professionals is one way Mr B. sees of changing the situation.

In many such cases the therapist will probably presume that the patient has a delusion. Nevertheless, in contrast to a patient with delusions, Mr B. knows very clearly that others do not accept his desire.

In one respect, experiences in sessions with transsexuals are very much like those with Mr B. At first Mr B. emphatically stated that he did not want psychotherapy: he wanted his body to adapt to the image that he is convinced will make him happy.

Throughout Mr B.'s history, simulating a leg stump has played an important role. The stump has been greatly eroticized but the desire for amputation has no erotic meaning. Although contact with amputated partners satisfies the erotic desires of Mr B., it has not changed his desire to be amputated.

Some argue that amputee fetishism is a 'deformative' fetish, whose genesis lies in early childhood experiences with caregivers who have a deformity. In the reported cases, however, early life experiences are inconsistent. One patient experienced a serious leg and foot burn when he was two years old and linked his fetish to this experience. Another patient was born with a club foot that drew much abuse from his father, who berated him for walking abnormally. One patient linked his fetish to early childhood observations of amputees in post-World War I Holland.

Although the fetish has also been linked to a domineering mother, in the present case there was no reported link of a traumatic event that led to an interest in amputees.

The clinically significant issue is how an individual with an amputee fetish evolves into a genital self-mutilator. Although the two phenomena may be separate, it is equally plausible to suggest that the fantasy of penile amputation is an upward displacement from the amputee fetish.

Transvestites may also become depressed in settings of loss and stress and subsequently attempt genital mutilation.[41] From a behavioural perspective, one could hypothesize that during puberty when the patient experienced nascent erotic arousal, his preferred masturbatory pattern developed from pictures of amputees in his father's textbooks; this was reinforced by subsequent masturbatory experiences with similar images. This is similar to what John Money has described as an individual's 'love map': a person's unique experience in discovering a preferred erotic stimulus.[42]

In summary, amputee fetishism may be more common than is reflected in the scant psychiatric literature available. It is not an innocuous behaviour if it can lead to genital mutilation and the onset of depression in such paraphilics may have serious consequences. Such cases raise the question of information that is offered over the Internet and how such data may be harmful to vulnerable individuals.

The vast majority of cases of male genital self-mutilation involved a diagnosed psychosis; however, most of the women did not have a psychotic illness. In female genital self-mutilators, three categories are noted: (1) self-induced abortors; (2) women with severe personality disorders or a factitious disorder; and (3) women with a psychotic illness. Indeed, it has been noted that, while self-mutilation in general is considerably more common in women, psychotically induced genital self-harm in females is a rarity.

As mentioned above, in female genital self-mutilation the presence of a psychotic illness is rare, but most of the women who deliberately inflict these injuries have severe personality disorders, again often characterized by dysmorphophobic features.

Dysmorphophobia (see p. 202) is the delusional or obsessive belief that there is something wrong with a part of the body. This leads to attempts to camouflage or change it through surgery. Perhaps the extreme logical extension of dysmorphophobia is transsexualism, where a patient believes that their whole body is wrong

– that they have been born into the wrong body in terms of gender.

A few transsexual patients have vainly sought surgical help to achieve genital mutilation and some have then proceeded to mutilate themselves. Non-psychotic self-mutilators are more likely to be disturbed in sexual identity. Such disturbance has been supposed to result from early loss of the father as the male figure of identification, or the predominance of the mother, but careful statistical analysis does not support this.

Because a proportion of those who genitally mutilate themselves do so for reasons linked to sexual identity disturbance, transsexualism became identified as a new 'disorder'. The treatment proffered is a surgical procedure; part of the justification of which is that it prevents self-mutilation occurring in the future.[43]

The first reported sex-change operation took place in Germany in 1931 but the procedure was not widely known until Christin (George) Jorgensen's much publicized surgery in Denmark in 1952.[44] The desire to be a member of the opposite sex had always been viewed by psychoanalysts as a perversion. In 1954, however, US hormone specialist Harry Benjamin asserted that Jorgensen's claim that he was a woman trapped within a man's body was indicative of a unique illness distinct from transvestism and homosexuality, perhaps conditioned by hormonal factors and not amenable to psychotherapy due to its fundamental biological nature. He named this non-psychopathic sexual disorder 'transsexualism'.[45]

Benjamin's discussion of diagnosis, aetiology and treatment provoked hostile reactions from psychoanalysts, who objected that it is one thing to remove diseased tissue and quite another to amputate healthy organs because emotionally disturbed patients request it.[46]

Professional opposition to sex-change surgery and disputes over its legality inhibited recognition of transsexualism as a disease for several years. In 1966, however, Johns Hopkins University physicians admitted performing experimental sex-reassignment surgery and claimed to be able to diagnose true 'Benjaminian' transsexuals. A 1965 survey showed that only 3 per cent of US surgeons would take seriously a request for sex-change surgery, yet by the early 1970s such operations were becoming commonplace.[47]

Gender identity disorder has two features: strong and persistent cross-gender identification and persistent discomfort about one's assigned gender or a sense of inappropriateness in the role of that gender. This disorder is manifested by cross-dressing and a search for hormonal and surgical reassignment of anatomic sex.[48]

Within the boundaries of our present scientific knowledge, the gender identity disordered patient is a physically, endocrinologically and genetically normal individual. All biochemical, radiological or other investigations are therefore negative. Consequently, the diagnosis emerges during the clinical interview.

There is a preoccupation or overwhelming desire on the part of the patient to acquire the anatomical sexual characteristics of their chosen gender and during adolescence there would be occasional masturbatory activities with fantasies of sexual contact with a person of the same anatomical sex, seen by the patient as a hetero-sexual scenario. Cross-gender identification of the adult primary transsexual almost invariably starts prior to puberty, and cross-dressing first practised in adolescence or adulthood makes the diagnosis at least questionable. The course in males is either a continuous unhappiness from childhood through adolescence into adulthood, or a late onset in early or even mid-adulthood, sometimes concurrent with transvestic fetishism.[49]

Anal intercourse, in the pre-operative phase of the male-to-female transsexual, is at times practised; it is explained as a wish for penetration and therefore femininity, and occasionally enjoyed. Marriage in the male-to-female transsexual is by no means un-common; reasons given are social pressure, loneliness or belief in a spontaneous cure for the condition. Almost invariably this ends in separation. It is rare in the female-to-male variant but sometimes initiated by the wish to have a child. It should, however, be added that the majority of male-to-female transsexuals who are attracted to males (approximately two-thirds of all male transsexuals) reject homosexual partners and desire virile, heterosexual males.[50]

Not infrequently the progressive, continuous course in the male-to-female transsexual is interrupted by a phase in early adulthood characterized by a return of gender identity to the anatomically 'correct' one. This is accompanied by exaggeratedly male, almost 'macho' behaviour and an occupational or recreational choice matching the return to masculinity (enlistment in the armed forces, professional car racing, buckjumping, mountain climbing). The desire for permanent femininity or even surgical reassignment in a middle-aged transvestite does not often represent a gender identity disorder. It may rather be a desire born out of diminishing sex drive, love of clothes or jewellery, or an attraction to a non-aggressive, 'feminine' existence.[51]

A recent development has been the arrival of a third gender – not male or female but 'transgendered'. The transgender movement is supposed to have started officially when in the summer of 1994 a group of transsexuals and their supporters set up camp outside the lesbian-feminist Michigan Womyn's Music Festival. Since 1991 when Nancy Burkholder was escorted off the land after coming out as a post-operative male-to-female transsexual, the festival's insistence on original female sex as the qualifying ground for gendered membership appeared to be openly used to exclude transsexual women.[52]

Despite the common notion that adult gender identity disorder is fixed and persistent once it develops, some reports describe transsexual patients who 'improved', sometimes even without treatment. Some, for example, eventually returned to their birth gender identity and role without treatment, but long-term follow-up data are unavailable. Improvements have also occurred after various psychological treatments.[53]

Professor Isaac Marks and colleagues from the Institute of Psychiatry in London have reported a case of adult gender identity disorder that remitted for four years in a man who was also sexually attracted to males from early adolescence and who developed severe obsessive-compulsive disorder (OCD) at age 40 after he became depressed when his mother died.[54]

If a form of transsexualism can turn out to be a temporary state and if conditions like obsessive-compulsive disorder can be linked to it, as is sometimes the case, then it is possible that some people diagnosed with transsexualism really have another disorder altogether. A prime candidate turns out to be multiple personality disorder.[55]

Psychiatrists Dr J. Modestin and Dr G. Ebner of the Psychiatric University Hospital in Zurich report the case of a young female patient who had symptoms of transsexualism and surgical intervention was considered.[56] When she was admitted to the hospital after having become depressed and suicidal, a thorough examination and observation revealed the presence of multiple personality disorder (MPD). Even though transsexualism and MPD are two different conditions, there are many similarities between them. The possibility of MPD should be considered in every case of transsexualism.

The transsexual who turned out to have multiple personalities

The patient, a 20-year-old female, was admitted to a psychiatric hospital because of a severe depression with pronounced suicidal thoughts. At admission, the patient declared that she was actually a man and asked to be called by a male name. The psychiatrist who had been treating her as an outpatient confirmed that he had given her the diagnosis of transsexualism and explained that her menstrual bleeding had strongly contributed to the development of the depression.

The patient said she had felt she was a boy since about five years old, that she had frequently behaved like a tomboy and had dressed accordingly. She had always felt uncomfortable and inappropriate being a girl even after puberty and she had been preoccupied for at least three years with getting rid of her female sex characteristics. After having learned about the possibility of an operation six months previously, she requested an operative sex reassignment.

At the inpatient unit the patient's behaviour was stormy and changeable. At times she was depressed, complained of not really being aware of herself, expressed feelings of emptiness, confirmed suicidal ideas and repeatedly slashed her arms. At other times she was relaxed, had good contact with some fellow patients and enjoyed playing the piano and ergotherapy sessions. Several times she left the hospital, but would call to say that she did not know where she was, or would return to the hospital asking the doorkeeper if he knew her name and where her unit was. The diagnosis of a dissociative disorder including multiple personality disorder was suspected.

The clinical exploration confirmed this diagnosis and the existence of three (later four) other personalities became apparent in repeated interviews. The first of the 'others' had appeared at the age of 4–5 years. A little later, another personality appeared: a boy, changing his age between five and 15, who had never been satisfied with his female body, who asked for the sexual reassignment surgery and who prompted the patient to take the appropriate steps. The individual personalities had limited knowledge of each other, none knowing all of them. The patient's original self, her original personality, she said, had died between the ages of seven and eight.

The patient admitted that even during those long-lasting periods when the boy clearly predominated, taking full control of her

329

behaviour and pursuing the idea of sex reassignment, the female personalities were also present, although they stayed in the background. The female personalities made the patient feel desperate and suicidal. During her treatment the patient came to realize that her transsexual feelings were only part of the complex problems she faced and she soon dropped the idea of sex reassignment surgery.

In this patient the diagnostic criteria for transsexualism were fulfilled. Beyond that, the characteristics defining 'core transsexualism' were present: namely an early age of onset of less than 13 years (so far known); lack of sexual arousal with cross-dressing; rather homosexual orientation and little sexual activity. These characteristics have been considered a better predictor for sex reassignment surgery. Indeed, surgery was considered. However, it turned out that the transsexual pathology was no more than a symptom of MPD, the underlying disorder.

The two disorders seem to be quite different. Whereas biological females are less likely to develop transsexualism than males, 90 per cent of patients with MPD are females. Transsexuals present their symptoms openly and ask for a specific intervention; in contrast, MPD patients frequently hide their symptoms so that they must be actively looked for. Transsexualism is usually a self-diagnosis and MPD frequently represents a delayed diagnosis. In spite of the high prevalence of other psychopathology, the transsexual patients present themselves with specific complaints demanding specific interventions, whereas a plethora of complaints is regularly presented by MPD patients. As a rule, childhood trauma, particularly sexual abuse, is found in patients with MPD. Abuse in childhood, including violence and neglect, occurs in female transsexuals less frequently than in MPD cases.[57]

Apart from these differences a more thorough study of both conditions reveals many similarities between transsexualism and MPD. Among others, these concern the frequency of occurrence which may also be influenced by wider social influences, psychopathology profiles and aetiology. Both MPD and – at least female – transsexualism have been considered primarily to be psychological disorders: a reaction to major psychic and/or physical trauma (MPD) and a result of chronic assaults on the patient's femininity and female sexuality (female transsexualism). These similarities do not appear by chance: both disorders have the same core problem, namely the disturbance of identity (a continuous coherent experience of the unique personal self, including bodily self). So the joint occurrence of both disorders in one patient does not come as a surprise, although no such case has yet been described in the literature.

What these cases do alert us to is the central role our sense of sexuality and gender occupy in our conception of our core identity.

13

Two's Company, Three's a Crowd: Multiple Personality Disorder

Was't Hamlet wrong'd Laertes? Never Hamlet.
If Hamlet from himself be ta'en away,
And when he's not himself does wrong Laertes,
Then Hamlet does it not, Hamlet denies it.
Who does it then? His madness.

Hamlet, V ii

Multiple personality disorder, MPD, is one of the most dramatic and controversial diagnoses in psychiatry and was made famous by books and films such as *Three Faces of Eve* (1957) and *Sybil* (1977) – in which Sybil claimed 16 different personalities. Patients contend that totally different personalities inhabit their minds and can completely take over their bodies from time to time.[1]

These personalities might exhibit a different gender, age, skill, hand preference, motivation and emotional style to the usual persona displayed. After a switch back to the base or core personality, the patient cannot remember the period during which any other personalities were in control.[2]

The theory is that in the face of some extreme trauma, often childhood sexual abuse, the mind deals with overwhelming stress by producing an alternative personality which experiences the shock, so protecting the core personality for whom the terrible event never occurred. British psychiatrists have always been more sceptical than their American counterparts over whether MPD properly exists. This cynicism follows its use as a defence in several legal battles over heinous crimes, where the perpetrator claimed that another personality in their minds was guilty, but not them.[3]

In the early 1980s Ken Bianchi, a US serial killer nicknamed the Hillside Strangler, claimed it was another personality inhabiting his body who had committed the murders. The evaluating psychiatrists suspected he was faking his supposed two personalities, and told him that in MPD there are usually at least three different personalities. Bianchi immediately produced another new personality.[4]

Examples like these render many experts deeply sceptical about MPD, but just because some cases may be examples of malingering does not mean that all are. More convincing cases exist, which ensures that MPD raises interesting philosophical questions about personal identity.[5]

The problem of personal identity revolves around the question: what makes you, you? What is it that makes up your personal identity so that even when you awake after a deep and long slumber, you still have a strong sense of personal continuity with the person who fell asleep the night before? These are not questions that normally impede our daily progress through life because our sense of apparent personal identity is so strong that it rarely seems a controversial issue. We also observe that those around us appear to demonstrate definable personalities with set tastes and attitudes, and this constellation of characteristics does not seem to vary widely in the one person from day to day.[6]

However, the striking psychiatric phenomena of dissociation, MPD and hysterical fugue all raise troubling questions about whether we should take our sense of personal identity quite so much for granted. What is especially intriguing about these phenomena is that they place our sense of memory, in particular memory of past personally significant events, right at the centre of our sense of who we are. Obviously we might regard memory as an important part of conscious life, but if it wasn't for these conditions, we might never have realized how essential memory is to personal identity.[7]

The phenomena popularly identified as evidence of 'multiple personality disorder' are also strangely attractive. The stories suggest that those who provide, who are, the evidence for this disorder are usually in acute distress, but those who wish to believe in it find the idea almost exhilarating. After all, most of us would prefer to think that we had undeveloped possibilities – that it would be exciting to be a married academic today, a celibate bus driver tomorrow and a teenage hooligan on Sundays.[8]

Some of us believe that 'multiple personality' reveals a truth about us all, that none of us is actually the simple, heroic self that we pretend: 'the self' is no more than an occasionally concordant swarm of impulses, easily divided.[9] The more sceptical suspect that it is a wish to avoid responsibility, and guilt, that causes some of us to pretend not to be the selves that actually we are.

The first characteristic of multiple personality disorder – or dissociative identity disorder (DID), as it is now called – is the 'presence of two or more distinct identities or personality states', usually referred to as 'alter personalities' or simply 'alters'. The second defining feature is that 'at least two of these identities or personality states recurrently take control of the person's behaviour'. The alter personality in control at a given time is referred to as 'out'; alters that are aware, yet not in control, of the individual's behaviour are termed 'co-conscious'. Often alters will be neither out nor co-conscious. In such cases, the individual may be amnesiac for what occurred during a period of time, and it is this amnesia that constitutes the third and final feature of the disorder, an 'inability to recall important personal information that is too extensive to be explained by ordinary forgetfulness'.[10]

Although this psychiatric condition is characterized by two or more distinct personalities within an individual, each with their own behaviour and complex social interactions, a controlling dominant personality is normally present (the usual self or host personality).[11]

This condition was first described in 1816 but with fewer than 300 case reports in the literature, it has always been a controversial diagnosis. It is included in disease classification systems under the category 'Dissociative disorders of memory'. Most diagnoses of MPD emanate from the United States and Canada, where up to 2 per cent of the general population are believed to meet the diagnostic criteria, yet it is treated with scepticism by European psychiatrists who regard it as iatrogenic in origin. In other words, the medical profession's belief in the disorder has created it.[12]

The increase in reported cases in the last three decades is believed to stem either from a growing awareness of the disorder and of its association with childhood trauma or from an interest in the disorder by writers and film-makers. Other theories are that this is a form of autohypnosis – people hypnotize themselves into the diagnosis by their firm belief in it. Perhaps there is also a learning theory element – by observing the phenomenon on film or in the papers people come to copy it.[13]

There are currently two primary positions: the traumagenic and the iatrogenic theories. Proponents of the traumagenic position state that DID develops in response to overwhelming trauma during childhood, primarily physical and/or sexual abuse, perhaps as a form of 'complex post-traumatic stress disorder (PTSD)' or 'disorders of extreme stress'.[14]

Proponents of the iatrogenic position maintain that DID is not post-traumatic in nature; they see it created by psychotherapy and/or the popular media. According to this theory, psychotherapists are usually responsible for the development of the disorder in their patients by suggesting the concept of multiplicity, using hypnosis to create symptoms, asking leading questions regarding symptoms in order to meet diagnostic criteria and then reinforcing behaviours consistent with the disorder. Several critiques of the iatrogenesis model of DID, based on the growing body of research on dissociative disorders, have seriously challenged this model.[15]

Perhaps the most widely held view in psychology is that dissociation is a single continuum, with 'highway hypnosis' as its mildest form and DID as its most extreme manifestation.[16]

In highway hypnosis you are lulled into a trance-like state by the repetitive scenery provided by prolonged driving. As a result your mind can be miles away thinking about something else while another part of your consciousness controls the car and attends to the road. Consequently you can reach the end of a long journey and suddenly become aware that you have no recollection of large parts of the trip although you were definitely there.[17]

Dissociation has been used to refer to memory losses, fragmentation of knowledge of the self and experience, and splitting of emotional aspects of experiences, numbing of feelings, psychological escape from unpleasant stimuli and trance-like states. The theory is that in the face of a very stressful situation you tend to dissociate so that only a part of you faces the stress. For example a soldier in the height of combat probably has to dissociate in order to accomplish violent tasks yet retain a sense of himself as a reasonable person and a family man.[18]

Dissociative experiences are altered sensory and consciousness states that draw attention away from some aspect of immediate awareness. In DID, the dissociation is so extreme that a completely separate personality evolves and splits away from the rest of the mind: one which the person might not be fully aware of.[19]

However, as noted earlier, the diagnosis of DID is extremely controversial. A highly critical editorial in the *British Journal of Psychiatry* in March 1995 suggested that the condition is largely generated within therapy.[20] The diagnosis, as the *New Scientist* (17 June 1995) reported, seems excessively subject to trends and fashions. Some interpret the disorder as one person having different strategies for dealing with a stressful world, rather than as the emergence of a plurality of persons.[21]

Certainly some dissociation is normal for anyone but the extreme forms are particularly linked to childhood sexual abuse. In this context dissociation is seen, at best, as necessary for survival in early life but problematic in adulthood. A child being abused by a carer or parent might usefully dissociate so that he or she is a different person during the abuse. This allows the child to maintain a more normal relationship with an abusing parenting figure – the abuse happened to another person, not the child. Also it might permit the child to forget the abuse altogether. Though this is useful to the child, at worst it is seen as highly disorganizing and disabling when manifested as DID in adulthood.[22]

A milder form of dissociation might not be the evolution of a different personality but simply the inability to recall an abusive experience. So dissociative amnesia is one variant of psychogenic amnesia or amnesia caused by psychological difficulties like stress.[23]

The most striking form of psychogenic amnesia is referred to by psychiatrists as hysterical fugue – the term 'fugue' comes from the Latin for flight – and fugue states are prolonged periods of amnesia associated with wandering, usually away from home. The amnesia lasts hours, weeks or occasionally years, and is usually seen as an escape from difficult or intolerable circumstances. The patient will wander often for long distances because the memory of who he is and therefore where he lives and works is completely gone, so the patient doesn't know where to go.[24]

Hysterical fugue might prove a useful escape from a personal difficulty because it inspires care in those around the victim, who might otherwise have been upset with the sufferer because of the original problem that provoked the need to escape.[25]

Dr Hans Markowitsch of the Department of Physiological

Psychology, University of Bielefeld in Germany recently reported the first case ever in the history of psychiatry where a case of hysterical fugue was brain-scanned using the latest technology. This allowed a visualization of the patient's brain as he attempted to recall personally relevant and therefore emotionally laden memories as opposed to more neutral facts.[26]

This research indicated that people suffering from fugue might be using the left brain hemisphere to access emotional memories while the rest of us use the right or emotional brain hemisphere. The brains of patients suffering from fugue appear to be handling memories of personal identity in a very unusual and different way to normal. The fact that brain scanning and psychological testing in this case did not suggest that straightforward malingering or deception was a factor also adds weight to the idea that fugue is a unique and real condition and its sufferers require special understanding.[27]

Since multiple personality disorder is thought to evolve most often in response to childhood sexual abuse there is a close link between the debate over the existence of MPD and recovered memory of childhood sexual abuse. In recovered memories a person goes to a therapist with a problem and during the therapy the counsellor makes the dramatic announcement that the client has in fact been abused as a child although the patient has no recollection of this 'fact'. The lack of memory is explained by the therapist as due to the memory being repressed so effectively that it is lost to conscious awareness but with the correct prompting it will return.[28]

But does this prompting retrieve a true memory or actually create a false one?

Some psychiatrists describe patients who were treated first by recovered memory therapy with poor results, and later by conventional psychiatric methods with good results. A study of individuals who had retracted false memories noted that, in the process of developing pseudomemories, the patients had felt more worthless, hopeless and suicidal than before.[29, 30]

Striking accounts of deterioration with recovered memory treatment have also been given in a number of books which criticized its use. One of the world's leading experts in the psychology of memory, Elizabeth Loftus, has presented data on a review of a random sample of 183 approved claims based on repressed memory made to the Washington State Crime Victims Compensation programme. Of 183 claims selected from 325 approved claims, 30 were randomly selected for closer examination. In this group, only three claimants thought about suicide, or attempted suicide, before recovering their first memory, but 20 did so *after* recovering memories.[31]

Magnetic image resonance brain scanning technology supports a theory that traumatic and narrative memory are physiologically distinct processes. Narrative memory is the everyday means of incorporating new experience within the linguistic frames of previous experience. Apparently, traumatic perceptions are not similarly processed in the amygdala of the brain. (The amygdala is the part of the brain that becomes active when strong emotions like fear or disgust are being experienced.) Instead of becoming integrated as verbal memories, they seem to remain frozen in time, retained as fragments. These fragments may manifest as bodily sensations, emotional state, vague images, words or phrases, sounds, mistaken identification of others, and intrusive thoughts. Using this information, treatment is focused on integrating the fragments so that the survivor has access to traumatic events.[32]

There are several examples of patients with a dissociative disorder who did not have a conscious recollection of an event yet showed signs of implicit transfer as evidenced by their behaviour. For instance, a woman who had no recollection of her identity was given a telephone and instructed to randomly dial a number, after which she dialled her own telephone number.

With Doris Fischer, one of the classic DID cases, among her five identities one could not read, write or speak.[33] This illiterate identity learned the linguistic skills with remarkable speed after one of the other identities taught her. However, that there can be signs of a more definite 'boundary' between personalities comes from signs of stress or other symptoms during switching. For example, patients with MPD often suffer from headache, which is sometimes precipitated or aggravated by the switch of personalities. Doctor Daniel E. Jacome from the Franklin Medical Center in Massachusetts reports the following case of a woman with MPD who experienced severe acute headaches without warning, solely during the transition between her host personality and her pain-prone personality. The link between headache and MPD was made only 15 years ago. A Holocaust survivor with an established diagnosis of MPD had recurrent, excruciating, acute ('thunderclap') headaches only when switching between her domineering personality and her personality who suffered from chronic back pain. None of her other personalities suffered from headaches.[34]

The woman with 19 personalities – and a headache

A 54-year-old woman was referred for neurologic consultation because of recurrent back pain, fatigue and headache. She had been diagnosed several years earlier with multiple personality disorder and had a total of 19 active personalities (16 women and 3 men) at the time of her initial evaluation. She had a domineering or host personality ('Joni') and an array of diverse personalities including a child, a soldier, a baby, a musician, a pair of twins forming one personality, and an observing reflective personality ('Bertha') that served as internal analyst.

For several years she had experienced excruciating ('exploding'), abrupt pressure headaches while switching between specific personalities. Her headaches could be brief, or might persist after the switch for variable lengths of time, but not for more than an hour or two. Headaches occurred when 'Joni' (the host personality) attempted to suppress the emergence of 'Anna' who held most of the psychological trauma and was prone to pain.

This woman was of Jewish-European ancestry and had been subjected to abuse both physical and psychological as a small child while living in her native country, which was occupied by the Nazis early in World War II. In the past she had suffered from asthma ('Carol') and chronic back pain ('Anna'). Eleven years earlier, she'd had a cyst successfully removed, alleviating her host personality's back pain but not that of 'Anna'. She complained of chronic fatigue and numbness in her right thigh. Her eyesight, she said, varied with each different personality: some required reading glasses, others used different glasses with different powers of refraction for reading. (Many similar optical differences have been documented in MPD cases, as have pain perception and arousal response differences.) Transition between personalities ('switching'), which normally occurs very quickly and dramatically in these patients, constitutes a stage of vulnerability and severe tension.[35, 36]

One case of post-traumatic-brain-injury MPD was reported by Professor Sergio Della Sala and colleagues at the Department of Psychology, University of Aberdeen. This is the case of a 32-year-old chef who suffered a traumatic head injury following a road accident. Several episodes of dissociative disorder, including multiple personality, were observed in him during the few months following his brain injury.[37]

The man who attacked himself

A.O. was first admitted to the orthopaedic ward, because of multiple bone fractures in his right lower limb and nasal septum. During his stay in hospital he became disorientated and even when he returned home both his mother and his general practitioner observed other episodes of psychic absence. He also began to sleepwalk. One night he wandered around his home, entered the bathroom and, apparently still keeping his eyes closed, attempted to shave himself with an electric razor, mumbling incoherently when questioned. The following morning, he had no memory of the episode.

A few days later, another notable episode was witnessed by A.O.'s general practitioner: the patient was very agitated and distraught, tried to hit himself and kept shouting in a sort of dialogue using two distinct voices, his own ('why are you beating me?') and a scolding falsetto voice ('you have been very bad'). These were his docile and blameworthy primary identity and the self-destructive one, which remained nameless. Throughout the episode, which lasted about two hours, A.O. swapped from one personality to the other every few seconds. This state was followed by partial memory loss. This account indicates the patient's apparent failure to integrate various aspects of his identity, memories and consciousness, a symptom typical of DID.

When subsequently asked about this episode, A.O. 'recalled' only that at the time he felt as if the left part of his body was awake, whilst the right (which had been in plaster for several weeks) was asleep. Similarly, he claimed that he could hear well through his left ear, but voices and sounds were 'delayed by several minutes in his right ear'. He said that he literally felt as if he was two distinct persons, like 'two loudspeakers of a stereo system which are disconnected and speak with different voices, that of an adult and that of a child'.

He also maintained that in that period of time he was enormously enjoying watching comic book character movies in which the superheroes were rescued by their *doppelgänger* (other self) – Batman freed by a bat, or Catwoman saved by a cat. A.O. also claimed that viewing these stories increased his sense of well-being.

Worried by the turn of events, A.O.'s general practitioner referred him to a psychiatrist who treated him with appropriate medication. When, after two months, the dosage of the drugs was reduced, A.O.

experienced another trance state and several instances of agitation. During one of these episodes he imperiously (and humourlessly) asked his father to provide him 'with a roasted chicken wrapped up in clingfilm to allow him to exercise his weak right leg by kicking the bird'. Pharmacological therapy was resumed and continued for eight months; no further episode has been reported since.

Professor Della Sala and his colleagues first saw the patient in March 1996, nine months after his brain injury. The neurological examination was unremarkable. A brain scan showed that blood flow was reduced mostly in the left hemisphere.

Two psychiatrists evaluated the patient independently, alone and with his relatives, on several occasions. During these interviews, which were audiotaped, the patient never appeared depressed or anxious. Both psychiatrists confidently excluded malingering; it is worth emphasizing that A.O. was not seeking financial compensation for his psychiatric symptoms, nor for the car accident, which did not involve other vehicles and did not give rise to litigation.

From the psychiatric assessments it emerged that A.O. had a normal childhood and his parents could recall only one isolated episode worth noting. In May 1995 (a month before the accident) his wife of three years asked for a divorce, apparently because she was fed up with the long periods A.O. spent working abroad, leaving her with her parents-in-law.

When asked, the patient talked about his relationship with his wife with some objectivity, manifesting sorrow and woe, sharing his emotions without showing pathological grief or any other abnormal reaction. In June 1996 (a year after his accident) A.O. went back to work, and the following January he started a new, satisfying relationship.

Many studies indicate that immediate or long-lasting behavioural changes, which may have personal, family and social consequences, are far from rare following traumatic brain injury (TBI). Among the problems most frequently bothering these patients one and five years after the accident are irritability, bad temper, mood changes and depression. These changes are often explained as resulting from injury to the frontal lobes. Personality and behavioural changes are thought to be such an obvious outcome of TBI that they are frequently used by film-makers to show the consequences of a head injury (for example in *Desperately Seeking Susan*, by S. Seidelman, 1985).[38]

Organic theories suggest that injury to the brain might act as a

341

'release mechanism' allowing some other aspect of our usual self to peep out of our mind. However, the fact remains that A.O. showed a clear-cut dissociative disorder, which he had never experienced before, following his brain injury, and studies suggest that TBI may be less rare than previously thought.

Certain case reports of DID or MPD suggest that dramatic childhood abuse or neglect is an inevitable accompaniment. For example, Dr Yukio Uchinuma and Yoshio Sekine of the Teikyo University School of Medicine in Tokyo and Tokyo University recently reported on a man who murdered four young girls between 1988 and 1989. The forensic psychiatric evaluation showed that soon after the sudden death of his dearest grandfather, who had been the one person he could rely on among his dysfunctional family, he developed dissociative symptoms. These included fugue and DID.[39]

His DID was thought to be manifest in at least four personalities: a host personality, a child personality, a 'cool' personality and a female personality.

The case is particularly significant because in Japan only five cases of DID were reported between 1919 and 1990, whereas more than 30 cases were reported in journals or at academic meetings from 1991 to 1997.

This 26-year-old man with no previous criminal record began his murders following the death of his grandfather, and this appears to have been of vital psychological significance. He excavated his grandfather's tomb at midnight, took out and ate his burnt bones and dedicated his victims to his grandfather after sexually abusing their corpses and eating parts of them. All this was done in the hope that his grandfather would be resurrected. He was arrested when attempting to kidnap a fifth girl.

The case of the man who changed into his victims

The personal history and clinical features of the case are quite complex, and only brief comment is made here. The subject was a low birthweight baby with congenital abnormalities of both arms, which made him unable to turn his palms upward and handicapped him in social activities. For example, in his childhood he could not hold small change in his palm and he was always careful to have small change with him. Once, when he had only notes in his pocket, he struck the cashier's hand and ran out of the shop. Similarly, he was incapable of receiving gifts with palms upwards, tending to grab at them, in his own words, 'like an eagle'. His parents, who appeared to be indifferent to his misery, were designated dysfunctional and 'dissociated' because such indifference is one of the dissociative mechanisms.

He was fed with artificial milk, chiefly by his grandfather and by a lodger with a slight degree of mental retardation. They had great difficulty in feeding and nursing such a low-weight baby, but his mother was too busy with the family business to take care of him.

After he entered kindergarten at the age of four, the boy always felt that he was being observed and ridiculed by his classmates, and was convinced that his teachers conspired in this. According to him, his life in kindergarten and school was 'a hell'. His only comfort was to spend his time with his grandfather.

His grandmother hated the grandfather and was sometimes violent towards him. His parents, whose marriage had been arranged by the grandmother, quarrelled constantly during his school years and were due to be divorced at the time of his first crime. Increasingly he sought comfort in collecting childish things such as cartoons. At senior high school in Tokyo, feelings that others were making fun of him became milder, but the collecting compulsion became stronger. He boasted of his voluminous collection, joining animation clubs and becoming acquainted with penpals all over Japan. These contrasted features were considered to be the precursors of his alter personalities: a 'child personality' and a 'cool personality'. During his childhood and adolescence, he had, on rare occasions, had fugues and a visual hallucination of a black shadow.

His family kept a bird, which he loved deeply. One day he was overwhelmed by an unexpected hatred of it and trampled on it, then buried it, dug it out again and caressed it tenderly. He repeated such acts several times.

When he was 20, the lodger whom he loved most next to his grandfather was taken away by a relative without notice. Soon afterwards he began to show paedophilic feelings towards little girls. This behaviour became compulsive, although he was sexually impotent. It is important to mention here that if the compulsive part of his personality was separated further from the other aversive part and became independently visualized, the former part could appear as an autoscopic phenomenon – he would view himself from outside, as in an 'out of body experience'.

The shock of his grandfather's sudden death caused him to lose feelings such as joy, sorrow and affection. He fervently desired to

343

look at every part of the corpse, but when he found that his grandfather had been cremated he began to be convinced that his grandfather was not dead but concealed. In a visual hallucination he saw his grandfather, who often said to him, 'I will soon come back', 'you will be able to see me before long' or 'you should pray more eagerly'. Once when he went to the cemetery at midnight along with his grandfather's favourite dog, his double, which was a little smaller than he, appeared in front of him and after excavating the tomb it began to take out and eat the burnt bones. Later he went and ate the bones several times a year. His stated reason for these acts was that unless he ate up all the bones, the bones of his grandfather would be doubled when his grandfather appeared again. Three months after the death of his grandfather the first murder was carried out. He dedicated each girl he had murdered, and the animals he had found dead on the roads or he himself had killed, to his grandfather in an attempt to resurrect him.

Many symptoms, including dissociative ones, were found. He no longer saw his parents and sisters as blood relations, and thought he must have been an adopted or abandoned child. His close friends became mere acquaintances. He showed dissociative amnesia: for example he was often surprised to find new videotapes in his car or in his room and could not remember how and where he had bought or stolen them. He would find himself, to his great surprise, in a strange street or a city, not knowing how and why he had come there.

About a year after starting the evaluation, it was realized that it was impossible to explain the whole clinical picture and the criminal facts unless DID was taken into account. Eventually he admitted that two distinct personalities, a 'child personality' and a 'cool personality', seemed to exist in his body; he had an uncanny impression of changing between the two. Sometimes he behaved quite differently, depending on the circumstances. He sent several letters confessing to having kidnapped and committed murder to a victim's family and to a newspaper. These letters were written using a female name, in handwriting quite different from his usual, which implied the existence of a 'female alter personality' who perpetrated the murders; he could barely remember writing and sending such letters. He even carried a box stuffed with a victim's bones to her home, at the risk of being arrested. Although he said that on these days he had a deep desire to see his grandfather's funeral once more (which seemed to be the reason why he had performed such daring acts), he had almost no memory of these acts.

It is possible that his desires were stirred by repeated broadcasting of the funeral of the Emperor Showa at the time. He kept a newspaper report on the state funeral as a precious thing, considering it as a report on the funeral of his own grandfather.

His testimony about his crimes illustrates his psychopathy and details of his first murder are abbreviated here (with the psychiatrists' comments in parentheses):

'I drove to a distant city and bought videotapes as usual. On my way back I stopped my car somewhere in a residential area and walked around there, where I saw a little girl who was alone. Such a lonely appearance reminded me of my having been alone in my childhood [a flashback], and curiously enough, I felt myself on the spot sweetly merging into her [change into a child alter-personality]. At the moment, my double, which was as small as she was, appeared in front of me [autoscopy]. The double approached her and asked her to accompany it. I observed the double acting very, very slowly with thrill and apprehension. She followed me as I came back to my car. When she got into my car, the double disappeared and I was filled with inexpressible sweetness, as if I were one with her. I drove with only a few words to her because it was unnecessary to talk a lot to her on account of our oneness with each other to the hill near my home where I used to go on a picnic with my grandfather in my childhood.

'After getting out of my car I sat down beside her on a hillside, remembering that I had had a good time with my grandfather around there [identification of the little girl with his grandfather] . . . All of a sudden, a number of rat-men with the faces of rats appeared behind trees, and came closer and closer [an innate tendency to visualize his affect, in this case his hatred toward the little girl who broke his oneness with her]. I thought for a moment, before being stunned with terror, that she must have beckoned them with her strange power to kill me, but when I came to myself I found her lying down on the earth "like a doll" instead of me. The rat-men must have become angry at her commander-like voice and have first knocked her down. Having a strong fear that I would be assaulted next, I ran away in a hurry. I had no memory of how and where I had made my way home. When I came to myself again I found myself at the entrance of my home [fugue]. It was already late in the evening. I greedily ate a lot of food, wondering why I could eat so much after running so long [orality]. After supper I engaged in recording TV programmes on videotape as usual, when my double appeared again because there remained the after-effect of fear about the rat-men. This time the double was a little smaller than I. I went to bed before I was aware of it.

'The next morning I awoke with a thought like this: "Last night I had a strange dream. I wonder whether it was a dream or a reality." Then an idea: "I'll go there to make sure that there must be a flesh-doll if it is a reality" occurred to me [autochthonous idea – ideas that arise suddenly, as if from nowhere, and that seem to be of vital importance].

'Following this idea, I went there with a video camera. I had no memory of where I had obtained it although the police insisted that I had borrowed it at a video shop before going there [dissociative amnesia].

'Anyway, I could find a flesh-doll [a curious but quite appropriate expression, corresponding to his double consciousness of thinking of the corpse as a dead human being and at the same time as a doll in a puppet show, which suggests his divided personality].

'Soon afterward another idea: "I'll make an offering to my grand-father." I began to film with a video camera the flesh-doll and my behaviour of inserting a finger or a screwdriver into the vagina along with my double. The double was coolly engaged in its work while I myself was observing the weird behaviour of the double with fear and aversion. Later in my room the double appeared again, and per-formed a ceremony of dedicating the videotape to my grandfather with two lighted candles fastened on the forehead, hoping that he would resurrect. I thought what a curious guy the double was. I suppose the double must be strange because it coolly performs weird things which I will never do in my usual state. I have a feeling that a cool guy in my body must have come out in such a figure [a cool alter personality].

'Later on, each time a similar idea occurred to me I went to the sweet hillside, which I had come to share with my grandfather again, to make sure whether the flesh-doll remained there. The last time I went there I found it changed into bones. After stroking them tenderly and eating some parts of them along with my double, I carried them to my home and placed them with care in the barn belonging to my grandfather.'

The subject experienced a variety of autochthonous or schizophrenic-like delusional ideas. Following these ideas, for example, he (and his double) lay down beside the corpse of a little girl with thankfulness because she reminded him of his grandfather, or he ate the hand bones of a little girl after burning them in order to keep in his body his precious reminiscences of his grandfather. Although he felt an aversion to the double's behaviour he could not refrain from these acts. Accordingly he admitted that he also had the same feeling as the double. In spite of his ambivalence, the moment an autochthonous idea occurred to him he behaved as if his personality had changed into a different one.

Apart from his detached attitude towards his family and his occasional violence towards them, he generally behaved normally in the other external aspects of his life. It seemed to him that the criminal and necrophilic cannibalistic acts (including vampirism) were merely a dream, and he denied his crimes, although through his testimony he appeared to admit them. According to him the crimes took place in 'another island', not in his territory. The little girls he had met were absolutely different from the real victims.

He recorded many television reports of his crimes as if they had been committed by other persons, although he had a very slight feeling of knowing his own crimes. Taking into account the letters admitting that he had kidnapped and committed murder, it can be said that he had a 'double consciousness' of his own crimes.

He had auditory hallucinations of a persecutory nature, in addition to hearing the voice of his grandfather (its content was restricted to his name and the word 'lynch'). Although these may occur in other conditions, we consider the possibility of schizophrenia. His behaviour was quite active and natural in some parts of his daily life, although he showed no interest in his work. No-one around him noticed his mental disorder. He grew to feel himself as an alien in this world after the death of his grandfather, far stranger and much more abandoned than the deformed person he was in his childhood. At his interview he revealed no mental disturbance, and one of his letters asking a victim's family to hold a funeral consisted of clear sentences filled with deep sorrow and anguish. These spoke against the possibility of schizophrenia. As a whole, the various contradictions could not be understood without the concept of DID.

As we've seen, a core feature of DID is the amnesia that exists between personalities. This phenomenon is a hallmark of the dissociation that reportedly occurs between memory structures in extreme dissociation.[40]

The nature and extent of the amnesia between personalities appear complex because a proportion of DID cases are reportedly aware of different personalities' experiences, and implicit learning occurs across personalities. It is commonly argued that DID patients dissociate their traumatic memories as a defensive function to minimize the distress these cause. However, little empirical investigation is reported on autobiographical memory in DID. In one study it was reported that DID was associated with poor recall of events occurring in early childhood. This finding may be considered consistent with the proposition that DID is associated with dissociation from early traumatic experiences. It is commonly claimed, however, that alter personalities have access to traumatic memories that are not available to the host personality.[41]

MPD/DID has posed a challenge to judges and juries. While the law has struggled to fit DID into its framework, no consensus has emerged on how standard rules of criminal responsibility should apply. The law's failure to fit it into traditional tests for responsibility is due largely to the nature of this unusual disorder.[42]

Perhaps the use of a new kind of scanner used by a group of doctors, led by Guochuan Tsai at Harvard Medical School, who have performed the first in-depth imaging study of brain activity in MPD, could in future solve these legal and psychiatric problems. This kind of advance in technology may finally resolve the issue of whether MPD really exists or is just an example of patients pulling the wool over the eyes of gullible psychiatrists.[43]

The advantage of the functional Magnetic Resonance Imaging technique is that it does not use radioactivity, unlike other brain scanning methods, so repeated scans on one subject over a period of time are possible without any medical hazard. MRI relies on an intense magnetic field to perturb the energy state of hydrogen atoms, and then measures the energy radiated as these nuclei return to their normal state.

This allows a precise visualization of low oxygenated blood, which indicates those parts of the brain being active, as these areas use up more oxygen from blood. Until this new imaging technique arrived, it was not possible to visualize brain activity so precisely during an actual personality switch in a patient before.

The investigators tackled the problem of pretence, which most British psychiatrists would suspect is at the root of MPD, by getting the patient to switch to a third 'pretend' personality as a control condition and compared this brain state with the real alternative personality she was plagued by.[44]

She confirmed the moment of a switch in personality by pressing a button while she was in the scanner, allowing these precise moments to be correlated with the images of her brain activity.

When the patient was changing from her normal everyday personality to the main 'alter' one, the part of the brain now thought to code for our memories and significant episodes in our past lives, the hippocampus, seemed to be inhibited and its activity significantly decreased. When she switched back from her 'alter' personality to her normal everyday one, the hippocampus was more activated than normal.

These results throw new light on where our sense of self is located in the brain. They suggest who we are is in fact strongly determined by memories of significant past events in our lives. It might even be that holding on to past turning points in our lives continues to define our outlook, and to change our personality we have to alter the focus of our memory of the past.[45]

These brain scanning results also converge with the current therapy for MPD which encourages the patient to recall, and perhaps even relive, the traumatic early event that produced the switch to another personality in the first place.[46]

It is particularly interesting that the activation is in the right hippocampus when the base or core personality is being switched back from the 'alter', as it is this right side which is generally implicated in emotional experiences. So it could be that recalling particularly emotional memories is vital to our sense of self, and denying them renders us prone to forgetting who we really are.[47]

But perhaps the most revolutionary aspect of this research is the fact that a definite difference in brain activity was demonstrated between different pathological personalities, but not when the patient was instructed to pretend to shift to a feigned personality. This means the new technique of functional MRI brain scanning could begin to persuade British psychiatry to take MPD more seriously. A redrawing of the map of disorders previously attributed to malingering and other dubious motivations could now be heralded by this study, for these new brain scanning techniques allow clinicians to look past the pretence, and directly into the brain.

MPD challenges the idea we have of ourselves – selves whose essential characteristics are simplicity, identity, transparency.

What is distinctive about the disorder is the possibility that there could be more than one person per body. At least some accounts of the condition represent alters as full-blown persons who may not suspect each other's existence. They can come to learn and have strong feelings about each other, discuss the others behind their backs; they can be introduced to one another and learn to live together. When confronted with the therapeutic aim of assimilation into each other, they resent the fact, as any sensible person would, that they are being asked to negotiate their own demise.[48]

Our problem, it can be argued, is that our present society is unusual in human history in that none of us can easily suppose that there is only one career or life available to us. We are confronted by choices, or the mirage of choices, that our ancestors did not need to trouble with. Long ago and far away most people were born into their destinies, and could live single, simple lives. We internalize, imagine all the possibilities (even the spurious possibilities) and somehow have to create our own single lives from chaos. Not surprisingly, we often fail, and so may either intuit a selfhood different from any particular ideal, or else imagine that the many different ideas are really different selves.[49]

14

DELUSIONS ABOUT WHO OTHER PEOPLE ARE: THE CAPGRAS DELUSION

All the world's a stage,
And all the men and women merely players.
As You Like It, II vii

The Capgras delusion or syndrome is one of the rarest and most colourful in neurology. The most striking feature of this disorder is that the patient – who is often mentally quite lucid in other respects – comes to regard close acquaintances, typically his parents, children, spouse or siblings, as 'impostors': he may claim that the person in question 'looks like' or is even 'identical to' his father, but really isn't. Although frequently seen in psychotic states, over a third of the documented cases of Capgras syndrome (CS) have occurred in conjunction with traumatic brain injury.[1]

Capgras delusion is one of a number of delusions involving person perception that are known collectively as delusional misidentifications (DMI). Until recently, misidentification syndromes were regarded as exotica in medicine, famous amongst doctors as much for their rarity as their extravagance. But over the past 20 years interest in them has grown, partly reflecting the greater number being reported and partly because a considerable proportion arise in patients with organic brain pathology. As many also arise in those without obvious neurological defects, they offer a direct link between the worlds of psychiatry and neurology; the vogue thinking is that psychiatric cases without identifiable brain injury are merely awaiting a technological advance that will finally allow such injury to be identified.[2]

The prevalence of Capgras syndrome is estimated at approximately one in 3,000 in the general population and is observed with a possibly higher frequency in female patients.[3]

One psychoanalytic hypothesis is that Capgras patients harbour overwhelming ambivalent feelings towards relatives and other love objects.[4] Unable to integrate their feelings of love and hostility, these patients experience delusional splitting of the object(s) into the good and genuine object and the bad and untrustworthy double. Hence the production of the Capgras delusion, which involves the belief that familiar people have been replaced by 'dummies' or impostors – even robots or aliens – allowing the victim to distrust or hate the double when in fact these are repressed feelings towards the real person.[5]

In recent years controversy has arisen over the precise cause of this syndrome, first mentioned by the German psychiatrist Kahlbaum in 1866 but more fully described by French psychiatrists Capgras and Reboul-Lachaux in 1923.[6] One reason for the increased interest is the hope that Capgras can tell us something about visual processing, the mechanism for face recognition and also the fundamental nature of psychosis.[7]

Capgras and Reboul-Lachaux described Mme M., a 53-year-old housewife, who developed a variety of delusions, including prominent ones, in which she asserted that her children and husband had been replaced by doubles. She even petitioned for a divorce on the grounds that the latter was not the man she married but that he had been murdered by the double (or rather 'doubles' – she counted at least 80 of them).

Since these first descriptions, observations have been published of many hundreds of Capgras delusion (CD) cases from many parts of the world and involving males and females aged from 9 to 90 years.[8]

Delusions, by their very nature, are bizarre – none more so than this one, where the victim makes odd mistakes about recognizing precisely who familiar and unfamiliar people are. This delusion raises issues about the way the brain and mind deal with identity.

What is so important scientifically, and what makes the Capgras delusion so fascinating, is that it suggests that identity is not a straightforward function of the brain and mind.[9]

Indeed, scientists like Hadyn Ellis and Michael Lewis of the School of Psychology at Cardiff University in Wales argue that the peculiar Capgras delusion fundamentally challenges our current general brain models for face recognition.[10] Because it seems to be about making a mistake in identifying someone, usually someone very familiar to the patient, it appears at first glance as though the syndrome might partly be explicable in terms of a dysfunction of the brain's visual system. But some, if not most, patients explicitly insist that the impostor resembles the original exactly.[11]

A well-publicized UK court case of Capgras delusion involved a teacher who, following a car crash, developed the belief that his wife had died in the incident and that the woman living with him was an impostor. He insisted that his real wife died in the accident and in court a consultant psychiatrist explained that his patient was suffering from Capgras delusion.[12]

Capgras delusion occurs in a variety of settings as a symptom of psychiatric illness (e.g. schizophrenia or mood disorders) or of disorders following structural brain damage or toxic-metabolic conditions, such as poisonings. However, some have described the syndrome as a memory disconnection between stored representations of familiar people and new information in which patients failed to take into account physical changes in their relatives which occurred after a period of separation or over time. After all, a long admission to a psychiatric hospital or perhaps even the isolation before admission produced by the psychosis could mean that many relatives have not been seen for some time.[13] The failure to adequately update episodic memories results in discrepancies between the new perception and the stored image. These proposals are valid, given the accounts from Capgras syndrome patients who have been able to identify currently misidentified relatives from backdated photographs.

CS could also be described in terms of the two brain hemispheres, right and left side, not connecting properly. This lack of connection might result from a failure adequately to integrate left and right hemispheric processing. According to this scenario, the two representations of a known face held by each hemisphere would fail to fuse, thereby producing a delusion of doubles.[14]

The propensity of CS to involve intimately associated persons and its apparent exclusivity to psychiatric illness encouraged many early investigators to adopt a psychoanalytic approach. Ambivalent feelings towards a familiar other which are not adequately repressed. The feelings of anxiety, guilt and anger resulting from such conflicts are then projected onto imagined impostor/s.[15]

Psychiatrists Dr Richard O'Reilly and Dr Ladi Malhotra of the University of Western Ontario recently reported a case of Capgras syndrome associated with extreme violent behaviour.[16] Here the patient's psychological dynamics support the psychoanalytic belief that the Capgras delusion initially arises from an altered emotional response towards one or more others and proceeds to intolerable ambivalent feelings. This ambivalence is neutralized through the imagined existence of doubles.

The case is important because, as mentioned, debate continues to rage over whether delusions like Capgras are biological or psychological in origin, as cases with obvious biological causes continue to be reported as well as cases with no brain abnormality at all.[17]

The woman who believed part of her body had been secretly replaced

Mrs M. was a 47-year-old divorcee, first seen by Drs O'Reilly and Malhotra when she was admitted to the forensic unit of a provincial psychiatric hospital in Canada. She was born in a small town, the oldest of four siblings. Her father worked as a motor mechanic and her mother as a housewife. There was no evidence of psychiatric illness in either branch of the family. The patient described her early childhood as relatively happy and uneventful until the age of eight, when her father started to drink heavily and to womanize. Mrs M. began to have nightmares, and at school was nervous and frightened of her teachers. Although her father continued drinking through her high school years, Mrs M. appeared to be well adjusted, had a group of female friends and took part in the usual adolescent pursuits, including dating. Educationally, she did well and left school at the age of 19 to work as a typist and secretary.

When she was 23 Mrs M. had a six-month courtship, during which she became pregnant. She had already experienced one psychotic breakdown by that time, and said that she married in order to avoid readmission to a psychiatric hospital. The couple's relationship was stormy; at the time of presentation Mrs M. had been separated from her husband for five years and divorced for two years. She had a daughter and son by her husband, aged 23 and 16 respectively, and an illegitimate child who was born one year after her son and adopted at birth.

Mrs M. was first admitted to hospital at the age of 22, following her conviction that her real father had gone off to Korea and that an almost identical double had come into the house to take his place. She had 11 subsequent admissions to psychiatric hospitals, and had been an inpatient in another hospital for four continuous years prior to the present admission. Mrs M. was diagnosed as suffering from paranoid schizophrenia and required a lot of psychiatric support, even when she was an outpatient.

Mrs M.'s delusion of doubles had always been central to her problems; her father, sisters and her husband, her two legitimate children, nursing staff and other patients had all been replaced by doubles at one time or another. In the case of her son and daughter she reported the existence of multiple doubles who frequently interchanged at various times during their lives. She believed that she had the ability to distinguish between these various impostors by spotting minor physical differences, such as in height, skin texture and length of nose.

Mrs M. also believed that some of the original people had disappeared permanently. She claimed that her father had never returned from Korea and that her real daughter had been murdered at the age of seven. In contrast, most of the other doubles alternated with the original people they were impersonating, although sometimes the originals remained absent for long periods of time: 'My son went off to explore the world when he was a toddler, only returning home a few years ago.'

It has been suggested that the Capgras syndrome is only manifested towards people with whom the patient has a strong emotional attachment. In fact, in the case originally described by Capgras and Reboul-Lachaux in 1923 this is not so, and in Mrs M.'s case she attributed doubles to many people whom she knew only slightly. For example, she had been on the unit for just one month when she stated that one of the male nurses had a double, and she also believed that one of the psychiatrists had a double who intended to murder her daughter. Mrs M. said that on one occasion, 10 years previously, she had seen a double of herself while in another psychiatric hospital. This experience only lasted a few moments and was not repeated, but she still believed in the existence of this self-double.

A consistent and fascinating phenomenon was her delusion of part-replacement: she reported that she had been aware for some time that a number of her bodily organs had been removed during the night and replaced by those of other patients. She explained that this involved an operation through her vagina, which enabled the organs to be exchanged without leaving a scar. She also claimed that her vagina, uterus, ovaries, liver, heart, stomach and brain had all been exchanged at some time or other. Occasionally messages arose from these organs. Some months previously a voice came from her stomach saying that it was going to kill her son. She felt that this was not her own voice, and then suddenly realized that the stomach belonged to another patient and had been exchanged for her own while she was sleeping.

Mrs M. demonstrated the unpredictability of some chronic schizophrenic patients and through the years had intermittently expressed aggressive and homicidal threats towards her family and fellow patients in various hospitals. At home there were occasional episodes of violence; when her eldest son was two years old she injured him by throwing him against a wall, and on another occasion she attacked her sister with a knife.

In the months before her admission to hospital, Mrs M. had remained relatively well. Though still deluded, she appeared to be functioning at a socially acceptable level, displaying neither overtly aggressive nor threatening behaviour. In the week prior to her transfer, however, she became convinced that another patient on the ward (Mrs V.) intended to murder her 'daughter's double'. Mrs M. believed that it was Mrs V. who had murdered the 'original daughter' 16 years previously, and also believed (incorrectly) that Mrs V. was about to be discharged from hospital. She came to the conclusion that the only way to save her daughter was to kill Mrs V. After ruminating on this for two days she then, while out on a pass from the hospital, obtained a large knife from a local shop and smuggled it into the hospital. During the night she entered Mrs V.'s bedroom and, while the patient slept, she cut her throat, killing her outright.

At her trial Mrs M. was found not guilty by reason of insanity. It was accepted that she felt the killing of this fellow patient was justified and morally correct on the basis of her delusional beliefs. She was ordered to be detained in a secure forensic unit.

This case report sheds further light on psychoanalysis of the Capgras syndrome. From interviews with Mrs M. it was clear that she had intense and ambivalent feelings towards a number of her family. She strongly resented her father's alcoholism and womanizing,

356

which disrupted the family stability. In her early twenties Mrs M. experienced an early schizophrenic disintegration. It appears that the intrapsychic regression that resulted allowed her to mobilize the primitive defence mechanism of splitting: the 'good father' was seen to be replaced by a double for whom she could more easily harbour aggressive feelings.[18]

Such dynamics have been suggested to explain the Capgras delusion. Others have expanded on this idea, suggesting that people become aware of changes in their usual mood responses to significant others and attribute these to changes in the other person. We might term this 'projected depersonalization'.[19]

Mrs M.'s hostile feelings towards her daughter may have been associated with her unexpected conception, which had forced the patient into an unwanted marriage. By employing the defence mechanism of splitting, she was able to experience these feelings as being directed at an unrelated double. Presumably even this did not allay her anxiety, and she then projected her homicidal wishes onto a number of people, including her psychiatrist and Mrs V., all of whom she accused of wanting to murder her daughter. Mrs M. then destroyed the person she perceived as wanting to harm her daughter. This had the incidental effect of sublimating her own homicidal impulses. Two pieces of evidence support this theory. First, Mrs M. was in a state of calm on admission, only 12 hours after the homicide. She stated that there was no further threat to her children, even though she had believed that a number of other patients in her previous hospital harboured similar feelings. Second, she had demonstrated projection of homicidal feelings previously, when a voice originating in her stomach spoke of killing her son. On that occasion she denied ownership of the stomach and voice, ascribing both to another patient.

Apart from the presence of the Capgras syndrome, this patient's behaviour resembles that of many chronic psychotic patients in long-stay hospital wards. It is worth bearing in mind that even chronic delusions can suddenly become invested with a high emotional charge, and that these patients can still act on their delusional beliefs in a violent way.

The psychoanalytic approach cannot explain the misidentification of people not characterized by negative or ambivalent feelings, such as health care workers or fellow patients; or reduplication of inanimate objects which carry no emotional valence, like road signs. Rather than offering an insight into the delusion's origins, these reports appear to indicate that potentially anyone with whom the psychotic patient interacts may become a target. Indeed, one patient's misidentification delusion involved the staff of a psychiatric unit and all of the unit's patients except the patient himself.

It is exceptional for there to be only one impostor. More often CS involves multiple person and/or animal misidentifications, the number of misidentified targets frequently increasing with the passage of time and even involving inanimate physical structures, such as hospital buildings which are believed to have been replaced by replicas. (This is known as reduplicative paramnesia.) Characteristically, the affected individual views impostors with anger and suspicion.

Doctor J. Arturo Silva and colleagues of San Jose, California, report the case of a patient with an unusual multifaceted delusion of misidentification including Capgras syndrome, in which people in the immediate environment, the other patients and hospital staff, were seen as hired actors in a stage production.[20]

The man who believed all the ward was a stage

Mr D., a 31-year-old homeless male, was admitted involuntarily to a psychiatric intensive care unit after he became verbally and physically threatening to citizens and police officers. During his stay, he manifested great suspicion and expressed extreme anger because he believed that all the ward's real patients had been evacuated from the premises prior to his admission and replaced with 'actors'. Mr D. stated that he arrived at this conclusion following a process in which he asked other patients a series of questions and carefully 'looked into their eyes'. When he confronted other patients about their status as actors playing patients, they responded with bewilderment and anger, feeling that Mr D. had dismissed their illnesses.

Because of his accusations, the other patients on the unit actively avoided Mr D.; he interpreted this as a strategy designed not to 'blow their cover'. When another patient repeatedly denied that he was mentally ill, Mr D. stated this was proof that the patient was an actor. In another instance, a manic patient claimed he was a famous actor, which Mr D. took as further substantiation of his misidentification delusions. Coincidentally, a movie company was filming on the hospital grounds, which Mr D. believed was the same company involved in the psychiatric unit's stage production.

More specifically, Mr D. recognized several of the patients, whom he had met during previous hospitalizations on the ward, and explained that whilst they may have been genuine psychiatric patients in the past, they had since been replaced by identical doubles who were well-paid actors. When he observed other patients leaving the ward for other clinical evaluations, he claimed that they were going to their 'makeup rooms' where they were made to look like psychiatric patients. He demanded to meet the director of the production and said, 'The whole ward is a stage and everybody plays the part.' He believed that 'the whole thing will be an Academy Award play' and would be shown on television. The reason for this play was to provoke him, the only 'authentic' patient, because essentially he had 'no mental problems'. The patient also believed that after his discharge, all the actors would leave the unit and be replaced by the real patients.

Mr D.'s delusions extended to the authenticity of the ward staff. He thought that the psychiatrists were simultaneously psychiatrists and actors, although the remainder of the unit's staff were actors only. He also believed that his grandmother and his father had been impersonated in the past by physically identical but psychologically different impostors. His delusions of misidentification had not been noted during previous psychiatric hospitalizations and there was no known history of mental illness in his first-degree relatives. There was also no history of head injury.

This patient had suffered for nine years from a psychotic disorder. His history included the development of chronic alcohol and cannabis abuse after the onset of psychotic symptoms. Mental status examination and psychological testing suggested he may also have been suffering from an organic mental disorder as a result of chronic alcohol usage. Despite medication, his delusion of misidentification and impaired judgement persisted.

Mr D. had spent many years interacting with mental health professionals and he had also spent several years living in an area of Los Angeles, in close proximity to movie studios. Long-term environmental exposure to this type of sociocultural milieu appears to have shaped the content of his delusions. These were also reinforced by factors such as the filming of a movie on the hospital grounds which was visible from the psychiatric ward. Grandiose statements by a manic patient who claimed to be an actor may have also served to support the patient's delusion.

Delusional misidentification in this case seems to have resulted from an interplay of psychological, organic and sociocultural factors. This case illustrates the value of a wider biopsychosocial focus in distinguishing Capgras from other delusions of misidentification and shows that emphasizing brain biological dysfunction alone is not sufficient.

However, there have also been case reports of Capgras occurring when there is no biological factor at all, perhaps as a result of extreme strain. Doctor Thomas Wenzel and colleagues from the University Hospital, Department of Psychiatry, in Vienna have recently reported the following history of a patient suffering from Capgras syndrome following extreme stress.[21]

The man who believed he was surrounded by impostors

The patient, a 37-year-old painter from an urban background in a Mediterranean country, had been imprisoned and tortured over several months in his country of origin 12 years before he arrived at the hospital. During torture he had been confronted with extreme violence by several perpetrators, disorientation techniques and the imminent threat of death. In a state of complete helplessness he expected torture to happen at any time.

A few weeks after release he developed symptoms of post-traumatic stress disorder, such as flashbacks, disturbed sleep, depersonalization and agitation. Irritable and depressed, he continued to live in a situation of permanent threat, continuously aware of the possibility that he might be captured and tortured again by secret police members. Psychotic symptoms including hallucinations, disorganized behaviour and speech in combination with mood swings were first observed by his family after he had been forced to continue working with a politically active group instead of settling down with a young woman he had intended to marry.

Only after emigration did the man become 'aware' that people in his surroundings had been exchanged for identical-looking doubles, though he could not ascertain why or by whom these changes had been made. During his first hospital interview he claimed that a discreet change could be observed in the impostors, but was unable to define his experience more precisely. He also stated that he was the subject of a 'cruel game' and felt helpless. These symptoms were accompanied by fear, tension and aggressive feelings.

During times when he discontinued medication, which was frequently the case when he was travelling back to his home country, he developed more pronounced psychotic symptoms, being convinced that his head was 'open' and that others, including psychiatrists, intended to 'perform manipulations on his body and brain' and could read his thoughts. He was given antipsychotic medication which stabilized his mood, though memories of torture continued to reappear.

Physical trauma, the psychological stressor of having experienced extreme and intentional cruelty over a prolonged period of time and, finally, forced migration contributed to this man's unstable condition; his delusions developed with the gradual loss of reality, the specific experience of persecution and the loss of trust in his identity and social interaction.

This case report illustrates how extremely stressful conditions and psychological or emotional disturbance can produce a Capgras delusion, again indicating that not all cases are caused by biological brain dysfunction. The situation of being tortured is also known to produce the well-known Stockholm syndrome where the hostages develop strong feelings of attachment to their persecutors. An explanation for this is that if your fate depends on the whims or moods of someone, you study that person in great detail and try to please them in order to avoid harm to yourself. If you survive the experience you believe you personally have had a major impact on them and this can lead to feelings of attachment. One way of dealing with the extremely stressful situation is to split the torturer into two people – one who can show mercy and another who is evil.

The essential paradox is that patients with Capgras delusion simultaneously recognize a face and, at the same time, deny its authenticity. This phenomenon can provide us with a fascinating clue to the very nature of normal face recognition.

Our understanding of how the brain recognizes faces has undergone many stages of evolution since the first basic sequential model was first described. The latest theory is that several different units of the brain, specializing in different aspects of information about a familiar person or his/her face, are accessed and the various bits of information are combined so that we recognize the face.

Capgras delusion raises many interesting issues concerning the interaction between cognitive processes underlying person recognition and the accompanying emotional responses. Not least is the basis of our sense of familiarity when encountering someone we know well, which can, as both the psychologist William James and the philosopher Bertrand Russell suggested, involve an automatic 'glow' of recognition.[22]

Doctor William Hirstein and V. S. Ramachandran of the Brain and Perception Laboratory at the University of California in San Diego recently reported a case of Capgras in a patient, D.S., who was unusual in that he claimed that his parents were impostors when he was looking at them but not when he spoke to them on the telephone.[23]

The suggestion is that in this patient connections from face-processing areas in the brain have been damaged. Apparently there are two components to the visual recognition of a familiar face, one of which is responsible for conscious recognition and the recall of associated information. The other is responsible for emotional arousal – the feeling of familiarity that accompanies conscious recognition of a familiar face.[24]

Yet this leaves two questions unanswered. First, why is the phenomenon most often found with close relatives? One possibility is that most usually with one's parents or spouse one expects a glow of arousal, so its absence leads to the delusion that one's parent is an impostor. With an emotionally neutral person on the other hand, such as one's postman, one does not expect such arousal, so there is no incentive for generating a delusion.[25]

A related question is: why does the mere absence of this emotional arousal lead to such an extraordinarily far-fetched delusion? Why doesn't the patient just think, 'I know that is my father but I no longer feel the warmth?' One answer is that some additional brain impairment or injury may be required to generate such extreme delusions.[26]

Although the Capgras syndrome is often regarded merely as a face recognition problem, perhaps it is part of a more general memory management problem.[27] When you or I meet a new person, our brains open a new file, as it were, into which go all our memories of interactions with this person. When the Capgras patient meets a person who is genuinely new to him, his brain creates a file for this person and the associated experiences, as it should. But if the person leaves the room for 30 minutes and returns, the patient's brain, instead of retrieving the old file and continuing to add to it, sometimes creates a completely new one. Why this should happen is unclear, but it may be that the emotional activation from familiar faces is missing and the absence of this 'glow' is a signal for the brain to create a separate file for this face (or else the presence of the 'glow' is needed for developing links between successive episodes involving a person).[28]

It is crucial to point out the patient has not lost his earlier episodic memories of the person; he remembers the 'other' person, but simply behaves as if he has met two different people, and creates separate files for them. Again, his problem is confined to the visual: the patient can recognize his parents over the phone. A problem of this kind may underlie not only Capgras syndrome but also the belief that objects have been replaced by duplicates.[29]

Perhaps the oddest aspect of Capgras patients' delusionary problems is their tendency to sometimes regard themselves as doubles, a tendency for which there are two possible explanations (which are not mutually exclusive).[30] First, photographs of themselves from the past do not evoke emotional activation and warm feelings, and the person in the photographs is therefore to be rejected as 'another person' (however bizarre that may seem to us with our intact brains). Second, his loss of emotional contact with people who matter to him most, such as his own parents, may lead him to say to himself: 'The reason I don't experience warmth is that they don't recognize me, and that in turn must be because I'm not the real person.' Indeed, on one occasion one patient made the following poignant remark to his mother: 'Mother, if the real person ever returns do you promise that you will still treat me as a friend and love me?'[31]

Philosophers have often emphasized that if there is any aspect of our lives that we can regard as axiomatic and beyond question, it is our own personal identity. This sense of a single, unified 'self' runs like a golden thread through the whole fabric of our experience. The Capgras patient, on the other hand, inhabits a strange no man's land between illusion and reality where even the enduring, unitary self can no longer be assumed. Studying these patients may not only allow us to observe the formation of new memories 'in slow motion' so to speak, but also give us insights into how the brain creates a sense of seamless unity from a lifetime of diverse sensory experiences.[32]

15

STRANGER THAN FICTION?

*I have never agreed with my other self wholly. The truth of the matter
seems to lie between us.*

Khalil Gibran, *Sand and Foam*

Neurologists Dr Hakan Ay and colleagues at Harvard Medical
School recently reported a case of an elderly lady who was admitted
to hospital complaining that her left hand was acting as if under
someone else's control; it hit her face and head, and she explained
she was afraid of it. She held her left hand with the right, claiming
to keep 'him' from hitting her, and said that her 'left hand tried to
strangle her'.[1]

The diagnosis turned out to be the extremely rare 'alien hand
syndrome', first reported in 1908 with only a few cases documented
world-wide since then. The sufferers believe their limbs have a mind
of their own, because they have usually, but not always, sustained
brain damage to the corpus callosum – the part of the brain which
joins the two cerebral hemispheres.[2] In this case, a stroke caused by
a blood clot brought about the distressing symptoms of this rare
condition.

Although the hand is most frequently affected, any limb or
combination of limbs might be involved. In the very first case ever

reported a 57-year-old woman felt that her left hand had a will of its own: at one point it grabbed and choked her throat and it took a great deal of effort, using her other hand, to pull it off. On one occasion another sufferer found that her left hand began to remove a cigarette from her mouth as she was about to light it with the right hand. She stated the left hand 'was trying to keep me from smoking'.

Another victim reported that her left hand would grasp her throat during sleep, so she slept with the arm tied down. One patient's right hand interfered with tasks being performed by her left hand, so she attempted to restrain it by wedging it between her legs, and by holding or slapping it with the left hand. While playing chequers on one occasion, the left hand of a male sufferer made a move that he did not wish to make, so he corrected the move with the right hand; however, the left hand, to the patient's frustration, repeated the false move.[3]

But alien hand syndrome may have significance beyond being a neurological curiosity; philosophers and brain scientists believe that the syndrome could reveal where 'free will' is located in the brain. The definitive cause of this fascinating syndrome is not yet known, partly because it is such a rare disorder and partly because the precise location of the damage in the brain that causes alien (or anarchic) hand syndrome varies between patients.[4]

Since a brain structure called the corpus callosum is all that connects the two cerebral hemispheres, perhaps if the two hemispheres become disconnected, activity in one part of the brain might not reach the awareness of another.[5]

The popular term for alien hand syndrome is Dr Strangelove syndrome, named after the Peter Sellers character in the 1963 Stanley Kubrick film *Dr Strangelove*. In the film a senior government military adviser, Dr Strangelove, has a hand which often fails to obey its master and acts as if possessed by a will of its own. At one point the hand makes a Hitler salute, which Dr Strangelove struggles to prevent. In fact, unlikely as it may seem, the syndrome as represented in the film is surprisingly neurologically and psychiatrically accurate, making one wonder if the film-makers had some direct experience of this disorder.[6]

Dr Strangelove sits in a wheelchair, indicating a disability of some kind – perhaps a stroke – and indeed, the vast majority of alien hand syndrome cases appear to be the result of a stroke or similar sudden leakage or blockage in the brain. Also, although the hand acts in a way that appears to oppose the will of its owner, there is a sense in which it actually represents what the owner would really want to do or express but is inhibited from doing for social or other reasons. So when the hand makes the Hitler salute, although at first this embarrasses Dr Strangelove and he struggles with it to stop the gesture, eventually he loses the battle and openly flaunts his previously hidden Fascist leanings. His body's behaviour comes into line with the hand, not the other way around.

This is one of the central questions that lie at the heart of any attempt to understand alien hand syndrome – where does the intention that drives the hand come from? Is it possible that the alien hand is really expressing a motivation of part of the brain that is normally suppressed? Does the hand reveal our hidden desires? Or is it so oppositional that it is difficult to conceive it reflects a hidden part of our personality? Furthermore, does this condition also raise fundamental questions about our sense of self, which is clearly linked to the experience of ownership?[7]

A possible illustration of this dilemma comes from a case of alien hand syndrome reported by neurologist Professor Sergio Della Sala from the University of Aberdeen.[8]

The woman who scolded her own hand

The woman in this case suffered a bleed into her brain following the rupturing of an aneurysm and afterwards reported that her left hand would uncontrollably reach out and grab nearby things and that it would not obey her. Emotional or stressful situations increased the likelihood of anarchic movements and she expressed dread and frustration with regard to these involuntary actions. Once during dinner her left hand had taken some fish bones from the leftovers and, much to her dismay, had put them in her mouth. On another occasion, while she was washing dishes her right hand had picked up a plate and at the same time her left hand had clasped another, making it impossible to carry out the task.

She never doubted that the wayward hand was a part of her own body, yet felt her left hand had a will of its own. She also had to contend with her left hand showing repetitive unwanted behaviour, such as scratching one of her legs or drumming her fingers on the table, which she could stop only by holding down the left hand with the right one.

The patient eventually reached the conclusion that her left hand's behaviour was completely beyond her control and took to talking to it in an attempt to influence it in some way. She tried talking to it nicely, scolding it or even attacking it with the other hand, saying, 'This hand does whatever it wants! This is what I have to do to get it to behave.' She also complained that she found it difficult to control her left leg. For example, she often felt that while walking, instead of rising to step forward, her left leg would press downwards. Whether or not this is an example of 'alien foot syndrome' is open to debate.

Studies on imitative behaviour suggest that awareness of body structure arises very early in the course of development.[9] Imitation of adults' movements by young babies has been widely described and this behaviour suggests an early ability to identify a body part as our own or as belonging to another person.[10] The recent discovery of neurones that become active during both observation and execution of a specific action might provide a neural basis for this mechanism.[11] This may mean that at the earliest stage of development a baby moves its own limbs to copy another person's movement, without at first being able to distinguish the ownership of the two.[12]

It is likely that this system undergoes continuous updating during development and adult life, and participates in the construction of what we will refer to as the internal body representation.[13]

The abilities to attribute an action to its proper agent, and to understand its meaning when produced by someone else, are basic aspects of human social communication. Several psychiatric syndromes, such as psychosis in general and schizophrenia in particular, seem to lead to a dysfunction of the awareness of one's own actions and the recognition of actions performed by others. For example, schizophrenics often believe an external agency is moving their limbs and so they feel they are not in control of their own bodies. This is referred to by doctors as passivity phenomena or by the patients as a sense of alien control.[14]

The psychotic also often feels they have special powers, and this could explain the high incidence of delusions relating to being the next Messiah or other powerful people. These special powers appear to derive from the experience psychotics have that they are in control of other people and events around the world.[15]

The feeling of losing personal control, or alternatively being in extensive control of external objects, suggests that the sense of personal agency breaks down in psychosis, as it does in a specific way with alien hand syndrome. Such syndromes, therefore, offer a framework for studying the determinants of agency: the ability to attribute actions to their proper source.[16]

A possible explanation for hallucinations is a confusion about whether or not your thoughts are your own. If you didn't realize your own mental 'internal conversation' was produced by yourself, then you could believe these thoughts were voices speaking at you.[17]

In early childhood we develop a sense of our own minds being separate from others', yet we also endeavour to work out what could be going on in other people's minds by using what is happening in our own, the so-called 'theory of mind'.[18]

The neuroscientist Christopher Frith, based at the Institute of Neurology in London, suggests that schizophrenics fail in monitoring their willed intentions, including those related to the expression of thought. The consequence is that they are unable to disentangle 'intentions' arising from external stimuli from those generated as a consequence of their own thoughts and intentions. Symptoms such as insertion of thought (believing your own thoughts are not your own but have been inserted into your mind from outside), hallucinations and delusion of control would directly derive from this difficulty. It would also seem that some system which monitors what is going on outside personal control breaks down, so although the psychotic person has caused an action, they believe the cause has arisen externally to them.[19]

Verbal hallucinations seem to fit this explanation. During verbal hallucinations in schizophrenic patients, the sensory areas relating to language remain active.[20] This suggests that their nervous system behaves as if it were actually processing the speech of an external speaker, hence their perception of their own thinking as originating from the outside world.[21]

In the cases of alien hand syndrome cited here, the patients attributed their own action to an external source. This tendency, however, corresponds to only part of the symptoms in schizophrenia. The same patients may experience the reverse as well, that is, they may experience the action of others as a consequence of their own intentions.[22]

So a sense of ownership is a vital brain and mind mechanism with bizarre consequences when it breaks down.[23]

The internal body can be severely affected by brain injuries such as strokes, giving rise to a wide variety of symptoms including denial of ownership of one's body part, and a failure to accept that your limb is paralysed following a stroke when it clearly is.[24]

In 1942 the neurologist Gerstman first introduced the term 'somatoparaphrenia' in order to describe cases of delusional elaboration in which the affected limb is involved in bizarre illusory ideas.[25] Milder forms of somatoparaphrenia have been described by stroke patients who report feeling that the paralysed limb is extraneous or that these limbs have departed from their body. In more severe forms of somatoparaphrenia, patients claim that the limb belongs to someone else. However, although alien hand syndrome at first glance appears somewhat similar to somatoparaphrenia, it is in fact a much stranger disorder.[26]

For example, Doctor T. M. Lewis and colleagues reported a particularly peculiar case of alien hand syndrome in a 90-year-old woman who had suffered a stroke.[27]

The woman who had a nickname for her hand

Following her stroke this patient developed alien hand syndrome; she demonstrated an unawareness that her left arm and hand were her own, treating the limb as a foreign presence that acted against her well-being. Sensation was moderately impaired on the left and the patient became frustrated by her inability to control her alien limb – frequently scolding it for 'being bad'.

Personification of the limb was clearly noted as the patient would refer to the limb as 'Gloria' or 'she'. She would then restrict the movements of her left arm by forcibly taking it and placing it firmly in her right armpit. The patient described episodes when her alien hand would remove her glasses or 'touch her in inappropriate ways'. When attempting to simulate drinking from a mug or using a fork, her alien hand grasped the item and thrust it towards her face. On each occasion the patient was perplexed by the action of her alien limb. She would often slap her hand and scold it; then she would apologize to it and gently stroke and caress it with her right hand.

When objects were presented blindly to the patient she could identify all items in the right hand but was unable to identify any in the alien hand. As a result of the problem the patient became frustrated and anxious. At one point during her rehabilitation she was placed on suicide precautions as she acknowledged being depressed and feared that her alien limb might try to hurt her with her cosmetic scissors.

Similarly, Doctor Ferdinando S. Buonanno and colleagues of the Department of Neurology at Massachusetts General Hospital in Boston recently reported the following case of an 81-year-old woman with an unremarkable medical history who developed spells of left face, arm and leg tingling.[28] On admission, she was confused and disoriented and misidentified her daughter as a nurse. She also complained that her left hand was acting as if under someone else's control; it hit her face and head and she said she was afraid of it.

The woman who was afraid of her own hand

On transfer to hospital, this patient occasionally scratched her left face and stroked her left forehead with her left hand. She made no attempt to look at her hand to correct the movements. She held her left hand with the right, claiming to keep 'him' from hitting her. When asked what trouble brought her to the hospital, she said that her 'left hand tried to strangle her'. She repeated that 'someone' was hitting and choking her neck, face and shoulder, and asked the nurse to restrain her left hand, fearful that 'hitting the breast will cause cancer'.

On examination, she was alert but showed the right hand when asked to show the left and could not distinguish her left hand from the examiner's. Her inability to copy simple diagrams was characterized by a series of irregular pen strokes.

During her first week in hospital, she was still afraid of her left hand and placed a pillow on her chest for protection.

In many cases patients do need to be protected from themselves. Their alien hand may attack them; as this woman's left hand had attempted strangulation as well as hitting her, her fear of it was understandable. Injuries have been caused – to others as well as to the patient – by hands that pour out scalding tea or shut the other hand in a drawer. Hands that operate independently in this way obviously need to be brought back under control if serious injury is to be avoided.

As we have seen, any attempt to understand alien hand syndrome usually starts from the anatomical fact that the brain is divided into two hemispheres – a left and a right. Due to the crossing of nerve fibres from the limbs in the spinal column and the brain stem near the neck, the brain's right hemisphere comes to control the left hand, and the left hemisphere the right hand.

However, when Wigan, the nineteenth-century English psychiatrist, attended the post-mortem examination of his best friend he was puzzled to find that his friend, who had lived a normal life, had only one cerebral hemisphere.[29] With this discovery, Wigan posed a question which has never been satisfactorily answered:

'Why are there two hemispheres when one is enough?' He also conjectured that the two hemispheres normally have a harmonious relationship with each other, and when this breaks down the result is insanity.[30]

To further demonstrate this theory, a case was reported in the 1980s by Dr Kurt Goldstein of a middle-aged woman who attempted to strangle herself with her left hand. On post-mortem examination she was found to have a brain tumour of the corpus callosum which had severed the connection between the two hemispheres. This meant that she was operating as two separate personalities.[31]

According to the late Professor Alan Parkin of the University of Sussex, the simplest explanation of alien hand is that the right brain hemisphere becomes freed from domination by the left hemisphere and decides to make its own way in the world. It is noticeable that most cases of alien hand involve the left hand which is controlled by the right hemisphere. It is also notable that the dominant brain hemisphere – controlling the right hand, which most of the population prefer to use – is the left one.[32]

But why does the right hemisphere appear to act so often in an anarchic and unhelpful way? Does our non-dominant hemisphere really build up an alternative view of the world and our actions in it?

A key problem with explaining alien or anarchic hand syndrome is that patients appear to vary in the extent to which they are depersonalized from the hand. Many patients regard their alien hand as 'it' but do not deny that it is part of them. In more extreme cases the patient denies the hand is theirs and suggests that it is under the control of someone else. Thus they shout commands and exclamations as the hand goes out of control. As we have seen, in some extreme cases the patient attributes a personality to the hand. Doctors Doody and Jankovic reported one case of a patient who believed that her left hand was a baby called Joseph and that actions to other parts of the body, such as nipple pinching, were a result of feeding.[33]

Yet another theory proposed by Professor Parkin is that in normal circumstances both hands co-operate in accomplishing tasks by suppressing each other as desired by the brain. In most actions the hands don't do exactly the same thing but complement each other. You would only use one hand to hold a table-tennis bat for example, while the other provides balance to the body; if both hands got directly involved in the task of holding the bat, chaos would ensue.[34]

So any movements planned in one brain hemisphere automatically suppress the other hemisphere and the hand under its control – perhaps via the connecting fibres of the corpus callosum. However, if the suppression mechanism goes wrong, as may be the case with alien hand, then it is possible for the other hand to become active and attempt to participate.

The apparently anarchic behaviour of the alien hand according to Professor Parkin's view has a much less sinister origin. If a task has a simple goal then any attempt by the alien hand to contribute positively is prevented because the other hand is already performing the task. The persistent re-selection of TV channels, the choosing of different shoes, pulling down of trousers that have just been pulled up, and so on, can in this view be interpreted as manifestations of the alien hand's inadequate attempt to make a positive contribution to achievement of the overall goal. The part of the brain controlling the alien hand does not realize it should co-ordinate with the other hand rather than attempting to act by itself. In trying to help it just gets in the way.[35]

What this disorder indicates is that our experience of being in charge of our bodies, and so initiating all personal action, has a neurological basis. In other words while the brain is the seat of all our actions and experiences, there is also a part of our nervous system which is responsible for our belief that we have free will in relation to our behaviour. Sufferers from alien hand syndrome feel they are no longer in control of a limb because the part of the brain that gives the sensation of control over their bodies has been damaged. When that happens, our limbs appear to act independently of us.[36]

But if there is a part of the brain designed to make us believe we are in control of our limbs, does the very fact that such a system has to exist mean we are not *really* in charge of our bodies?[37]

Research conducted in the 1980s found that the same electric brain wave changes that characteristically precede all limb movements occur several hundred milliseconds *before* we appear to consciously decide to move a limb. If our conscious decision to act is *preceded* by brain changes that anticipate action, then our 'decision' to choose how to behave, or 'freedom' (as in free will) is in fact illusory. Our choices have in a sense been decided beforehand by our brains.[38]

In an experiment where subjects were tracking by hand an unpredictably moving target, the change in their hand trajectory occurred as early as 100 milliseconds following the target jump, whereas the vocal signal by which they reported their awareness of the jump was not observed until more than 300 milliseconds later.[39]

In another study researchers instructed subjects to perform simple hand movements at will and to report the instant at which they became aware of wanting to move. The time of awareness was found to lag behind the onset of readiness by about 350 milliseconds. In the researchers' terms, 'The brain "decides" to initiate, or at least to prepare to initiate the act before there is any reportable subjective awareness that such a decision has taken place.'[40]

The implications of this view of the link between brain and consciousness are revolutionary, not least because they introduce a whole new defence for criminal lawyers. So how confident are the neurologists of this new perspective?

Doctor Sean Spence, a research fellow in brain scanning at London's Hammersmith Hospital, argues that whether we have free will has to be reconsidered in the light of alien hand syndrome.[41] He suggests that this position is supported by a famous experiment conducted in the 1960s where neurosurgical patients had electrodes implanted in the parts of their brains that initiate limb actions. They were instructed to look at slides on a carousel and to advance the shutter by pushing a control button. In fact, the latter was bogus and the slides were advanced by an amplified signal originating from the electrodes in the subject's own brains (as they prepared to press the button).[42]

The patients were apparently astounded by the effect. It seemed to them that the slide projector was anticipating their decisions. What was really happening was a concrete demonstration that our brain appears to know what we are going to do next, and *before* we ourselves become consciously aware of our decision.[43]

Our sense of control would seem, therefore, illusory and it follows that most of us share in common the useful delusion that we have free will. Patients suffering from alien hand syndrome, however, have lost this experience in relation to a particular limb. In a sense, therefore, people suffering from this disorder are closer to the reality of how much we are really responsible for our actions than the rest of us.[44]

Because they have lost the function of the part of the brain that normally works to make us believe we have conscious freedom of will, they develop the experience of becoming remote spectators to the actions of their bodies.

Defenders of human 'free will' argue that what happens *before* the brain itself decides to act is still unknown, and there may be a role for our own autonomy there. But even these free will guardians concede that the neurological research indicates that whatever happens before the brain is roused must occur below our conscious awareness.

It appears that one of the prices we have had to pay for conscious awareness of ourselves to evolve as a function of the brain is the delusion that we are responsible for all our actions. If we had conscious awareness of ourselves but no sense of free will, our bodies would feel alien to us. After all, think what your hand is doing right now. Did you consciously put it there?[45]

But delusions like alien hand syndrome can only help us understand the brain if we drive a distinction between the form of the delusion and the content. The distinction between form and content is not always easy to make, however, as we have seen.

To psychiatrists, the form and the content are the two key components of the psychotic state. The form is the kind of symptom that a psychotic experience takes – it might be a hallucination that God is speaking to you directly and issuing commands that you do his work. Otherwise, the form could be a delusion – the belief that you are God or have direct access to his or her mind. Delusions and hallucinations are two distinct forms of psychotic experience – one is a belief, the other is a sensation, usually visual or auditory.

The reason for driving a distinction between form and content is that form, very generally speaking, appears universal across cultures and throughout history. People appeared to have heard voices in the distant past and in remote parts of the planet. In contrast, the content of their delusions and hallucinations has differed.

The content of the psychosis is what God says to you or what you believe is your mission plan from the deity. While many people may share the same delusion that they are God or an agent of God, the precise content of each delusion is usually unique. This raises the puzzling question of why and what determines the content of the disordered thinking that constitutes psychosis.[46]

One important clue comes from evidence that the composition of delusions seems to be influenced by the immediate environment of the psychotic patient. As our environments change, so naturally do the contents of delusions that psychiatrists observe.[47]

The more strange a delusion appears to be, the more likely the underlying diagnosis is schizophrenia. Schizophrenia is one of the two major psychoses with no obvious biological cause yet found, the other being manic-depressive psychosis. Schizophrenia starts some time after puberty with the loss of integrated personality, which often continues as a chronic symptom. In most cases it is a psychosis from which some psychiatrists believe there is little or no chance of recovery, with patients falling into a state of mental decay. Others, like myself, believe that with early and vigorous treatment the prognosis is excellent.[48]

With schizophrenic patients, the following symptoms can be noted: (1) *auditory hallucination*, in which patients hear imaginary voices; (2) *delusion*, false, bizarre beliefs about the world; (3) *gemachtes erlebnis*, a sense of being manipulated by the will of someone or something other than oneself; (4) *autism*, in which patients detach themselves from the real world and live in their own world; (5) the *blunted affect*, a lack of emotion in response to any stimuli; and (6) *abulia*, a lack of will and desire and the inability to make decisions.

So schizophrenia is characterized by abnormalities of thinking, perception and emotion. Paranoid schizophrenia is the commonest sub-type and early symptoms typically include bizarre delusions, auditory hallucinations and interference with thinking. In the chronic form, blunting of emotion, social withdrawal and avolition can become more obvious. Age at onset is usually the late twenties or early thirties and both sexes are equally affected. Current cultural beliefs appear to determine the content of delusions in schizophrenia and there is often a religious theme ('I am God'). However, a common secular delusion is that of being pursued by secret agents.

So although personality problems, schizophrenia and manic depression may be universal and may determine the form of the symptom – whether you hear voices or not – the content of what the voices say to you or the content of your delusion appear to be heavily influenced by your environment.[49]

For example, computer technology and the Internet are new features of modern society and sure enough these have begun to make an appearance in reported delusions. Intriguingly – and there has yet to be proper formal research into this point – it seems that any change in society has to be established for some time before it makes an appearance in a delusion.

Although the Internet has begun to feature in psychopathology, most usually in the form of Internet addiction, the debate amongst psychologists is whether in itself it could spawn an entirely new gamut of illnesses or merely feature as a new item in older disorders. Addictions are as old as the hills, so the fact that the Internet should begin to feature as a form of an addiction does not mean that an entirely new disorder has now surfaced.

However, Dr Glenn Catalano and colleagues from the Department of Psychiatry at the University of South Florida College of Medicine report two recent cases of delusions involving the Internet which provide intriguing clues as to what determines the content of delusions.[50]

The man with a web-site delusion

The patient was a 40-year-old man who had a self-inflicted gunshot wound to the face as a result of a suicide attempt. He shot himself in response to an embarrassing prank he believed had been played on him by friends. He said they had placed photographs of him masturbating, and videos of him and his girlfriend having sex, on the Internet.

He reported that a friend in the Central Intelligence Agency had placed Internet bugs in his ears so that they could read his mind and control his thoughts. He also believed his friends had placed a link between his web page and his extremities and by hitting different keys, web browsers could make his extremities jump.

The man who believed he was a webmaster

The second patient was a 41-year-old man who said that he was a witch and that he ran an online service that gave advice to new witches. He reported that he was a webmaster and that he created web pages for others. He believed that his powers were so strong that he could surf the net using only his mind. He also said that he received magnetism from the Internet at certain times each day, just as it said on the bottle of a famous soft drink.

In both these cases and, as mentioned before, in all delusions the precise genesis of delusional thinking remains a mystery but can be shaped by current cultural and political experiences; there are many case reports of patients' delusions being influenced by topics covered in the media or by recent emotionally charged events.

In the cases of the two patients detailed here, it could be that they felt so threatened by the Internet that it became one of the new tormentors in their paranoid delusions. Both patients had minimal if any personal experience of computers or the Internet and were of less than average intelligence. However, their ignorance may have intensified their fantasies of the Internet and caused an amplification of their fear. Such delusions may become more prevalent as Internet use continues.

There have also been patients whose delusions were based on their concern about being influenced by products of super-modern science. These patients were so focused on the possible effects of new technologies (either real or imagined) that they incorporated these fears into their delusional system.

Patients with schizophrenia have described being controlled by and entwined with the Internet, and others have perceived themselves as characters in a film, with their life played out for the cameras. Doctor Shubsachs and Dr Young, psychiatrists at the Royal Edinburgh Hospital, call this the Hollywood Phenomenon[51] and psychiatrists Dr Tomison and Dr Donovan of the Langdon Hospital in Exeter reported a case of this phenomenon.[52]

The man who thought he was being held by the SAS

G.W., a 23-year-old unemployed man who had had two previous admissions for acute schizophrenic psychosis was remanded in custody on charges of malicious wounding, burglary and possession of an offensive weapon. For five months he had felt that he was being filmed by hidden cameras and that newspaper articles had a special significance for him. He also believed that people spoke to him in codes.

Prior to committing the offences he had not slept and felt 'high and excited'. He felt that he was performing, that he had been hypnotized and that codes had been put into his mind. On the night of the offences he smashed windows, believing it was part of the filming exercise. He defecated in a bin, returned to his flat, and cooked some stew. He then left the flat in stockinged feet and festooned three young men with the stew. He also felt compelled to ring a doorbell that said 'this one'. When a young man answered the door, G.W. entered, claiming to be a member of the Drug Squad. He ransacked the flat, played a guitar, picked up a Stanley knife and made the two male occupants take off their trousers. He then cut one of the occupants on the arm and made them walk to a telephone box. In the process he cut the other man on his back. He forced the men to telephone the police, who arrived and arrested him. G.W. continued to claim to be a member of the Drug Squad, was abusive and attempted to drive the police car.

When seen in custody, and after admission to hospital, he maintained that the staff and the interviewing doctor were members of the SAS. He also believed that the sequence of events was part of an SAS training exercise which was being filmed.

A similar phenomenon is described by Dr Rachel Forsyth and colleagues from the University of Bristol Division of Psychiatry, who recently reported the case of a computer game as the basis for a delusion.[53]

The man who took playing a video game very seriously

A young man was admitted from prison to a psychiatric facility after reports that he had been acting in a bizarre manner. He had been arrested for stealing motor vehicles and for assaults with weapons. At interview he was found to be experiencing the delusion that he was a player inside a computer game in which points are scored for stealing cars, killing assailants and avoiding police vehicles.

Psychotic symptoms had emerged slowly over two years. His family had noticed him becoming increasingly withdrawn and isolated from social activities and he developed delusions that strangers were planning to kill him. He also experienced auditory hallucinations, constantly hearing an abusive and derogatory voice. A computer enthusiast, he began to play computer games incessantly and felt that the games were communicating with him via the headphones. He also came to believe he was inside one of these games and had to steal a car to start scoring points. He broke into a car and drove off at speed, believing he had 'invulnerable' fuel and so could not run out of petrol. To gain game points he chose to steal increasingly powerful vehicles, threatening and assaulting the owners with weapons. Later he said he would have had no regrets if he had killed someone, since this would have increased his score.

After arrest and while in prison he continued to believe he was in the game, and when he was admitted to hospital six weeks later, part of ward management was to deny him access to computer games. Nothing abnormal was found on physical examination, but he was diagnosed as suffering from paranoid schizophrenia. He responded well to further treatment with anti-psychotic medication.

In this report it was not suggested that computer games can be the cause of psychosis, but it does seem likely that with the growing use of computers for relaxation, game scenarios will be incorporated more often into delusional systems. A worrying aspect is that in many of these games points are scored for acting violently, and killing people is often a feature. If the game is transposed into the real world by someone in a delusional state, the risk of subsequent violence is high – particularly if violence is not perceived to be illegal or morally wrong.

Doctor S. A. Spence of the Academic Department of Psychiatry, University of Sheffield, argues that such cases may be understood within a broader context – the content of psychotic phenomenology incorporating elements of the patient's psychosocial environment, while the form of a psychotic symptom (e.g. 'delusion') represents an underlying biological 'signal'. In 1993 he reported a patient with paranoid schizophrenia whose auditory hallucinations derived from a computer game.[54] These hallucinations underwent delusional interpretation with the patient believing that they 'meant' she was homeless. In that report he predicted that 'similar cases will arise as video games become more widely accessible'.

But even Dr Spence could not have foreseen the extremely worrying case of the man who delusionally hijacked a plane as a result of being influenced by a computer game.[55]

Doctor Atsushi Ichimura and colleagues at Tokai University School of Medicine, and the Tokai University Medical Research Institute in Japan report a case of what they define as Chronic Alternate-World Disorder (CAWD), which they argue is a symptomatic behaviour in which a person becomes fanatically engrossed in a virtual-reality (VR) world to the extent that he or she can no longer distinguish between the actual world and virtual reality.[56]

The case in question involves a man who hijacked a jumbo jetliner in order to fly the aeroplane on his own after developing CAWD from the use of light-simulator software. Doctor Ichimura and colleagues believe cases of CAWD will increase as VR spreads throughout our society and in view of this, propose precautionary and preventive measures be taken by providers of VR systems for patients with schizophrenia or personality disorders.

Symptoms of this condition include the inability to distinguish VR space from the real world, which becomes a chronic state even when the person is out of VR space. When this chronic state continues, it is commonly referred to as a 'cognitive disorder', and it stems from a mental predisposition rather than organic psychosis (psychic trauma/injuries, inflammation, tumour, degeneration, vascular disorder, ageing and drug use).

There are instances in which, after a family member is afflicted with psychosis, similar symptoms can be seen in other family members who haven't been afflicted with psychosis.

Most popularly available computer games are not yet at the stage of sophistication where virtual reality is replicated. However, Dr Ichimura and colleagues feel that such games can be considered VR devices by young users who can achieve a sensation of unreality in spite of the relatively unsophisticated VR technology. It could be said, therefore, that CAWD could potentially be acquired from all visual-imaging devices – which, by representing spurious experiences and space through the use of their multi-media capabilities, could be implicated in VR pathology.

The computer game player who hijacked a plane

This case report concerns a young man who developed CAWD on a flight simulator and proceeded to actually hijack a jumbo jet and attempt to fly the plane.

The patient attended prestigious private junior and senior high schools, and graduated from university. His graduation thesis was based on 'Transportation Economics', and it was his dream to become a pilot. His medical records showed that he had received psychiatric out-patient therapy and according to statements given by his neighbours, high-pitched laughter could be heard coming from his house at night. Four days prior to his attempted hijacking, he purchased a kitchen knife which was taken away by his father.

In his spare time he used a flight simulator, which was set up in his bedroom, and this served to increase his desire to fly and be around aeroplanes.

The following is part of a transcript of the aircraft to tower radio transmissions during the episode on the plane:

'The man commanded the co-pilot to leave the cockpit, saying, "Get out! You're in my way." The man seated himself in the co-pilot's seat, took hold of the control stick, and commanded the captain to head for Yokota airbase from the plane's present location above Ohshima . . . The man demanded that he sit in the captain's seat, saying, "It's harder to fly a real plane than in those games."

'The captain, unwilling to comply, said, "You want to sit in my seat? I don't think I can let you do that . . . There are many other planes up here, so it could be dangerous." The man acknowledged the captain's advice and obediently replied, "Yes (I understand)."

'The captain said to the man, "I'd like to increase our altitude so that we don't crash into anything." Although the man obediently acknowledged the captain's words and said, "Yes (I understand)", 22 seconds after this conversation, the man fatally stabbed the captain in the neck.'

At this point, only the young man was at the controls in the cockpit. He fumbled with the instruments in an attempt to disengage the autopilot, but was unable to do so and shortly after he forced the control stick forward and the aircraft's nose pointed down over Sagamihara City. The aircraft descended to an altitude of 1,000 feet (approximately 300 metres above sea level), which was less than 200 metres above the ground. Seven members of the flight crew then rushed into the cockpit, seized the man, and regained control of the aircraft. Had they waited one more minute the aircraft would have crashed into Yokota airbase.

This is what the young man said after the incident:

'I couldn't be satisfied with games any longer. I had done it so well on games, I thought that if anybody could land the aircraft, I could. I'm sorry about the captain. If we had crashed, I would have done a terrible thing to the passengers and the residents of the area. I wanted to fly at low altitude, but the captain didn't want to tell me how to disengage the autopilot and I couldn't fly the plane the way I wanted to . . . so I stabbed him. I chose to land at Yokota instead of Haneda because the landing strip is longer. I wanted to demonstrate to the public that planes are safe.'

While it appears that he went to great lengths to develop a detailed plan, its execution was haphazard and game-like. As a result of his obsession with his flight simulator and his resultant difficulty distinguishing between VR and the real world, the life of the captain was lost and the lives of 503 passengers were put in jeopardy.

The significance of this case lies in the fact that electronic instruments such as VR devices, which are proliferating in our society, influenced the nature of the incident and the events leading to the development of his psychosis.

But if your environment, for example the Internet or Hollywood films, can influence delusions, can an actual place induce psychosis?

The answer could be 'yes' in relation to the so-called Jerusalem syndrome.

Psychiatrist Dr Yair Bar-El and colleagues from the Kfar Shaul Mental Health Centre in Jerusalem, Israel, recently reported that Jerusalem's psychiatrists are encountering an ever-increasing number of tourists who, upon arriving in Jerusalem, develop a psychotic illness.[57]

They argue this is because Jerusalem is a city that conjures up a sense of the holy, the historical and the heavenly; it holds a unique attraction for people of several of the world's faiths and religions – especially Jews, Christians and Muslims. When people dream of Jerusalem, they do not see the modern, politically controversial Jerusalem, but the holy biblical city.

In view of the consistently high incidence of this phenomenon, it was decided to channel all such cases to one central facility (the Kfar Shaul Mental Health Centre) for psychological counselling, psychiatric intervention and, if deemed necessary, admission to hospital.

Over the course of 13 years, some 1,200 tourists with severe Jerusalem-generated mental problems have been referred to this facility. Of these, 470 were admitted to hospital. On average, 100 such tourists are seen annually and 40 of them require admission to hospital.

On the basis of clinical experience, Dr Yair Bar-El and colleagues identified three main types of patient with Jerusalem syndrome.

Type I refers to individuals already diagnosed as having a psychosis before their visit to Israel. Their motivation in coming to the country is directly related to their mental condition and to the influence of religious ideas which often reach delusional levels. They feel compelled to come to Jerusalem and do 'something' there. They identify with biblical characters from the Old or New Testament. They are often convinced that they are one of these characters. Jewish tourists generally identify with characters from the Old Testament, and Christian tourists with characters from the New Testament. Men and women generally identify with male and female personalities respectively.

For example, an American tourist in his 40s who was suffering from paranoid schizophrenia began to identify with the biblical character Samson. He started to work on his body image by exercising and weightlifting, and felt compelled to visit Jerusalem in order to move one of the giant stone blocks forming the Western

(Wailing) Wall which, in his opinion, was not in the right place. On arriving at the Western Wall, he attempted to move one of the stones and instigated a terrible commotion, culminating in police intervention and his admission to hospital.

Contrary to the usual accepted practice, the duty psychiatrist challenged the patient's delusional ideas, telling him that he could not possibly be Samson and that, according to the Bible, Samson had never been in Jerusalem. The patient reacted to this with rage, broke a window, and escaped through it. A team was sent out to look for him, and a student nurse eventually found him standing at a bus stop. Demonstrating commendable wisdom, she told him that he had proved that he possessed qualities similar to Samson's and that he could now return to the hospital, which he did of his own volition. A hospital examination showed him to be in an acute psychotic state; he was still convinced that he was Samson and that he had a mission to accomplish. After receiving anti-psychotic medication, he calmed down and was able to fly back home, escorted by his father.

Type II relates to groups of people with mental disorders (such as personality disorders) or obsessions with fixed ideas, who nevertheless do not have a clear mental illness. Type II probably accounts for a relatively large number of Jerusalem syndrome sufferers. In groups, they are highly visible; they stand out in public places, especially holy ones and are occasionally featured in the media but do not, on the whole, reach professional psychiatric agencies.

However, within this type fall various Christian groups who settle in Jerusalem in order, for instance, to bring about the resurrection of the dead or the reappearance of Jesus Christ. Such groups usually consist of no more than about 20 members. One group, previously located in Jerusalem, is now settled near Jericho, another is located in the Jerusalem Forest and yet another is based in the centre of Jerusalem. The members of these groups wear distinctive clothing which, according to them, is similar to that worn in the days of Christ.

Members of these groups do not usually undergo psychiatric examination because they cause few problems and do not endanger others or break the law.

The third type in this syndrome is perhaps the most fascinating, in that it describes individuals with no previous history of mental illness who fall victim to a psychotic episode while in Israel (and especially while in Jerusalem), recover fairly spontaneously and then, after leaving the country, apparently return to normal.

Numerically, type III is a relatively small category: in the 13 years of the study there were only 42 cases fitting the main diagnostic criteria.

Type III does not usually involve visual or auditory hallucinations. Patients know who they are and do not claim to be anyone else. If questioned, they identify themselves by their real name. However, they ask not to be disturbed in the completion of their mission. Their condition usually returns to normal within 5–7 days; in other words, it is a short-lived episode. These individuals often clearly need treatment, and receive it, but recovery is usually spontaneous and not necessarily due to treatment. Experience has taught that improvement is facilitated by, or dependent on, physically distancing the patient from Jerusalem and its holy places.

Upon recovery, patients can usually recall every detail of their aberrant behaviour. They are inevitably ashamed of most of their actions, and feel that they have behaved foolishly or childishly. They sometimes describe their conduct as akin to that of a 'clown' or a 'drug addict'. However, most are reluctant to talk about the episode, and so it has been difficult to gain a deeper understanding of the phenomenon. Those who do talk often speak about a sense of 'something opening up inside them'. After this sensation, they feel an obligation to carry out certain actions or to replay their message.

In seeking out distinctive background features of type III patients, it was discovered that, of the 42 cases, 40 were Protestants, one was Catholic, and one was a Jew who had lived as a Protestant while in hiding during World War II. All 40 Protestants came from what can be described as 'ultra-religious families'. The Bible was their most important book, and the family would read it together at least once a week. It also served as the source of answers to seemingly insoluble problems – especially for the father, the head of the family. For fundamentalist believers of this type, Jerusalem assumes the highest significance; such people possess an idealistic subconscious image of Jerusalem, the holy places and the life and death of Jesus. It seems, however, that those who succumb to type III of the Jerusalem syndrome are unable to deal with the concrete reality of Jerusalem today – a gap appears between their subconscious idealistic image of Jerusalem and the city as it appears in reality. One might view their psychotic state, and particularly the need to preach their universal message, as an attempt to bridge the gap between these two representations.

Several explanations have been offered to account for psychotic breakdown among travellers. Some of these suggest that the change of routine involved in travel influences the mental state to a considerable extent. A number of factors are involved, such as unfamiliar surroundings, proximity to foreigners or strangers, inactivity, a sense of isolation and culture clash. Compounded by the special significance of Jerusalem to Jews, Christians and Muslims, these factors may serve to trigger an acute psychotic episode. The 'existential' mode of travelling (this mode refers to journeys to a spiritual centre) is a modern metamorphosis of the pilgrimage. It is worth noting that Freud reported having experienced a sense that the world around him was no longer real while visiting the Acropolis.

The possibility that other place-oriented syndromes and the Jerusalem syndrome may share a common denominator, even though they appear to be fundamentally different, should not be dismissed. For instance, in the case of airport wanderers' or 'airport syndrome', a condition found among tourists who get lost and who experience psychotic episodes in airports, it has been suggested that airports symbolically highlight pre-existing problems. However, unlike victims of the Jerusalem syndrome, people who develop airport syndrome forget their identity, are unaware of where they have come from or where they are going to.

But if a place can play a role in inducing psychosis, can a particularly evocative moment do so as well? For example, what about the turn of the millennium?

In December 1999, psychiatrists Dr J. S. E. Hellewell and P. M. Haddad from Trafford General Hospital, Manchester, wrote to over 60 general psychiatrists in the North-Western Region requesting that they provide details of all of their patients who appeared to be affected clinically by the millennium.[58] A sizeable proportion described having encountered one or more patients within this category and a number of patients with established psychiatric disorders were reported to have incorporated millennial themes into their symptoms.

Examples of delusions with a millennial content included becoming the Messiah, being destined to change the world on New Year's Day, and the belief that the world would change irrevocably at midnight. Several patients with psychoses appeared to have taken warnings regarding the 'millennium bug' rather literally, describing this in terms of physical infestation.

Another key influence on delusions is mood. If you are clinically depressed then your thinking becomes very negative. The most extreme manifestation of this is Cotard's syndrome – believed to be the most profound delusional end point of severe depression. In Cotard's syndrome you simply believe that you no longer exist! It is referred to by psychiatrists as the ultimate nihilistic delusion.

A German doctor, R. P. Stolk, reported a case in which an 18-year-old suddenly felt that the world had changed and he became convinced that he had died – an experience he quite naturally found strange and terrifying. He felt that his insides were rotting and nothing was functioning. He also thought that his relatives had died and although they were still walking about, they had risen from the dead or were merely doubles. He was very anxious and repeatedly tried to commit suicide. However, he recovered after a few weeks of treatment and was profoundly puzzled by his experiences.[59]

Stolk commented that this psychotic experience could reflect the emotional changes that can occur in severe depression when some people remark that they can't experience anything any more, as if their emotional life has been paralysed. They make comments to the effect that 'I was living dead'.

The notion of the living dead has had a powerful appeal down the centuries and still exercises the imagination of people drawn to horror movies and science fiction. However, the basis for the idea of the living dead could come from psychiatric experiences.

In the eighteenth century Charles Bonnet described the case of an elderly lady who probably suffered a stroke, but when she recovered the ability to speak she demanded to be dressed in a shroud and placed in a coffin, saying that she was already dead. The attempts of her daughter and servants to talk her out of this delusion only made her agitated and annoyed that they would not offer her this last service. Finally, they began to dress her in a shroud and lay her out to calm her down. The old lady supervised this activity carefully, checking the arrangement of the shroud and the whiteness of the linen. When she fell asleep, she was undressed and put into bed, but on awakening still insisted that she was dead and should be buried. This delusional belief lasted a long time.

In 1880 Cotard's original description of the condition was introduced as *délire de négation*; it was described as having various degrees of severity, from mild states characterized by feelings of despair and self-loathing to more severe forms in which the patient experiences a feeling of change both inside and outside himself. In the most severe cases, denial of the very existence of self occurs.

Cotard's first case was a 43-year-old woman who believed that she had 'no brain, nerves, chest or entrails, and was just skin and bone'. The psychiatrist was of the opinion that he had identified a new type of depression characterized by anxious melancholia, ideas of damnation or possession, suicidal behaviour, insensitivity to pain and delusions of non-existence and immortality.[60]

In 1995 the psychiatrists Berrios and Luque reviewed more than 200 articles containing reports of cases of Cotard syndrome. Using complex statistical techniques, they argued that there was a group of patients who showed no outward signs of depression but still believed they were dead or did not exist. Nevertheless, they did confirm that depression was reported in the vast majority (89 per cent) of the subjects, and among the nihilistic delusions the most common were those concerning the body (86 per cent) and existence (69 per cent).[61]

Despite the fact that most patients recover, Cotard's syndrome appears to have wider significance. According to psychiatrists Enoch and Trethowan, it 'brings us face to face with the very meaning of existence itself'.[62]

Proof of one's existence is an important strand in philosophy, dealt with especially by René Descartes (1596–1650), who was perhaps the greatest doubter of all time, given his need to reject any belief of which he could not be absolutely certain. Born in La Haye, a small town in France that has since been named after him, Descartes lamented the lack of precision he found in the philosophy of the day compared to the rigour and absolute certainty of mathematical proof. His chronic uncertainty about anything outside of mathematics led him eventually to doubt his own existence and to wonder how he could be sure he even existed. Indeed, if he could not be sure of *that*, then what could he be sure of? Perhaps his existence was only a kind of dream.

Descartes's momentous discovery was that if he doubted, then *something or someone* must be doing the doubting, so the very fact that he doubted proved he existed. Hence the most famous quotation in philosophy, 'Cogito, ergo sum' (I think, therefore I am). Strictly speaking this should really be 'I doubt, and because I doubt, I know I exist.'[63]

At first sight Cotard patients are merely bad philosophers because even though they say they are dead or do not exist, they maintain that they can think. But what they often give as evidence of their non-existence or death is that they don't have proper feelings. According to Bertrand Russell, this is actually close to what

Descartes intended; that is, 'cogito' should be interpreted not just as 'I think' but as 'I think and feel'.

If the Cotard syndrome arises out of a fundamental change in feeling, then there appears to be a link here with the Capgras syndrome. In this syndrome one believes that close relatives have been replaced by impostors. As we saw in Chapter 14, currently the most popular theory to explain this relates to the possibility that due to brain dysfunction in facial recognition, the pathway linked to emotional responsiveness is impaired, but not the pathway associated with object recognition. So whilst the patient realizes that the person they are viewing is identical to their relative in appearance, due to the absence of the usual emotions and the lack of a sense of familiarity, they assume that this cannot be the relative and must therefore be an impostor.

Recently, it was psychologists Dr Andrew Young of Cambridge University and Dr Kate Leafhead of Durham University who first intriguingly proposed that the Capgras and Cotard syndromes were linked.[64]

They argued that in both syndromes there is a problem with emotional responsiveness and a deduction is then made from this experience. In Capgras it is that relatives have been replaced by impostors, while in Cotard's syndrome, since the person has no feeling, they are dead or do not exist.[65]

Perhaps another key link is that depressed people tend to attribute negative events to internal causes; they shoulder undue responsibility and therefore guilt for whatever happens to them. In contrast, the paranoid or people with persecutory delusions attribute whatever happens to them to external causes. Any change in themselves is attributed to a change in others ('they must be impostors') while the depressed assume it is all down to them ('I must be dead').

This theory also explains the direction of aggression which tends to follow these two syndromes. In Capgras cases the altered perception is externalized and so is the violence, with some Capgras patients threatening or harming the supposed impostors. In Cotard patients, on the other hand, where an internal attribution is made for the perceived abnormality, violence is directed towards the self.

At first sight it appears paradoxical that people who say they are dead should try to kill themselves. The resolution to this paradox is that Cotard patients believe that although they are dead, they are in a unique situation of still having thoughts and feelings. To these patients, suicide may represent a final solution to their discomfort, even if the possibility of suicide is, ultimately, proof of their existence.

With this strange delusion we have finally returned – with a possible explanation of where the idea of zombies and the living dead could have come from – to the states of being that are not dissimilar to vampires and werewolves, and with which we began this journey through some of the most extraordinary experiences possible.

16

WOULD YOU KNOW WHAT A DELUSION IS –
EVEN IF YOU HAD ONE?

In modern science, unfortunately, the boundaries of the brain are being extended and the mind is getting progressively smaller.
Solms, a psychoanalyst working in a neurosurgical unit

So what do these extraordinary states of mind, linked to bizarre thinking that produce fantastic delusions, tell us about the mind and brain? I believe they show that if delusions did not exist, we would be left without access to a crucial understanding of ourselves. Knowing when we or others get things fundamentally wrong in terms of beliefs can help us sharpen up our own act by making us more accurate in our perceptions of reality.

Delusions can be viewed as individuals' attempts to make sense of events: as incorrect explanations of experiences.[1] Typically, delusions are defined as fixed, false beliefs. This begs the question: if the beliefs are false, why do they persist? The answer to this question is not just important for the medically certified deluded, but has the potential to liberate the rest of us from personal behaviour and attitudes which could be binding us to an unhelpful or a distorted view of reality.

A belief may persist as a result of two processes: obtaining confirmatory evidence and discarding disconfirmatory evidence. So why do persecutory delusions remain when every day their central predictions are contradicted? Part of the answer may lie in the research field of anxiety disorders. A crucial factor in the maintenance of anxiety disorders is 'safety seeking behaviour'. An example of safety seeking would be the flight phobic who avoids flying or those who fear heights by avoiding tall buildings.

So if the fear of heights leads to the avoidance of tall buildings the victim of this phobia might continue to believe that they have survived the danger by avoiding these buildings. Those who fear spiders might believe they have survived encounters with what they believe to be dangerous creatures by avoiding them or squashing them. The only way the spider phobic could learn that spiders are not as dangerous as they believe is by allowing an encounter with a spider. Their safety or avoidance behaviour precludes the very possibility that might cure them.

Similarly, it could be that a belief produces behaviour likely to protect the belief from disconfirmation or the truth. This is a hugely important notion as it generalizes to the rest of our lives. For example, it may be that we give up working hard because we believe that hard work will not get us anywhere, yet the consequence is that our belief is never exposed to personally disconfirmatory evidence.

Doctor Freeman and colleagues from the Institute of Psychiatry in London recently proposed that safety behaviours also contribute to the maintenance of persecutory delusions, and perhaps their model can be generalized to delusions in general.[2] Persecutory delusions are threat beliefs that share with anxiety disorders the theme of 'anticipation of danger'.

Individuals with persecutory delusions may also take preventative action in order to obtain safety. Such action may render disconfirmatory evidence ineffective by turning the situation into a 'near miss'. In short, safety behaviours are likely to result in potentially disconfirming evidence being discarded, and thus contribute to delusion maintenance.

In their research Freeman and colleagues also found that all those with persecutory delusions reported at least one safety behaviour in the last month. Avoidance was the most common type of safety behaviour; most frequently these people avoided meeting others or attending social gatherings, walking on the street, being far from home or being in enclosed spaces. Other strategies included protection, invisibility, vigilance and resistance. Protection behaviours included not answering the front door; checking all the locks of the house; only going outside accompanied by a family member; and placing a chair against the bedroom door at night. To decrease their visibility, and hence the chances of being attacked, individuals would, for example, wear a hat or cycle helmet, shop or walk down the street quickly, alternate routes and time of their return home and 'keep eyes to the ground'.

Many of the participants in Freeman's research believed that the safety behaviours had a degree of success, which is consistent with the hypothesis that safety behaviours are a maintenance factor.

The more anxious the participant, the more often safety behaviours were used. This confirms the finding that individuals who feel frightened or anxious act upon delusions, and it has important implications for the postscript at the end of this chapter on what you should do if you meet someone with a delusion. Check how they feel about the delusion – if they appear anxious or frightened then there is a distinct possibility that they will act on their delusion.

If actions associated with persecutory delusions are often attempts to reduce the perceived threat and consequent feelings of anxiety, this explains the previously puzzling connection between safety behaviours and the negative symptoms or withdrawal often found in psychosis and schizophrenia.[3] It is easy to see how a false belief can be maintained if the person never performs actions that directly test the belief because they are so fearful that those precise actions could place them in great danger. This goes some way to explaining how many incorrect beliefs arise – the behavioural consequence is the vital issue, not the inherent plausibility of the belief itself.

Yet it is true that many delusions contain content so bizarre that most people would dismiss them out of hand. If someone told you aliens from another planet were bombarding the streets with a death ray and it was dangerous to go outside it is unlikely that you would consider taking avoidance action. A vital issue these cases raise is about the nature of delusion or false belief. What is the difference between false beliefs (which surely we all labour under from time to time; yes – even doctors) and the medical symptom of delusions?

We must start with the technical definition of delusion, which is a neglected issue in the field but is perhaps the foundation of all psychiatry and clinical psychology. I want to argue that the most widely accepted definition of delusion within psychiatry is technically and fundamentally flawed. The current definition emphasizes content of belief – it says that you are deluded if the content of your belief fits certain criteria. I propose instead that the content is irrelevant. The crucial issue is how you got to your belief – the reasoning process that took you to where you are in the land of conviction.

This issue is vital, as the arrival process explains why the content is bizarre and also why the belief is maintained in the presence of problematic evidence. So when a patient arrives in my clinic and informs me that he is the Pope, according to current psychiatric lore I should focus on the content of the belief and establish for example whether this is false or not. But for me the key point is why he concludes this and the vital question then is, 'Why do you believe you are the Pope?' – or, 'How did this idea come about?' If the patient replies, 'I saw the gulls fly south for the winter this morning and that means I am the Pope,' I am saved my phone call to the Vatican to check if their leader is missing. I can deduce that the statement is a delusion because the reasoning process involved is so out of kilter with accepted forms of deduction in our culture.

My view reveals a common error when people discuss ideas they find incredible: the issue isn't *what* others believe but *how* they came to their conclusions. The journey to belief reveals much more of their state of mind than the final creed.[4]

Part of the problem for psychiatry is that it has long wrestled with the deep problem of how a belief could be a symptom of an illness. For example, in defining a delusion there is usually a 'cultural condition': a key feature of a delusion is that it should not be representative of a set of beliefs widely held in the culture the patient comes from. So, for example, if the patient comes from a country where most people believe him to be the Pope, then his belief can no longer be considered delusional (even if he really isn't the Pope).

Yet this immediately means that delusions as symptoms are expressly relativistic – they depend on the culture the patient comes from and can only be judged within that context. They also appear to depend on the moment in history when you interview a patient. A patient interviewed a thousand years ago would not be diagnosed as deluded for expressing the belief that the world is flat, but she would be if she expressed the same belief in the twenty-first century.[5]

So a pattern of beliefs presented by one person may be evidence of mental illness, whereas the identical set of ideas presented by another person in a different cultural or historical context may not be. On a superficial level, this makes it hard to conceive of delusional ideas as a medical condition. After all, a heart murmur is evidence of a heart abnormality whether it is diagnosed in London or in Timbuktu. The patient's condition presumably is not affected by where they live. Therefore, a potential paradox in establishing delusions as a medical problem emerges if the same person can be diagnosed correctly in different and mutually incompatible ways simply because of his or her social or historical context.

Consider *folie à deux*, the delusion shared by two people discussed in Chapter 2, 'It Takes Two to Tango'; also millennial cults, national hysteria and most, if not all, organized religions. If psychiatric diagnostic manuals can consider *folie à deux* as a shared delusion, then why not allow *folie à trois*? Or *folie à trente*, for that matter? If these manuals can consider that families can share in delusions, then why not several families or entire groups of people who are genetically unrelated but who consider themselves to be family? For that matter, why should the number of people who share a symptom be theoretically relevant at all?[6]

The person with heart disease still has heart disease if his entire town does as well.

On the other hand, we can plausibly define a 'functional heart' as one that permits an organism to go out and perform the activities that are required to sustain that organism. Similarly we can plausibly define a 'functional rational structure' as one that preserves truth-value enough of the time to allow the individual to survive physically and to communicate socially, the two usually being linked.[7]

If we use whether a belief allows adequate or basic functioning in a society as our definition of delusion then it is easy to see that believing you are the Pope, when no one else thinks this, is likely to lead you into conflict with the rest of society. On this basis, 'beliefs that are socially maladaptive' appears a useful way of defining delusions.

Except there are, of course, many minorities who hold beliefs that lead them into conflict with the larger majority. Does that always mean the majority is right and the minority deluded? In the old Soviet Union political dissidence was defined as mental illness partly for these precise reasons.

No – beliefs are not something that should purely be put down to democracy – we surely cannot take a vote on what is truth – for the scientist making an original discovery would always then be outvoted before he could persuade us of his new finding.

It seems more useful to return to my argument that the content of the belief is less important than how you got there. For how you got there tells us something about your ability to form accurate judgements about reality. If you only ever believed something because the majority of others did so first, although this could certainly keep you out of an asylum for a while, if you took it to its logical conclusion and never made a decision without consulting others, a psychiatrist could soon be knocking at your door.

Dr Mujica-Parodi and Dr Sackeim at the New York State Psychiatric Institute and Columbia University, New York, agree with me that what we should be looking at is something much more fundamental than the content of beliefs; it is the ability to think in a manner that preserves truth-value. The connection between thinking in ways that preserve truth-value and our two desiderata of minimal functioning (physical survival and social communication) is commonsensical. Individuals who have true knowledge that they are in front of a hole are less likely to fall into it. Having true knowledge of the fact that winter will inevitably follow summer can help one plan ahead and stockpile food. By extension, a group of individuals who have true knowledge have a shared frame of reference that will allow them to communicate.[8]

One point about delusions as opposed to widespread false beliefs is that the delusional usually have huge problems persuading even just one other person to agree with their highly idiosyncratic ideas. Yet it seems odd to define a delusion as merely a belief which you cannot persuade anyone else to share; in practical terms it appears that a delusion is most reliably a judgement you cannot persuade your psychiatrist to share. We can easily imagine a large group of people who have false knowledge that acts as a shared frame of reference – cults and fringe political groupings are good examples – so the problem remains how to reliably define delusions in the face of widespread non-rational or false beliefs.

Consider two cases. The first is a student who believes that he will perform well in his exams only if he is in possession of a certain 'lucky' charm during these exams. Since he owns the charm, bringing it to his exams does not present a problem. He continues to hold this belief even though his performance in exams varies in direct correspondence to the amount of time that he spends studying in preparation for these exams and is not related to whether the charm is in his possession. Instances in which he has the charm and does well reinforce his belief, but instances in which he does well without the charm or does poorly with the charm are discounted as insignificant.[9]

The second case concerns another student who believes that she will perform well in her exams only if she sees nine black cats on the day that she takes her exam. This belief causes problems for the student for she often spends hours before her exams running around trying to find the nine black cats, and sometimes is unable to find them. This student also continues to hold on to her belief in spite of the fact that her performance varies in direct correspondence to the amount of time she spends studying in preparation for these exams and is not related to whether she has, in fact, found the nine black cats. Again, instances in which she has found the nine black cats and does well reinforce her belief, while instances in which she cannot find the nine black cats but does well, or finds the nine black cats but does poorly, are perceived as aberrations.[10]

Both students hold false beliefs in spite of evidence to the contrary. The first student's false belief is not uncommon, while the second student's is considered extremely odd. The first student's belief improves his level of functioning by providing an easily attainable (false) sense of security. The second student's belief impairs her level of functioning by making the object of (false) security beyond her control. So, is one case delusional and one not delusional because of considerations of cultural acceptance, or because of considerations of functionality?[11]

A distinction between beliefs that are *arational* and beliefs that are *irrational* might be helpful here. Arational beliefs are those that are held in the absence of information to support them. Irrational beliefs are those that are held in spite of evidence to the contrary; the problem here is not lack of information, but the refusal to acknowledge it. Delusions might be restricted to examples of irrational thinking.[12]

A potential difficulty is that many 'bizarre' delusions (i.e. delusions whose content is not physically possible) seem to evade diagnosis on similar grounds. For the patient who considers himself to be an ambassador from another planet, what counts as a relevant counterexample? And the patient who believes that her thoughts are being controlled by an outside source? For many delusions, the intuitive problem is not that we have reason to believe that they are false, but rather that we have no reason to believe that they are true. Yet such beliefs seem to be 'arational' and so by our earlier description would not be considered to be 'delusional'.[13]

Bizarre delusions are not just of low probability; more interestingly, the deludeds' 'investment' in these beliefs is disproportional to their probability of being true. Thus, a woman who believes that her guru can perform miracles is not necessarily delusional if this belief does not prevent her from taking steps to act on her own behalf. The same believer, on the other hand, might very well be recognized as delusional if she gives away all of her possessions and takes to sea in a leaky boat in the expectation that she will be saved.

Again we come back not to the content of the belief but to how the conviction makes you act and how helpful these actions are to your functioning.

Another reason why false content is not the issue is that it is possible with good reason to hold false ideas.

Rational false beliefs are always considered to be non-delusional, regardless of functional or social considerations. Rational false beliefs are defined here as those that are likely to be true given the reasonable premises the individual holds and if no counterexample has yet been presented. An example is the parent who believes that his child is in school because the child is usually in school during the day, unaware of the fact that the child has been taken to a hospital.

This is a false belief firmly held, but is reasonable to hold it given the premises of the parent and the fact that no one has yet provided any evidence to the contrary. The parent has a strongly held false belief – this does not mean he is deluded.

However, you begin to wonder about the parent's mental state if on providing good evidence that their original belief is wrong (for example a phone call from the hospital) the parent refuses to give up the original conviction that the child is still at school. In their immunity to evidence that contradicts their point of view the deluded start to part company with the rest of us. The critical issue is how much information must be ignored in order to maintain the belief. The amount of contradictory information one must ignore is directly proportional to the severity of the delusion.

Availability of counterexamples accounts for our perception that bizarre delusions are symptoms of a more severe illness than non-bizarre delusions. To believe that the streets are being sprayed with a death ray by aliens is open to numerous bits of evidence against it without our having to go far looking for such data.[14]

This revised view shifts the focus from whether the belief is true and culturally accepted to the question of how the belief was arrived at and how it is maintained. It is only the latter issue that is dictated by brain function. Let us consider the following example:

A 19-year-old college student in London is diagnosed with mania. He believes that his girlfriend, a student in Scotland, is cheating on him. He states his reason for this belief: 'The colour of the petals on this flower prove to me that my lover is betraying me.' The flower in question is a rose that she has given him during a visit. The girlfriend confides privately to the psychiatrist that she is, in fact, having an affair with a classmate and that she has not told her boyfriend.[15]

This case qualifies as a delusion by my criteria, but not by standard psychiatric criteria (because the content of the belief is true). This example points out the limitations of the standard requirement that a belief be false.

We have seen that just defining and recognizing a delusion is far from easy. The debate about the causes of delusions is similarly complex.

Some authors have argued that delusions are caused by a malfunction of the brain: for example in those with delusions of misidentification, specific neural pathways involved in creating a feeling of familiarity may be damaged, as we saw in the debate about Capgras.

Researchers in the cognitive psychology tradition have looked at possible errors or biases in reasoning; those with delusions may have a rapid 'jump-to-conclusions' style and somehow do not seem to use knowledge of everyday situations.[16] Recent research has emphasized that this is a tendency not to seek evidence, as opposed to a lack of ability to use it. Others see delusions as the attempt to account for strange experiences, for example hallucinations.[17]

The conflict arises because most delusions don't seem to make sense, and this explains why we look for brain dysfunction as causes. Perhaps if we looked deeper, delusions actually might begin to make some kind of sense at a psychological level. So is the perspective that attempts to explain delusions by disordered biochemistry too reductionist or simplistic?

Jung, developing suggestions made by Freud, presented work in which he asked schizophrenic patients to free-associate.[18, 19] By this means he thought he could show that much delusional talk in fact related to such issues as sexual desire and wish-fulfilment. 'These symptoms immediately became comprehensible when considered from the standpoint of the individual's previous history,' he argued. He describes a woman who saw herself as superior and yet unjustly imprisoned, and who thought that Socrates had experienced the same: 'Therefore she is Socrates. This, as you see, is a simple metaphor based on an obvious analogy.'

Grandiose delusions in particular might relate to self-esteem. In contrast, ideas of persecution perhaps develop in a context of isolation, misunderstanding and anger. Cognitive therapy with a considerable number of individuals suffering from delusions suggests that often the content of the delusion seemed to relate in various ways to aspects of a person's life and concerns.[20] These areas could be termed 'motivational' and it would be useful to explore them, even if these motives were not being conceived as causes of the delusions.

If goals are things individuals pursue or avoid and are concrete manifestations of our more general motivational drives, then do delusions really tell us something about underlying goals?

Psychologists John E. Rhodes and Simon Jakes of the Department of Psychology, St Ann's Hospital, London, recently presented the following cases with the aim of suggesting that goal analysis can illuminate delusional thinking.[21]

The man who talked to aliens

P.A. firmly believed that he could communicate with aliens and that he had special powers, for example that he could change his character. He said: 'I can travel through time . . . like a time worm . . . Some aliens are mouldy characters, and yet some others are intellectual. Aliens might take over the world.' He would go off with them, he explained, since 'I have no purpose in this world.' At the age of 17 he saw a light in the sky which he thought was following him. He assumed it must be a spaceship.

P.A. had failed at college and had to leave: his brothers, however, have successful professional careers. He said that throughout his life he had had either too little or too much sex and had problems in being a competent person. He said he would like to find a goal, that 'something is missing . . . something spiritual'. He then added: 'before, I wanted to be a leader, to rule the world.' Now, he said he would like to 'get a job, get married, get more advanced, that is, more educated and have more self-achievement'.

A paraphrase of P.A.'s delusional statements might be: I have thoughts which seem to come from elsewhere ('aliens'), not from this everyday world. My personality seems unusual – is this a special power?

The major theme seems to be the belief or wish to possess extraordinary ability or competence. Having ability superior to that of most others might suggest that P.A. had issues relating to social role evaluation.

The major themes shared by his delusion and his life are competence and evaluation: his delusion is perhaps a type of wish-fulfilment. Other themes seem secondary, that is, if he were competent then he would have a purpose and hence have direction. P.A. has great difficulties with language, and this may also contribute to the theme of communications.

From this case it does seem possible to show that delusions suggest themes which reflect persistent and serious concerns of the patient. The pattern of correspondence does not seem to be random, but whether this is true for all cases and types of delusion is unknown. This view coincides with the ideas of Jung and Freud.[22, 23] The cases presented here demonstrate that a link can be made between delusional themes and themes related to personal goals. Clearly, this does not imply that this meaning is the cause of the delusion or the cause of its content.

However, according to biological psychiatrists delusions are meaningless and random and links should not exist. Any links found would be coincidental and the observer might be inventing them in an 'effort after meaning'.

Talk and verbal communication in general have many functions, but one crucial function may be that they provide the individual with the opportunity to describe the world from a personal perspective. Some psychiatrists have suggested that delusional talk is somehow 'empty'; however, the assumption that delusional talk makes reference to experience contradicts this.

If delusions relate to motives, do general classes of delusion relate to more general motives? Some well-recognized types of delusion do seem to point in this direction: delusions of pregnancy and love as a desire for attachment; grandiose delusions as a desire for achievement or power; persecutory delusions as an expression of the feeling of being an outsider. So, perhaps most, if not all, mental illness involves the frustration of fundamental human needs.

Even if there are themes that link a delusion to what is going on in someone's life, the fact that we have to work so hard to uncover the theme is where the real problem lies with the delusional.

In other words, the essential predicament of the person who believes they are the Messiah placed on Earth is not the actual belief itself. It is the fact that they don't have the guile to stop the 'Messiah talk' temporarily when being interviewed by a psychiatrist. All of us have internal states and beliefs which we know may be socially unacceptable and know that voicing these ideas will result in ostracism, or worse. We may believe we are right but we know we must often keep our beliefs to ourselves for tactical reasons.

So my Messiah patient will avoid the inconvenience of an involuntary stay in hospital if they simply avoid mentioning this delusion. The key point may be the inability to understand the impact of an idiosyncratic belief system on others. The Messiah patient wants to be followed or worshipped, but instead gets carted off to an asylum.

This argument is about the notion that the fundamental deficit in delusion formation is centred on a relatively new concept in psychology and psychiatry called 'theory of mind'.[24]

Theory of mind, or so-called Machiavellian intelligence, is the capacity to infer the mental states of other individuals and to manipulate them in order to maximize social success.[25] This probably emerged during human evolution in response to the need to cope with an increasingly complex social environment. Perhaps disturbance in the understanding of others' mental state is fundamental to psychiatric disorders.[26]

It may be that the deluded are so overwhelmed by their internal states that they take little heed of what is going on around them, and as a result end up in trouble with medical services, society at large, or even the law. Or perhaps the problem the deluded have is more their inability to persuade others to take them seriously or at least not withdraw from them. The issue of delusions then becomes in fact the way the deluded deal with them.[27]

Some scientists have interpreted psychotic symptoms as impairments in the processes that underlie a 'theory of mind', including the ability to represent beliefs and intentions.[28] For example, when asked to describe photographs of people, schizophrenics described more the physical appearance, rather than the mental states.[29, 30]

We need a long period of development before achieving adult status because of the difficulty of acquiring social skills, and in particular the ability to read other people's minds effectively.[31] The evolutionary extension of the juvenile period may have been crucial in enabling humans to acquire a vast amount of possible social strategies (procedural rules), such as co-operation, tactical deception, exploitation of the expertise of other individuals (deliberate manipulation), and in developing the understanding of *when to employ the strategies*.[32] The latter is known as meta-learning.[33] This process is not merely time-consuming, but opportunities to test the consequences of social interaction strategies are limited.[34]

Hence, social interactions are simulated in the mind, to assist the evolution of social intelligence.[35] Trial and error, pretence play and learning by imitation may be essential.[36] Social cognition is closely associated with face recognition and perception of other social signals and, particularly in humans, is connected with affective states, suggesting that these may have evolved as internal signals in response to the social environment.[37]

It is notable that most psychoses tend to start during late adolescence or early adulthood when perhaps the need to read minds effectively becomes most pressing and confusing.

Delusional misidentification syndromes have been associated with theory of mind deficits, because clinical observation suggests that affected persons are incapable of experiencing a link to the mental life of familiar individuals, leading to the delusional belief that a person is replaced or duplicated, as we saw in Capgras syndrome.[38] Disturbances of social reasoning appear almost always to be involved in psychiatric disorders.[39]

The emergence of social intelligence in primate evolution denotes a decisive step in the evolution of humankind. Perhaps some aspects of mental illness may be regarded as the evolutionary 'cost' to humankind of the development of this (relatively) advanced capability of mind-reading.[40] In other words, one may be tempted to say that mental disorders are unique to humans because of their extreme specialization on social cognition – the need to understand each other's minds.[41]

This is a fascinating theory but is there any definite evidence in its favour?

Evolutionary psychologists and anthropologists propose that human behaviour and cognition have been shaped by the natural selection that occurred when humans lived in hunter-gatherer societies.[42] Humans are social animals, and social factors have therefore been a powerful selective force during recent evolutionary history, exerting profound effects upon psychological architecture.[43] These differences may be reflected in the nature of psychiatric illnesses.

In hunter-gatherer societies, ancestral male alliances were typically formed among blood relatives, and hostile threats came mainly from alliances of male strangers. In contrast, a major hostile threat among women might be exclusion from a circle of female mutual assistance, and denigratory gossip might lead to a damaged reputation. The difference in the nature of threats to the sexes may be expected to lead to differences in men and women's perception of threat, which in turn might be expected to lead to a sex difference in the content of persecutory delusions.[44]

A sex differential ought to be apparent both in the identity of the putative hostile group and the nature of their hostile intent. The prediction would be that men with persecutory delusions will tend to identify physically violent male strangers as their persecutors, especially strangers organized into gangs. Women, by contrast, would identify their persecutors as being familiar females (such as family members, friends and neighbours) and verbal hostility as the form of persecution.[45]

Florence Walston and colleagues from the Department of Psychology, University of Newcastle upon Tyne, indeed found that delusions in contemporary patients are consistent with this prediction: 73 per cent of deluded women identified familiar people as their persecutors, whereas 85 per cent of deluded men identified strangers as their persecutors.[46]

The possibility remains that the sex differences observed are primarily 'cultural' and are caused mainly by differences in the modern social experiences of men and women. But what is fascinating about this evidence is that if theory of mind is a fundamental issue in psychosis and the different genders have particular specializations to fit their differing roles in society, then this difference in delusional content fits this hypothesis perfectly.

This intriguing idea means that the truth content of delusions is no longer the issue: rather it is how delusions affect your relationships with others.[47]

The advantage of this theory is that delusions are unlikely to represent a defect in truth deciphering.[48] How one tells whether something is true or not is still hotly debated by scientists and philosophers. Truth determination seems to be an active process involving the testing of ideas, which most of us don't do routinely in our lives. If truth determination has something to do with delusion formation then how is it that delusions don't appear to be more common?[49]

Popper, a British philosopher of science born in Vienna, asserted that your ideas are only truly scientific and correspond to reality if they are testable in some independent manner. This leads to the trenchant position that you deserve intellectual respectability only if you can specify the conditions under which you will give up your beliefs, and then actively seek to set up those conditions. This is the essence of the experiment – the procedure that is the bedrock of science. But how many of us routinely think this way? Popper says that arriving at the truth is about having an idea when relentlessly trying to prove it wrong with experiments. Most people do the opposite – when they have an idea they dwell on the evidence in favour of it, not against it.[50]

In conversation how often do you meet someone who argues against themselves? Indeed, this in itself appears slightly unbalanced.[51]

It was reading Popper's *Logic of Scientific Discovery* that led me to start asking the main speakers at psychiatric conferences, 'Could you please specify the conditions under which you are willing to give up your beliefs?' This only got me strange looks and requests to sit down.[52]

Popper leads us to the view that science is not a body of facts or data, but merely a method; my definition of science is the systematic attempt to detect error in our ideas. A good experiment is one whose methods and results effectively eliminate viable competing theories. Reading Popper leads one inevitably to the astonishing and disturbing conclusion that most scientists do not themselves understand what science is, and are actually confused about why they are using the procedures they employ.[53]

When teaching the junior doctors at the Maudsley I would start by asking for a definition of science, only to receive very odd and incoherent answers. Yet these doctors arrived after studying science A levels for two years, plus five years of scientific medical school and often several years of a higher science degree.

The antidote to Popper is Thomas Kuhn's *The Structure of Scientific Revolutions,* in which Kuhn argues that actually you can't test everything, and scientists can only work by making some basic assumptions which are not challenged. This set of beliefs, common to a community of scientists, guides their endeavours but can come unstuck when results become increasingly incoherent – leading to a 'paradigm shift'. This is a period of turmoil when it becomes necessary for old assumptions to be questioned, then abandoned and new ones take their place.[54]

We desperately need a paradigm shift in psychiatry today as never before.

For example, biological psychiatry continues on the assumption that reliable physiological differences will eventually be found amongst the mentally ill, even if they cannot yet be demonstrated. This basic assumption is not amenable to testing because no amount of failure to confirm it would count as adequate disconfirmation for the committed biologists. There could be no experimental result that would stop biologists looking for the cause of mental illness in the brain, raising the question of whether the driving force behind their thinking is strictly scientific in the Popperian sense.[55]

The problem is that most approaches to the understanding of delusion, brain and mind remain reductionist.[56]

Perhaps the most famous anti-biologist of the mind is Descartes, who postulated that we are composed of two different substances, body and mind, with mind not being explainable by or reducible to the material. This is known as 'Cartesian dualism'. Gilbert Ryle, Waynflete Professor of Metaphysical Philosophy at Oxford, mocked this view as 'the dogma of the ghost in the machine'.[57]

Ryle argued that the Cartesians were as erroneously reductionist as the materialists in trying to diminish mind to a single ethereal substance rather than a physical one. His thesis is that the many and various ways we speak about 'the mind' are potentially misleading, and that mind is an emergent property of the brain. It would be impossible therefore to look closely at the brain and 'find' the mind located somewhere specifically in there. Talking about mind as different from the body, Ryle argues, is a bit like – after having been shown around Oxford University with its various colleges, laboratories and offices – asking precisely where the University is. The University is an emergent property of its various components – it is not located anywhere specifically, but could not exist without the constituent offices, colleges and laboratories.[58]

Some accused Ryle of providing a philosophical justification for abandoning the need to acknowledge the existence of mind altogether – a kind of extreme behaviourism. Ryle vigorously denied this. But he would agree that the problem for psychiatrists is that we are the only doctors who have no direct access to our subject matter – the mind. No matter what the brain-scanning boys might try to tell you, whenever we interact with our patient, our research and clinical activity are based on inferences we are constantly making about what is really going on in the patient's mind.[59]

A common confusion is to assume the patients' answers to our questions, or their behaviour – the only materials we usually have to work with – are a reliable indicator of what's inside the 'black box'. This notion is a useful dose of humility whenever my clinical decisions or research suppositions seduce me into the delusion that I can read minds. A delusion I see all around me on the ward – in my colleagues.[60]

But if scientific facts are publicly observable data – demonstrated by experiments – then one problem of mind is that your experiences are inside your mind with a kind of 'insidedness' that is vastly different from the way that your brain is inside your head. Someone else can open up your head and see what's inside but no one can open your mind and look into it – at least not in the same way that any other phenomena in the universe can be observed. So it looks as though your experiences and other mental states can't just be physical states of your brain. There has to be more to your mind than your body with its nervous system.[61]

There is a view that is different from both dualism and physicalism. (Dualism is the view that you consist of both a body plus a soul, and that your mental life goes on in your soul. Physicalism is the view that your mental life consists of physical processes in your brain.) Another possibility is that your mental life goes on in your brain, yet all those experiences, feelings, thoughts and desires are not physical processes. This would mean that the grey mass of billions of nerve cells in your skull is not just a physical object. It does have lots of physical properties – great quantities of chemical and electrical activity go on in it – but it has mental processes as well.[62]

This view that the brain is the seat of consciousness, but that its conscious states are not just physical states, is called dual aspect theory and is what I personally subscribe to. I teach it to junior doctors and medical students by making this comparison: the mind is to the brain what a painting is to a canvas. You need a canvas to support a painting – but studying the canvas will reveal much less about the painting than an understanding of art would.[63]

This artistic analogy serves well to explain my final conclusion about delusions. This comes from Friedrich Nietzsche's existential philosophy. The importance of Nietzsche for me is his view that truth is not something we discover 'out there' as separate from us, but is a vision we impose upon the world, driven as we are by our egos.[64] Our systems of understanding the world, therefore, have less to do with logic and more with artistic creation. Nietzsche also very strongly urges that we take relentless responsibility for the consequences of our decisions and our understandings.

It is the lack of ability to accept that we are accountable for our own lives and choices that I see daily in my clinic as one of the major causes of psychological disturbance.[65] Yet this is not a perspective one finds advocated much within our field and I do feel that psychiatry frequently chooses to shoulder an impossible burden when we take on individual responsibility for our patients' contentment and stability.[66]

Nietzsche's views could of course be turned against himself, as he did appear to suffer some kind of psychotic breakdown for the last 11 years of his life, possibly assisted by abuse of chloral hydrate and the tertiary symptoms of syphilis. He was probably veering towards psychological disturbance before then, as he often publicly lamented that few contemporaries could understand his greatness. Three chapters of his autobiography *Ecce Homo*, completed in 1888, were entitled 'Why I am so clever', 'Why I am so wise' and 'Why I write such good books'.

Nietzsche has always suffered from an undeserved reputation for being a supporter of Fascism, but this is due to the posthumous unscrupulous re-editing of his notes by his sister and nurse Elizabeth, who was married to an anti-Semite. So the idea of a master race in fact has little to do with Nietzsche's famous concept of the 'superman' who is able to face chaos and still impose order upon it through the sheer force of his 'Will to Power'.[67]

I know of no better description of what we do when we discuss our ideas with others. We all want to have an impact but the problem arises when we misjudge our impact and provoke undesirable reactions from those around us. This is why we monitor reactions to our ideas and modify them to assist our journey through life's relationships. We can only survive by successfully negotiating connections with others. The amazing thing about the deluded is their inability or intransigence in modifying their ideas in the face of overwhelming negative feedback from society.[68]

The 'theory of mind' idea I advocated earlier places emphasis on this as the crucial problem for the deluded – their inability to assess the reaction they will provoke.[69]

We have yet to understand fully why this is. But according to Nietzsche you fully embrace existence not by always concurring with what others tell you or want for you in life, but instead by trying to impose your will on the universe. By trying to make a difference to it.

By this measure we should be judged not on how many people

agree with us, but more on the scope of our ambition. By this standard the attempt of the deluded to persuade us of their ideas deserves more than just medication. It deserves respect.

POSTSCRIPT

Psychotic phenomena are very common in the general population – some estimates are that one in three people will have experienced at least one psychotic symptom, such as hallucination or a vision, in their lifetime.[1] So it is highly likely you will encounter sooner or later a person who appears to be delusional. How you react to that person could have profound implications for you as well as for them.

Such encounters are precarious and intricate because (a) there are few conventional social rules governing such a complex situation, and (b) the consequences for either party if the event is not handled well could be more severe than usual. For example, ostracism, altercation, severe upset or an admission to the local psychiatric unit can follow the display of delusional phenomena.[2]

The first important point to emphasize is – as I hope the people populating this book have illustrated – that the vast majority of people suffering from, or even delighting in, delusions are not dangerous to others.[3]

Encountering delusional thinking or other psychotic phenomena can be frightening, not least because of the apparent unpredictability of sufferers. However, I have written this book and presented these cases because I believe dialogue with the delusional has much to offer us. It will not only assist in the specialized scientific enterprise of understanding the brain and mind, but such people's experience should inform our personal understanding of what it is to be human. Many who behave in ways we find reprehensible are actually suffering from a view of the world we don't share. Often we can't see past the behaviour to the ideas behind it – yet it is the perspective people subscribe to which is the engine that drives problematic actions. If we can grope towards some understanding of the most bizarre and incomprehensible ideas of all, then surely there is more hope for us to understand what each other thinks.[4]

Many have said the most complex entity in the known universe is the human brain, but in fact there is something much more intricate and elaborate: human society – or groups of brains interacting. What is produced when minds try to understand and manipulate each other is where the real mystery and excitement of the human sciences lie.[5]

Yet delusions seem to represent such an obstacle to mutual understanding that they appear the one phenomenon which defies evolutionary, social or biological purpose.

I advanced the argument in the last chapter that delusions and psychotic experiences could be uniquely human phenomena, so the breakdown of supposedly normal experience and rationality is an inevitable consequence of our evolutionary journey. This could mean that the deluded are paying a price for the benefits the rest of us have accrued from recent evolution of the brain and the mind. If so, we have an obligation to look after them if they need society's assistance.

This leads naturally to the first issue in any encounter with delusional thinking, which is not to confuse the ideas people might express with what they really believe. Behaviour is a much better guide to what someone really subscribes to than merely what they say. I have encountered many patients who claim to be the next Messiah but who continue to act exactly as they did before the delusion emerged. They get on with their jobs, with their relationships and the rest of their lives as though nothing has changed at all. However, they persist with 'delusional talk' when they come to see me. So the question is: do they really subscribe to these sentiments when nothing they do in life reflects this altered perspective?

So an essential issue is not what people say – no matter how alarming this may sound – but rather what they are doing about their ideas. The behaviour is the key. Patients who firmly believe they have been swindled out of their rightful place on the throne and are brought back to me by the police after trying to get into Buckingham Palace have delusions that are clearly more salient to them than those whose ideas produce no discernible change to their lives.

My own view, which is controversial within psychiatry, is that treating someone with a delusion that has no negative impact on his life is probably not at all helpful to him. Medication usually has some side-effects, so a cost-benefit analysis of treatment often leads me to support people with delusions but not to formally intervene.

However, for those whose symptoms are troubling them, the usual first-line treatment for patients with psychotic symptoms such as hallucinations and delusions is antipsychotic medication. The finding that this type of medication was effective in the treatment of psychosis during the 1950s brought about a revolution in the care and management of people with schizophrenia. Modern and older antipsychotic medications reduce or even banish completely what doctors refer to as 'positive' symptoms during acute crises and prevent subsequent relapse.

'Positive' symptoms are problems like hallucinations and delusions, while 'negative' symptoms are the lack of motivation, apathy and withdrawal that many psychotic people also exhibit. There is no clear-cut reliable evidence that any antipsychotic medication is helpful for negative symptoms. Antipsychotic medication also has some limitations with regard to its efficacy on psychotic systems. For example, a substantial number of patients will continue to experience persistent and distressing hallucinations and delusions or will be subject to periodic relapse of these symptoms despite appropriate doses of antipsychotic medication; it must also be said, however, that the reluctance to increase doses temporarily explains why many are left with persistent symptoms.

Although the introduction of newer 'atypical' antipsychotic medications has gone some way to improve the situation, medication still does not provide full remission for large numbers of patients. The discovery of drug therapies that will eradicate psychotic symptoms has remained elusive since the 1950s when chlorpromazine, a drug still widely in use in the United Kingdom today, was first introduced as a possible treatment for psychosis.

As a result of the limitations in drug treatments, many clinicians and researchers also pursue complementary approaches that can enhance the effectiveness of medication and improve the outcome of psychosis. The main areas investigated are those that involve some form of psychotherapy, although by the mid-1980s most researchers and clinicians interested in schizophrenia were familiar with large-scale studies showing little or no efficacy of supportive or Freudian-type psychotherapies in the treatment of the disorder and its symptoms.

Early research into other psychological methods of treating schizophrenia emerged predominantly from the behavioural school and focused on modifying symptoms and the behaviour associated with the disorder. These approaches particularly concentrated on using external reinforcers to modify observed psychotic behaviour, such as talking to oneself. The therapists reinforce non-delusional speech using social approval and punish delusional speech verbally. Delusional speech significantly decreases, and the results are maintained both inside and outside treatment sessions.

This behavioural approach ignores the mental processes behind a delusion and instead focuses on any unhelpful behaviour it produces. The patients' expression of delusions is seen as 'delusion talk' and it is the verbal exposition that is seen as the problem, not the delusion itself. After all, if you keep your strange ideas to yourself then you are unlikely to get into trouble with others.[6]

The theory behind this approach is that you will get so involved with the rest of normal life and be positively reinforced for this that you will eventually forget your delusions. Implicit in some distraction approaches such as this is the reasoning that the impact of experiencing delusions will decrease if attention is redirected through the introduction of competing stimuli. This is hypothesized to occur as a result of the person's concerted ability to direct attention away from the delusion.

However, as many scientists in the field would argue, the weakness with the behavioural approach is that it ignores the fact that something pretty fundamental has surely gone wrong with brain and mind function for the delusion to have arisen in the first place.

Studies evaluating the effect of a number of different approaches on the severity of schizophrenic patients' hallucinations find that cognitive modification of the patient's beliefs is most effective at reducing the duration and frequency of his hallucinations.[7] The cognitive interventions involve helping the patient to examine her beliefs regarding the origin of the voices and their meaning.[8] The intervention focused on helping her to consider the possibility that her voices were originating from a negative or harmful source. The emphasis is on helping the patient to reach her own conclusions rather than those of the therapist. The patients change their beliefs about their voices, and their hallucinations reduce in severity.[9]

Patients should also be given a 'normalizing rationale' to reduce the stigma of mental illness and the fears and anxiety evoked by their symptoms. Comparisons can be made between psychotic symptoms and phenomena that occur in the normal population in extreme circumstances, such as under conditions of sensory deprivation or high levels of stress. The normalizing strategy also includes teaching individuals anxiety management techniques, plus techniques designed to increase self-esteem and reduce depression.[10]

The approach that I have pioneered for delusions is a particularly robust approach and based directly on the idea that confrontation and challenge are fundamentally unhelpful. Instead, I take a patient's delusional ideas and examine with them the implications of those ideas. In other words my focus is more on where your ideas take you and what they mean that you should be doing next in your life. I believe it is only by examining the implications of the ideas that people may begin to see how helpful or otherwise their thinking is.

Let's take a practical example. Say a patient resistant to all other treatment approaches declares to me that the CIA are following him, are bugging his home and office and are out to 'get' him. A Freudian analysis might suggest that paranoia like this is based on a grandiose defence of low self-esteem. The fact that the CIA are out to get you must mean you are a special person; after all, why are they picking on you? It could also explain why the rest of the world has not recognized your specialness as a person and you have not achieved what you should have done – there is a conspiracy holding you back from claiming your rightful place in society.

But all that analysis, in my experience, is not helpful to getting people to change such ideas. I believe instead that a more radical approach is required, which often appears to mean that you take the patient's delusion more seriously than they do themselves. An important point is that at no time do I collude or agree with delusional thinking while with a patient. Instead I say something like 'Let's assume for a moment that you are right – I am not saying I know you are right – I am not sure from what you have told me that what you say is true or not, but just let me go along with your ideas for a moment. If the CIA really are following you and they are intent on killing you, then surely you are doomed? The CIA are a multibillion-pound organization and they usually get their man. I

413

don't know why you think telling an impoverished NHS psychiatrist like me is going to help.

'If the CIA are out to get you, then it might be better for you to give yourself up to them and ask them if there is anything you can do to help them in order to prevent them killing you. Otherwise, maybe you should move out of your family home to prevent your family being injured in the cross-fire and head for a remote place and hide out for a while. Perhaps you should invest a lot of money in security protection, though I am not sure how much good that is going to do for you . . .' etc., etc.

The point about attempting to illuminate for the client the consequences of their ideas is that when a person sees that the direction they are heading in is contradictory, frightening or a dead end, they are more likely to reverse and reconsider the original idea.

Where my treatment is different from belief modification is that I do not distract a patient from their delusion by asking them to examine the evidence; I distract them from the central idea by asking them to assess what the future may hold if their concepts are correct. If the natural consequences of their thinking raise their anxiety sufficiently, this will usually provide the necessary drive for a reconsideration of their philosophy.

Robust though this approach is, it is done with great concern for the client; it is important not to make fun of them or belittle their ideas. Indeed, I consider their notions more earnestly than they do themselves, which is why I see implications they themselves have not considered. So I believe we should take delusions very seriously, and not just dismiss them as the epiphenomena of disordered biochemistry in action.

So if you encounter someone with a delusion the steps to take are:

1   Investigate whether the delusion is leading to actual problematic behaviour – focus not so much on what someone thinks but on what they have done about it. Are they planning to do something dangerous to themselves or others as a result of their delusion? Only if dubious behaviour has occurred, or is in the offing, should you take action to intervene in the life of a person with delusions.

2   If the person is definitely suffering as a result of their delusions, encourage them to see a doctor or specialist. In the vast majority of cases treatment is effective and medication, as we have seen throughout this book, is helpful.

3   Make sure that people close to the deluded person are aware of

their thinking. It is possible for even those who know you well to be totally unaware that you hold delusions. Also, since the thought processes of the psychotic are not necessarily intact, their reassurance to you that they are all right or that they are indeed seeking treatment may not be a reliable reflection of reality.

Abstract ephemeral ideas are important because they are the fundamental basis for action in our lives. Delusions are fascinating and significant in the study of mind and brain because they are a bizarre bridge between strange thinking and odd behaviour. Delusions underpin the most remarkable actions we will ever witness. From flying planes into skyscrapers to climbing into lions' cages in zoos, the most dramatic action in life is the result of extraordinary thinking.

The grandeur of delusion is not just that somehow the brain and mind construct such phenomenal architecture or belief that it appears to stand without visible support from the rest of our cognitive processes, but also the grandeur involved in the fantastic behaviour that it produces.

But perhaps the most vital lesson to learn from those on the edge of the couch is that we should take all ideas seriously, even if they are not true, because they reveal another kind of reality – not one pertaining to the external world, but a truth about our internal realms. Given how difficult the study of brain and mind continues to be, research into delusions offers a window into an obscure domain. So analysing the stories of the people who have populated these pages, remarkable and often tragic though they may be, is a vital part of the effort to understand ourselves.

Since the darkest place in the universe remains the inside of the human skull, those who pursue the study of delusion are like early explorers entering uncharted territory for the first time. This journey is one I see undertaken by my patients every day in my clinic, yet it remains the most intriguing in human endeavour, for there is no stranger trip than that to, and back from, the edge of the couch.

NOTES

INTRODUCTION

1. S. L. Murray, H. G. Holmes, D. W. Griffin (2000), 'What the motivated mind sees: Comparing friends' perspectives to married partners' view of each other', *J. Experimental Soc. Psychology*, 36, 600–20.

2. S. Freud (1950), *Collected Papers*, vol. 4 [translated by J. Riviere] (Hogarth Press, London).

3. W. S. Anglin, J. Lambek (1995), *The Heritage of Thales* (Springer Verlag, New York).

4 M. Enquist, O. Leimar, J. Ljungberg, Y. Mallner, N. Segerdahl (1990), 'A test of the sequential assessment game: Fighting in the cichlid fish', *Nannacara anomala: Animal Behavior*, 40, 1–14.

5. O. Hasson (1994), 'Cheating signals', *J. Theoretical Biology*, 167, 223–38.

6. R. W. Elwood, K. E. Wood, M. B. Gallagher, J. T. A. Dick (1998), 'Probing motivational state during agonistic encounters in animals', *Nature*, 393, 66.

7. G. A. Parker (1974), 'Assessment strategy and the evolution of fighting behaviour', *J. Theoretical Biology*, 47, 223–43.

8. Y. G. Kim (1995), 'Status signalling games in animal contests', *J. Theoretical Biology*, 176, 221–31.

9. S. David (1997), *Military Blunders: The How and Why of Military Failure* (Carroll and Graf, New York).

10. R. Gabriel (1986), *Military Incompetence: Why the American Military Doesn't Win* (Noonday Press, New York).

11. R. Wrangham (Jan. 1999), 'Is military incompetence adaptive?', *Evolution & Human Behavior*, 20 (1), 3–17.

12. C. Boehm (1992), 'Segmentary "warfare" and the management of conflict: Comparison of East African chimpanzees and patrilineal-patrilocal humans', in H. A. Harcourt, F. B. M. de Waal (eds), *Coalitions and Alliances in Humans and Other Animals* [137–73] (Oxford University Press, Oxford).

13. J. H. Manson, R. W. Wrangham (1991), 'Intergroup aggression in chimpanzees and humans', *Current Anthropology*, 32, 369–90.

14. R. W. Wrangham, D. Peterson (1996), *Demonic Males: Apes and the Origins of Human Violence* (Houghton Mifflin, Boston, MA).

15. M. Enquist, O. Leimar (1983), 'Evolution of fighting behavior; decision rules and assessment of relative strength', *J. Theoretical Biology*, 102, 387–410.

16. J. Goodall (1986), *The Chimpanzees of Gombe: Patterns of Behavior* (Harvard University Press, Cambridge, MA).

17. B. B. de Mesquita, D. Lalman (1992), *War and Reason: Domestic and International Imperatives* (Yale University Press, New Haven).

18. L. H. Keeley (1996), *War Before Civilization* (Oxford University Press, New York).

19. R. A. Hinde (1993), 'Aggression and war: Individuals, groups, and states', in P. E. Tetlock, J. L. Husbands, R. Jervis (eds), *Behaviour, Society and International Conflict* [8–70] (Oxford University Press, Oxford).

20. J. Popp, I. DeVore (1979), 'Aggressive competition and social dominance theory', in D. A. Hamburg, E. R. McCown (eds), *The Great Apes* [317–38] (Benjamin/Cummings, Menlo Park, CA).

21. R. L. Trivers (1991), 'Deceit and self-deception: The relationship between communication and consciousness', in M. H. Robinson, L. Tiger (eds), *Man and Beast Revisited* [175–92] (Smithsonian Institution Press, Washington, DC).

22. M. K. Surbey, J. J. McNally (1997), 'Self-deception as a mediator of cooperation and defection in varying social contexts described in the iterated Prisoner's Dilemma', *Evolution & Human Behavior*, 18, 417–35.

23. S. E. Taylor (1989), *Positive Illusions: Creative Self-Deception and the Healthy Mind* (Basic Books, New York).

24. C. S. Raps, C. Peterson, K. E. Reinhard, L. Y. Abramson, M. E. P. Seligman (1982), 'Attributional style among depressed patients', *J. Abnormal Psychology*, 91, 102–8.

25. J. E. Starek, C. F. Keating (1991), 'Self-deception and its relationship to success in competition', *Basic & Applied Social Psychology*, 12, 145–55.

26. L. Rue (1994), *By the Grace of Guile: The Role of Deception in Natural History and Human Affairs* (Oxford University Press, New York).

27. G. M. Stephenson (1984), 'Intergroup and interpersonal dimensions of bargaining and negotiation', in H. Tajfel (ed.), *The Social Dimension: European Developments in Social Psychology*, vol. 2 [646–67] (Cambridge University Press, Cambridge).

28. R. Dawkins, J. R. Krebs (1978), 'Animal signals: Information or manipulation?', in J. R. Krebs, N. B. Davis (eds), *Introduction to*

Behavioural Ecology: An Evolutionary Approach [282–309] (Blackwell, Oxford).

29. E. S. Adams, M. Mesterton-Gibbons (1995), 'The cost of threat displays and the stability of deceptive communication', *J. Theoretical Biology*, 175, 405–21.

30. A. R. Mele (1997), 'Real self-deception', *Behavioral Brain Sciences*, 20, 91–136.

31. N. Dixon (1976), *On the Psychology of Military Incompetence* (Jonathan Cape, London).

32. N. Dixon (1988), *Our Own Worst Enemy* (Futura, London).

33. G. Regan (1993), *Snafu: Great American Military Disasters* (Avon, New York).

34. G. Regan (1987), *Someone Had Blundered: A Historical Survey of Military Incompetence* (B. T. Batsford, London).

35. J. Perry (1996), *Arrogant Armies: Great Military Disasters and the Generals Behind Them* (John Wiley, New York).

36. H. A. Sackeim, R. C. Gur (1997), 'Flavors of self-deception: Ontology and epidemiology', *Behavioral Brain Sciences*, 20, 125–6.

37. T. O'Reilly, R. Dunbar, R. Bentall (2001), 'Schizotypy and creativity: An evolutionary connection?', *Personality and Individual Differences*, 31 (7), 1067–78.

38. H. J. Eysenck (1993), 'Creativity and personality: Suggestions for a theory', *Psychological Inquiry*, 4, 147–78.

39. K. R. Jamison (1989), 'Mood disorders and patterns of creativity in British writers and artists', *Psychiatry* 52, 125–34.

40. A. M. Ludwig (1995), *The Price of Greatness: Resolving the Creativity and Madness Controversy* (Guildford, New York).

41. F. Post (1996), 'Verbal creativity, depression and alcoholism: An investigation of 100 American and British writers'. *Brit. J. Psychiatry*, 168, 545–5.

42. N. C. Andreasen (1987), 'Creativity and mental illness: Prevalence rates in writers and their first-degree relatives', *Am. J. Psychiatry*, 144, 1288–92.

43. K. R. Jamison (1993), *Touched by Fire: Manic-depressive Illness and the Artistic Temperament* (Free Press, New York).

44. J. A. Keefe, P. A. Magaro (1980), 'Creativity and schizophrenia: An equivalence of cognitive processing', *J. Abnormal Psychology*, 89, 390–8.

45. J. L. Karlsson (1984), 'Creative intelligence in relatives of mental patients', *Hereditas* 100, 83–6.

CHAPTER 1: WEREWOLVES, VAMPIRES AND WITCHES

CHAPTER 1: WEREWOLVES, VAMPIRES AND WITCHES

1. T. Fahy, S. Wessley, A. David (1988), 'Werewolves, vampires and cannibals', *Med. Sci. Law*, 28 (2), 145–9.
2. P. E. Keck, H. G. Pope, J. I. Hudson, S. L. McElroy, A. R. Kulick (1988), 'Lycanthropy: Alive and well in the twentieth century', *Psychol. Med.*, 18, 113–20.
3. P. M. Jackson (1978), 'Another case of lycanthropy', *Am. J. of Psychiatry*, 135, 134–5.
4. F. G. Surawicz, R. Banta (1975), 'Lycanthropy revisited', *Can. Psychiatr. Assoc. J.*, 20, 537–42.
5. F. Hamdy Moselhy (1999), 'Lycanthropy: New evidence of its origin', *Psychopathology*, 32, 173–6.
6. H. A. Rosenstock, K. R. Vincent (1977), 'A case of lycanthropy', *Am. J. Psychiatry*, 134.
7. M. M. Innes (1955), *The Metamorphosis of Ovid* (Penguin, London).
8. R. J. Gorlin (1983), 'Facial folklore', *Mead Johnson Symp. Perinat. Dev. Med.*, 22, 43–8.
9. N. Jardine, J. A. Secord, E. C. Spary (eds), *Cultures of Natural History* (University of Cambridge Press Syndicate, Cambridge).
10. S. Ferracuti, R. Sacco, R. Lazzari (1996), 'Dissociative trance disorder: Clinical and research findings in ten persons reporting demon possession and treated by exorcism', *J. Pers. Assess.*, 66, 525–39.
11. S. Pereira, K. Bhui, S. Dein (1995), 'Making sense of "possession states": Psychopathology and differential diagnosis', *Brit. J. Hospital Medicine*, 53, 582–6.
12. P. E. Keck, H. G. Pope, J. I. Hudson, S. L. McElory, A. R. Kulick (1988), 'Lycanthropy: Alive and well in the twentieth century', *Psychol. Med.*, 18, 113–20.
13. M. Benzech, N. Witt, J. J. Etcheparre, M. Bourgeois (1989), 'A lycanthropic murderer', *Am. J. Psychiatry*, 146, 942.
14. T. Fahy, S. Wessley, A. David (1988), 'Werewolves, vampires and cannibals', *Med. Sci. Law*, 28 (2), 145–9.
15. A. D. Gaines (1995), 'Culture-specific delusions: Sense and non-sense in cultural context', *Psychiatr. Clin. North Am.*, 18, 281–301.
16. P. G. Coll, G. O'Sullivan, P. J. Browne (1985), 'Lycanthropy lives on', *Brit. J. Psychiatry*, 147, 201–2.
17. T. R. Dening, A. West (1989), 'Multiple serial lycanthropy', *Psychopathology*, 22, 344–7.

18. R. K. Chadda, N. Ahuja (1990), 'Dhat syndrome: A sex neurosis of the Indian Subcontinent', *Brit. J. Psychiatry*, 156, 577–9.

19. A. R. Kulick, H. G. Pope, P. E. Keck (1990), 'Lycanthropy and self identification', *J. Nervous Mental Disorders*, 178 (2), 134–7.

20. P. H. Salmons, D. J. Clarke (1992), 'Vampires, werewolves, and demons: Twentieth-century reports in the psychiatric literature', in R. Noll, *Cacodemonomania* (Brunner/Mazel, Philadelphia, PA).

21. T. Fahy (1988), 'Lycanthropy: A review, *J. R. Soc. Med.*, 82, 37–9.

22. M. Summer (1966), *The Werewolf* (University Books, New York).

23. P. H. Salmons, D. J. Clarke (1992), 'Vampires, werewolves, and demons: Twentieth-century reports in the psychiatric literature', in R. Noll, *Cacodemonomania* (Brunner/Mazel, Philadelphia, PA).

24. *Ibid.*

25. G. Zilboorg, G. W. Henry (1941), *A History of Medical Psychology* (Norton, New York).

26. L. Illis (1964), 'On porphyria and the aetiology of werewolves', *Proc. R. Soc. Med.*, 57, 23–6.

27. L. E. Figuera, M. Pandolfo, P. W. Dunne, *et al* (1995), 'Mapping of the congenital generalized hypertrichosis locus to chromosome Xq24–q27.1', *Nat. Genet.*, 10, 202–7.

28. K. Rao, B. N. Gangadhar, N. Janakiramiah (1999), 'Lycanthropy in depression: Two case reports on psychopathology', *Psychopathology*, 32, 169–72.

29. B. Ackner (1954), 'Depersonalization. I. Aetiology and phenomenology', *J. Mental Science*, 100, 838–53.

30. H. F. Moselhy (1999), 'Lycanthropy: New evidence of its origin', *Psychopathology*, 32, 173–6.

31. T. R. Dening, A. West (1990), 'The Dolittle phenomenon: Hallucinatory voices from animals', *Psychopathology*, 23 (1), 40–5.

32. H. A. Rosenstock, K. R. Vincent (1977), 'A case of lycanthropy', *Am. J. Psychiatry*, 134, 1147–9.

33. P. H. Salmons, D. J. Clarke (1987), 'Cacodemonomania', *Psychiatry: J. for Study of Interpersonal Processes*, 50 (1), 50–4.

34. E. Schendel, R. F. C. Kourany (1980), 'Cacodemonomania and exorcism in children', *J. Clinical Psychiatry*, 41, 119–23.

35. L. A. Sharp (1994), 'Exorcists, psychiatrists, and the problems of possession in northwest Madagascar', *Soc. Sci. Med.*, 38, 525–42.

36. F. D. Whitwell, M. G. Barker (1980), '"Possession" in psychiatric patients in Britain', *Brit. J. Medical Psychology*, 53, 287–95.

37. A. S. Hale, N. R. Pinnit (1994), 'Exorcism resistant ghost possession treated with clopenthixol', *Brit. J. Psychiatry*, 165, 386–8.
38. A. Furnham, P. Bower (1992), 'A comparison of academic and lay theories of schizophrenia', *Brit. J. Psychiatry*, 161, 201–10.
39. L. Alonso, W. D. Jeffrey (1988), 'Mental illness complicated by the santeria belief in spirit possession', *Hospital Community Psychiatry*, 39, 1188–91.
40. I. O. Vlachos, B. Stavroula, P. Hartocollis (1997), 'Magico-religious beliefs and psychosis', *Psychopathology*, 30, 93–9.
41. M. Risso, W. Boker (1968), 'Delusions of witchcraft: A cross-cultural study', *Brit. J. Psychiatry*, 114, 963–72.
42. E. Schendel, R. F. Kourany (1980), 'Cacodemonomania and exorcism in children', *J. Clinical Psychiatry*, 41 (4), 119–23.
43. R. J. Castillo (1994), 'Spirit possession in South Asia, dissociation or hysteria?', *Cult. Med. Psychiatry*, 18, 1–21.
44. J. Iida (1989), 'The current situation in regard to the delusion of possession in Japan', *Japanese J. Psychiatric Neurology*, 43, 19–27.
45. D. C. Goff, A. W. Brotman, D. Kindlon, M. Waites, E. Amico (1991), 'The delusion of possession in chronically psychotic patients', *J. Nervous Mental Disorders*, 179, 567–71.
46. S. Pfeifer (1994), 'Belief in demons and exorcism: An empirical study of 343 psychiatric patients in Switzerland', *Brit. J. Medical Psychology*, 67, 247–58.
47. J. L. Saver, J. Rabin (1997), 'The neural substrates of religious experience', *J. Neuropsychiatry & Clinical Neurosciences*, 9 (3), 498–510.
48. V. S. Ramachandran, S. Blakeslee (1998), *Phantoms in the Brain* (William Morrow, New York).
49. A. B. Newberg, E. G. d'Aquili (2000), 'Cognitive models and spiritual maps: Interdisciplinary explorations of religious experience', in J. Andresen, R. K. C. Forman (eds), *The Neuropsychology of Religious and Spiritual Experience* [251–66] (Imprint Academic, Thorverton, England).
50. D. Birnbacher, R. J. Seitz (2001), 'Neural correlates of religious experience', *European J. Neuroscience*, 13 (8), 1649–52.
51. M. A. Persinger (1993), 'Paranormal and religious beliefs may be mediated differentially by subcortical and cortical phenomenological processes of the temporal (limbic) lobes', *Perceptual & Motor Skills*, 76 (1), 247–51.

52. M. A. Persinger (1991), 'Canonical correlation of a temporal lobe signs scale with schizoid and hypomania scales in a normal population: Men and women are similar but for different reasons', *Perceptual & Motor Skills*, 73 (2) 615–18.

53. M. A. Persinger (1991), 'Preadolescent religious experience enhances temporal lobe signs in normal young adults', *Perceptual & Motor Skills*, 72 (2), 453–4.

54. A. B. Newberg, E. G. d'Aquili (2000), 'Cognitive models and spiritual maps: Interdisciplinary explorations of religious experience', in J. Andresen, R. K. C. Forman (eds), *The Neuropsychology of Religious and Spiritual Experience* [251–66] (Imprint Academic, Thorverton, England).

55. A. A. N. Marusich (1997), 'Religious conversion: Explorations in biogenetic structuralism', *Dissertation Abstracts International (Humanities and Social Sciences)*, 57 (8-A), 3535.

56. J. L. Saver, J. Rabin (1997), 'The neural substrates of religious experience', *J. Neuropsychiatry & Clinical Neurosciences*, 9 (3), 498–510.

57. A. Palmer Pol, J. J. Montano Moreno, A. Calafat Far (2000, Spanish), 'Prediction of ecstasy consumption based on the use of artificial neural networks, *Adicciones*, 12 (1), 29–41, (Sociedad Cientifica Espanola de Estudios Sobre el Alcohol, Spain).

58. C. L. Krumhansl, J. Louhivuori, P. Toiviainen, T. Jaervinen, T. Eerola (1999), 'Melodic expectation in Finnish spiritual folk hymns: Convergence of statistical, behavioral, and computational approaches', *Music Perception*, 17 (2) 151–95 (University of California Press).

59. H. Prins (1992), 'Vampirism: A clinical condition', in R. Noll, *Vampires, Werewolves, and Demons: Twentieth-century Reports in the Psychiatric Literature* (Brunner/Mazel, Philadelphia, PA).

60. T. A. E. Kamla (1985), 'A. Hoffmann's vampirism tale: Instinctual perversion', *American Imago*, 42 (3), 235–53.

61. H. Prins (1990), '*Bizarre Behaviours: Boundaries of Psychiatric Disorders*' (Tavistock/Routledge, New York).

62. L. Alonso, W. D. Jeffrey (1988), 'Mental illness complicated by the santeria belief in spirit possession', *Hospital Community Psychiatry*, 39, 1188–91.

63. M. Yvonneau (1990), 'Matricide and vampirism', [French], *Evolution Psychiatrique*, 55 (3), 575–85.

64. F. Cro, M. Peronti, G. Margherita, G. Bersani (1997), 'A case of auto-vampirism in a patient with borderline personality disorder and chronic multiple substance abuse', [Italian] *Rivista di Psichiatria*, 32 (4), 165–72.

65. I. O. Vlachos, B. Stavroula, P. Hartocollis (1997), 'Magico-religious beliefs and psychosis', *Psychopathology*, 30, 93–9.

66. R. Noll (1992), *Vampires, Werewolves, and Demons: Twentieth-century Reports in the Psychiatric Literature* [xxv, 244] (Brunner/Mazel, Philadelphia, PA).

67. P. Wilgowicz (1991), 'Off the subject', [French] *Revue Française de Psychanalyse*, 55 (6), 1763–7.

68. J. Gomez-Alonso (1998), 'Rabies: A possible explanation for the vampire legend', *Neurology*, 51 (3), 856–9.

69. R. Noll (1992), *Vampires, Werewolves, and Demons: Twentieth-century Reports in the Psychiatric Literature* (Brunner/Mazel, Philadelphia, PA).

70. B. D. Kelly, Z. Abood, D. Shanley (1999), 'Vampirism and schizophrenia', *Irish J. Psychological Medicine*, 16 (3), 114–15.

71. A. Bourguignon (1997), 'Vampirism and autovampirism', in L. B. Schlesinger, E. Revitch (eds), *Sexual Dynamics of Antisocial Behavior*, 2nd edn (Charles C. Thomas, Springfield, IL).

72. *Ibid.* 1147–9.

73. P. D. Jaffé, F. DiCataldo, (1994), 'Clinical vampirism: Blending myth and reality', *Bulletin Am. Academy Psychiatry & Law*, 22 (4), 533–44.

CHAPTER 2: IT TAKES TWO TO TANGO

1. M. Mazzoli (1992), 'Folie à deux and mental retardation', *Canadian J. Psychiatry*, 37, 278–9.
2. C. Laseque, J. Falret (1877), '*La folie à deux ou folie communiquée*', *Annals of Medical Psychology*, 18, 321.
3. M. H. Sacks (1988), '*Folie à deux*', *Compr. Psychiatry*, 29, 270–7.
4. A. O. Schmidt (1949), 'A case of *folie à deux*', *J. Abnormal Psychology*, 44, 402–10.
5. M. Ghaziuddin (1991), '*Folie à deux and mental retardation*', *Canadian J. Psychiatry*, 36, 48–9.
6. D. H. Ropschitz (1957), '*Folie à deux*: A case of *folie imposée à quatre* and *à trois*', *J. Mental Science*, 103, 589–96.
7. M. D. Enoch, W. H. Trethowan (1979), *Uncommon Psychia Syndromes* (John Wright, Bristol).
8. R. Howard (1994), 'Induced psychosis', *Brit. J. Hospital Medicine*, 51, 304–7.
9. R. Tabarés-Seisdedos, R. Corral-Márquez (2001), 'Images in psychiatry: Miguel de Cervantes, 1547–1616, *Am. J. Psychiatry*, 158, 1392.
10. S. R. Cajal (1972), *La Resurrección del Quijote, in La Psicología de los Artistas,* 3rd edn (Espasa-Callpe, Madrid).
11. E. Freud (ed.) (1960), *Letters of Sigmund Freud* (Basic Books, New York).
12. S. J. Kiraly (1975), '*Folie à deux*: A case of "demonic possession" involving mother and daughter', *Canadian Psychiatric Assoc. J.*, 20 (3), 223–7.
13. A. Pulver, M. Brint (1961), 'Detection of hostility in *Folie à deux*', *Arch. Gen. Psychiatry*, 5, 257–65.
14. J. M. Silveira, M. V. Seeman (1995), 'Shared psychotic disorder: A critical review of the literature', *Canadian J. Psychiatry*, 40, 389–95.
15. A. Munro (1986), '*Folie à deux revisited*', *Canadian J. Psychiatry*, 31, 233–4.
16. L. S. Tucker, T. P. Cornwall (1977), 'Mother–son *folie à deux*: A case of attempted patricide', *Am. J. Psychiatry*, 134 (10), 1146–7.
17. A. D. Neagoe (2000), 'Abducted by aliens: A case study', *Psychiatry: Interpersonal & Biological Processes*, 63 (2), 202–7.
18. E. Bourguignon (1974), *Culture and the Varieties of Consciousness* (Addison-Wesley, Reading, MA).
19. M. Chan, W. C. Kee (1983), 'Epidemic hysteria: A study of high risk factors', *Occupational Health and Safety*, 52, 55–64.

20. R. A. Bryant (1997), '*Folie à famille*: A cognitive study of delusional beliefs', *Psychiatry: Interpersonal & Biological Processes*, 60 (1), 44–50.

21. R. Cawthra, G. O'Brien, F. Hassenyeh (1987), 'Imposed psychosis', *Brit. J. Psychiatry*, 150, 557–71.

22. E. H. Norman (1945), 'Mass hysteria in Japan', *Far Eastern Survey*, 14, 65–70.

23. B. Radford, R. Bartholomew (2001), 'Pokemon contagion: Photosensitive epilepsy or mass psychogenic illness?', *Southern Medical J.*, 94, 197–204.

24. Kwan Weng Kin (1997), 'Fit-inducing cartoon affected nearly 12,000 Japanese children', *The Straits Times* (Singapore).

25. Agence France-Press (1998), 'Flashing-light cartoon series to resume', *New York Times*.

26. T. Abdul Rahman (1987), 'As I See It . . . Will the hysteria return?', *The New Straits Times* (Malaysia).

27. R. E. Bartholomew (1994), 'The social psychology of "epidemic" koro', *Int. J. Social Psychiatry*, 40, 44–60.

28. R. M. Albrecht, V. Oliver, D. Poskanzer (1964), 'Epidemic neuromyasthenia: Outbreak in a convent in New York State', *J. Am. Med. Assoc.*, 187, 904–7.

29. S. M. Benaim, J. Horder, J. Anderson (1973), 'Hysterical epidemic in a classroom', *Psychological Medicine*, 3, 66–73.

30. M. J. Colligan, L. R. Murphy (1979), 'Mass psychogenic illness in organizations: An overview', *J. Occupational Psychology*, 52, 77–90.

31. R. W. Metzger (1989), 'Report of an illness outbreak at the Harry S. Truman state office building', *Am. J. Epidemiology*, 129, 550–8.

32. H. S. Faust, L. B. Brilliant (1981), 'Is the diagnosis of "mass hysteria" an excuse for incomplete investigation of low-level environmental contamination?', *J. Occupational Medicine*, 23, 22–6.

CHAPTER 3: THE PHANTOM LOVER SYNDROME

1. J. W. Lovett-Doust, H. Christie (1978), 'The pathology of love: Some clinical variants of de Clérambault's syndrome', *Soc. Sci. Med.*, 12, 99–106.

2. M. V. Seeman (1978), 'Delusional loving' (Archives of General Psychiatry), *Am. Med. Assoc.*, 35, 1265–7.

3. P. Brown, P. Lloyd (1986), 'A disorder of falling in love', *Sexual & Marital Therapy*, 1, 1.

4. M. Zona, K. K. Sharma, J. Lane (1993), 'A comparative study of erotomania and obsessional subjects in a forensic sample', *J. Forensic Sciences*, 38, 894–903.

5. H. F. Harlow, M. K. Harlow (1965), 'The affectional systems', in A. M. Schrier, H. F. Harlow, F. Stollnitz (eds), *Behavior of Nonhuman Primates: Modern Research Trends 2* [287–334] (Academic Press, New York).

6. K. K. Kienlen, D. L. Birmingham, K. B. Solberg, J. T. O'Regan, J. R. Meloy (1997), 'A comparative study of psychotic and nonpsychotic stalking', *J. Am. Acad. Psychiatry Law*, 25, 317–34.

7. G. De Clérambault (1921), 'Les psychoses passionelles', in *Oeuvre Psychiatrique* (Presses de France, Paris).

8. E. A. Zarrouk (1991), 'The co-existence of erotomania and Capgras Syndrome', *Br. J. Psychiatry*, 159, 717–19.

9. M. O. Enoch, W. H. Trethowan (eds) (1991), *De Clérambault's Syndrome in Uncommon Psychiatric Syndromes*, 3rd edn [24–50] (Butterworth-Heinemann, Cambridge).

10. M. V. Seeman (1978), 'Delusional loving' (Archives of General Psychiatry), *Am. Med. Assoc.*, 35, 1265–7.

11. M. Bergman (1987), *The Anatomy of Loving* (Columbia University Press, New York).

12. J. W. Lovett-Doust, H. Christie (1978), 'The pathology of love: Some clinical variants of de Clérambault's syndrome', *Soc. Sci. Med.*, 12, 99–106.

13. L. B. Raschka (1979), 'The incubus syndrome: A variant of erotomania', *Canadian J. Psychiatry*, 24 (6), 549–53.

14. A. C. Pande (1981), 'Co-existence of Incubus and Capgras Syndromes', *Br. J. Psychiatry*, 139, 469–70.

15. A. Munro (1995), 'The classification of delusional disorders', *Psychiatric Clin. North America*, 18 (2), 199–212.

16. M. Bergman (1987), *The Anatomy of Loving* (Columbia University Press, New York).

17. T. Manschcreck (1998), 'Delusional disorder', in B. J. Sadock, H. Kaplan (eds), *Synopsis of Psychiatry*, 8th edn [517–23] (Lippincott, Williams & Wilkins, Baltimore).

18. G. B. Leong, J. A. Silva, E. S. Garza-Trevino, D. Oliva, *et al* (1994), 'The dangerousness of persons with the Othello syndrome' [American Society For Testing and Materials ASTM], *J. Forensic Sciences*, 39 (6), 1445–54.

19. A. Munro (1991), 'Phenomenological aspects of monodelusional disorders', *Br. J. Psychiatry* 159 (14), 62–4.

20. M. Marks, P. de Silva (1991), 'Multi-faceted treatment of a case of morbid jealousy', *Sexual & Marital Therapy*, 6 (1).

21. R. R. Mowat (1966), *Morbid Jealousy and Murder* (Tavistock, London).

22. L. J. West (1968), 'The Othello Syndrome: A fresh look at the Oedipus complex', *Contemporary Psychoanalysis*, 4, 103–10.

23. P. V. Butler (2000), 'Reverse Othello syndrome subsequent to traumatic brain injury', *Psychiatry: Interpersonal & Biological Processes*, 63 (1), 85–92.

24. J. H. Segal (1989), 'Erotomania revisited: From Kraepelin to DSM-III-R', *Am. J. Psychiatry*, 146, 1261–6.

25. R. L. Goldstein (1986), 'Erotomania in men', [letter to editor] *Am. J. Psychiatry*, 143, 802.
R. L. Goldstein (1987), 'More forensic romances: De Clérambault's syndrome in men', *Bulletin of Am. Acad. of Psychiatry Law*, 15, 267–74.

26. J. T. Okimura, S. A. Norton (1998), 'Jealousy and mutilation: nose-biting as retribution for adultery', *Lancet*, 352, 2010–11.

27. N. Phelan (1958), *Atoll holiday* [145] (Angus and Robertson, Sydney).

28. H. P. Lundsgaarde (1974), 'Transactions in Gilbertese law and justice', *J. Polynesian Soc.*, 83, 192–222.

29. D. E. Lewis Jr (1990), 'Tungaru conjugal jealousy and sexual mutilation', *Pacific Studies*, 13, 115–26.

30. A. Brewis (1996), *Lives on the Line: Women and Ecology on a Pacific Atoll* [48–50] (Harcourt Brace, Texas).

31. G. B. Leong, J. A. Silva, E. S. Garza-Treviño, D. Oliva, M. M. Ferrari, R. V. Komanduri, J. C. B. Caldwell (1994), The dangerousness of persons with the Othello syndrome', *J. Forensic Sciences*, 39 (6), 1445–54.

32. G. Goodwin (1942), *The Social Organization of the Western Apache People* [341] (University of Chicago Press, Chicago).
     M. E. Opler (1941), *The Economic, Social, and Religious Institutions of the Chiracahua Apache* [410-11] (University of Chicago Press, Chicago).

33. J. P. Boyd (1950), *The Papers of Thomas Jefferson*, vol. 2 [497] (Princeton University Press, Princeton).
     M. Twain (1981 edn), *The Adventures of Tom Sawyer* [176] (Bantam, Toronto).

34. R. L. Stevenson (1900), *In the South Seas* [268–9] (Chatto, London).
     K. Bhanganada, T. Chayavatana, C. Pongnumkul, *et al* (1983), 'Surgical management of an epidemic of penile amputations in Siam', *Am. J. Surg.*, 146, 376–82.

35. H. E. Book (1971), 'Sexual implications of the nose', *Comp. Psychiatr.*, 12, 450–5.

36. D. M. Buss, R. J. Larsen, D. Westen, J. Semmelroth (2001), 'Sex differences in jealousy: Evolution, physiology, and psychology' [143–9], in W. Gerrod Parrott (ed.), *Emotions in Social Psychology: Essential Readings* [xiv, 378] (Psychology Press/Taylor & Francis, New York).

37. J. N. Mackenzie (1898), 'Physiological and pathological relations between the nose and the sexual apparatus in man', *Johns Hopkins Hosp. Bull.*, 82, 10–17.

38. D. M. Buss (2000), *The Dangerous Passion: Why Jealousy Is As Necessary As Love and Sex* (The Free Press, New York).

39. D. M. Buss, R. J. Larsen, D. Westen, J. Semmelroth (2001), 'Sex differences in jealousy: Evolution, physiology, and psychology' [143–9], in W. Gerrod Parrott (ed.), *Emotions in Social Psychology: Essential Readings* [xiv, 378] (Psychology Press/Taylor & Francis, New York).

40. *Ibid.*

41. D. M. Buss, N. Malamuth (eds), *Sex, Power, Conflict: Evolutionary and Feminist Perspectives* (Oxford University Press, New York).

42. D. M. Buss, R. J. Larsen, D. Westen, J. Semmelroth (2001), 'Sex differences in jealousy: Evolution, physiology, and psychology' [143–9], in W. Gerrod Parrott (ed.), *Emotions in Social Psychology: Essential Readings* [xiv, 378] (Psychology Press/Taylor & Francis, New York).

43. W. J. Winslade, J. W. Ross (1983), *The Insanity Plea: The Uses and Abuses of the Insanity Defense* (Scribner, New York).

44. *Ibid.*

45. T. Reik (1949), *Of Love and Lust: On the Psychoanalysis of Romantic and Sexual Emotions* (Farrar, Straus & Giroux, New York).

46. D. de Rougement [translated by M. Belgion] (1983), *Love in the Western World* (Princeton University Press, Princeton).

47. D. M. Buss (1994), *The Evolution of Desire: Strategies of Human Mating* (Basic Books, New York).

48. K. O. Ferris (2001), 'Through a glass, darkly: The dynamics of fan–celebrity encounters', *Symbolic Interaction*, 24 (1), 25–47.

CHAPTER 4: SEXUAL DELUSIONS

1. M. Hirschfeld (1956), *Sexual Anomalies* (Emerson Books, New York).

2. R. I. Simon (1997), 'Video voyeurs and the covert videotaping of unsuspecting victims: Psychological and legal consequences', *J. Forensic Sciences*, 42 (5), 884–9.

3. M. W. Braaioraj, J. Boulet, A. Pawlak (1992), 'The paraphilias: A multiplicity of deviant behaviours', *Canadian J. Psychiatry*, 37, 104–8.

4. S. J. Hucker (1985), 'Self-harmful sexual behavior', *Psychiatric Clinics North America*, 2, 323–36.

5. C. Gosselin, G. Wilson (1980), *Sexual Variations* (Simon & Schuster, New York).

6. K. M. Beier (1994a), *Weiblichkeit und Perversion – Von der Reproduktion zur Reproversion* (Fischer, Stuttgart).

7. K. M. Beier (1994b), 'Gibt es eine weibliche Analogie zur Perversion?', *Psychotherap. Psychosom. Med. Psychol.*, 44, 137–43.

8. C. Brezinka, W. Biebl, J. Kinzl, O. Huter (1991), 'Spät Erkannte und Negierte Schwangerschaft – Psychopathologie der Verdrängungsmechanismen und Auswirkungen auf die Geburt', *Arch. Gynecol. Obstet.*, 250, 1039–41.

9. S. Freud (1905), *Drei Abhandlungen zur Sexualtheorie* (Deuticke, Leipzig).

10. L. J. Kaplan (1991), *Weibliche Perversionen* (Hoffmann und Campe, Hamburg).

11. K. Püschel, G. Hasselblatt, H. Labes (1988), 'Kindermörderinnen: Meist geistig unreif eine Analyse unter kriminologischen Aspekten', *Kriminalistik*, 10, 525–8. G. Rendueles (1989), *El Manuscrito Encontrado En Ciempozuelos* (Ediciciones Endymion, Madrid).

12. H. Thomsen, M. Bauermeister, R. Wille (1992), 'Zur Kindestötung unter der Geburt. Eine Verbundstudie über die Jahre 1980–1989', *Rechtsmedizin*, 2, 135–42.

13. C. Gosselin, G. Wilson (1980), *Sexual Variations* (Simon & Schuster, New York).

14. J. Wessel, J. W. Dudenhausen, J. W. Schönegg, K. Schmidt-Gollwitzer (1990), 'Abgewehrte Schwangerschaftswahrnehmung. Zum Bild der Schwangerschafts-verdrängung', *Münch Med. Wschr*, 132, 374–80.

15. R. J. Stoller (1979), Perversion. Die Erotische Form von Haß (Rowohlt, Reinbeck). D. H. Strauss, R. L. Spitzer, P. R. Muskin (1990), 'Maladaptive denial of physical illness: A proposal for DSM-IV' *Am. J. Psychiatry*, 147, 1168–72.

16. R. Wille, K. M. Beier (1994), '"Verdrängte" Schwangerschaft und Kindestötung: Theorie-Forensik-Klinik', *Sexuologie*, 2, 75–100.

17. E. Trube-Becker (1975), 'Zur Kindestötung', *Ärztin*, 10, 3–14.

18. J. D. Lichtenberg (1991), 'Psychoanalyse und Säuglingsforschung', in *Female Analogies to Perversion* [93] (Springer, New York).

19. R. S. Shiwach, J. Prosser (1998), 'Treatment of an unusual case of masochism', *J. Sexual & Marital Therapy*, 24 (4), 303–7.

20. J. Hirschmann, E. Schmitz (1958), 'Strukturanalyse der Kindesmörderin', *Z. Psychother. Med. Psychol.*, 8, 1–20.

21. F. Morgenthaler (1987), *Homosexualität – Heterosexualität – Perversion* (Fischer, Frankfurt).

22. S. Mentzos (1990), 'Neurotische Konfliktverarbeitung. Einführung', in *Psychoanalytische Neurosenlehre Unter Berücksichtigung Neuer Perspektiven* [207] (Fischer, Frankfurt).

23. P. de Silva, A. Pernet (1992), 'Pollution in Metroland: An unusual paraphilia of a shy young man', *J. Sexual & Marital Therapy*, 7, 3.

24. S. Rachman (1966), 'Sexual fetishism: An experimental analogue', *Psychological Record*, 16, 293–6.

25. R. Dewaraja (1987), 'Formicophilia, an unusual paraphilia, treated with counseling and behavior therapy', *Am. J. Psychotherapy*, 41 (4), 593–7.

26. B. Knight (1979), 'Fatal masochism: Accident or suicide', *Med. Sci. Law*, 19, 118–20.

27. R. Caplan, J. Komaromi, M. Rhodes (1996), 'Obsessive-compulsive disorder, tattooing and bizarre sexual practices', *Br. J. Psychiatry*, 168 (3), 379–80.

28. N. Buhrich (1983), 'The association of erotic piercing with homo-sexuality, sadomasochism, bondage, fetishes and tattoos', *Archives Sexual Behavior*, 12, 167–71.

29. B. E. McGuire, G. L. Choon, P. Nayer, J. Sanders (1998), 'An unusual paraphilia: Case report of oral partialism', *J. Sexual & Marital Therapy*, 13 (2), 207–10.

30. R. W. Byard, S. J. Hucker, R. R. Hazelwood (1990), 'A comparison of typical death scene features in cases of fatal male and female autoerotic asphyxia with a review of the literature', *Forensic Sci. Int.*, 48, 113–21.

31. R. Blanchard, S. J. Hucker (1991), 'Age, transvestism, bondage, and concurrent paraphilic activities in 117 fatal cases of autoerotic asphyxia', *Br. J. Psychiatry*, 159, 371–7.

32. G. T. Gowitt, R. L. Hanzlick (1992), 'Atypical autoerotic deaths', *Am. J. Forensic Med. Pathol.*, 13, 115–19.

33. R. W. Byard, P. Botterill (1998), 'Autoerotic asphyxial death – accident or suicide?', *Am. J. Forensic Med. Pathol.*, 19, 377–80.

34. R. R. Hazelwood, P. E. Dietz, A. W. Burgess (1983), 'Investigation of autoerotic fatalities', in R. R. Hazelwood, P. E. Dietz, A. W. Burgess (eds), *Autoerotic Fatalities* [121–38] (D. C. Heath, Lexington, MA).

35. J. Johnstone, R. Huws (1997), 'Autoerotic asphyxia: A case report', *J. Sexual & Marital Therapy*, 23 (4), 326–32.

36. S. Tough, J. Butt, G. Sanders (1994), 'Autoerotic asphyxial deaths: Analysis of nineteen fatalities in Alberta, 1978–1989', *Can. J. Psychiatry*, 39, 157–60.

37. J. Uva (1995), 'Review: Autoerotic asphyxiation in the United States', *J. Forensic Sci.*, 40, 574–81.

38. R. Book, G. Perumal (1993), 'Sexual asphyxia: A lesser epidemic', *Med. Law*, 12, 687–98.

39. S. Hucker (1990), 'Sexual asphyxia', in R. Bluglass, P. Bowden (eds), *Principles and Practice of Forensic Psychiatry* [717–21] (Churchill Livingstone, Edinburgh).

40. W. Friedrich, P. Gerber (1994), 'Autoerotic asphyxia: The development of a paraphilia', *J. Am. Acad. Child Adolesc. Psychiatry*, 33, 970–4.

41. P. Haydn-Smith, I. Marks, H. Buchaya, D. Repper (1987), 'Behavioural treatment of life-threatening masochistic asphyxiation: A case study', *Br. J. Psychiatry*, 150, 518–19.

42. P. E. Dietz (1989), 'Television-inspired autoerotic asphyxiation', *J. Forensic Sci.*, 34, 528–9.

43. R. O'Halloran, J. Lovell (1988), 'Autoerotic asphyxial death following television broadcast', *J. Forensic Sci.*, 33, 1491–2.

44. R. Hazelwood, P. Dietz, A. Burgess (1983), *Autoerotic Fatalities* (Lexington Books, Lexington, MA).

45. W. Ober (1984), 'The sticky end of Frantisek Koczwara, composer of "The Battle of Prague"', *Am. J. Forensic Med. Pathol.*, 5, 145–9.

46. S. Innala, K. Ernulf (1989), 'Asphyxophilia in Scandinavia', *Arch. Sex. Behav.*, 18, 181–9.

47. M. Diamond, S. Innala, K. Ernulf (1990), 'Asphyxiophilia and auto-erotic death', *Hawaii Med. J.*, 49, 11–24.

48. C. Wessellus, R. A. Bally (1983), 'Male with autoerotic asphyxia syndrome', *Am. J. Forensic Med. Pathol.*, 4, 341–5.

49. J. Cooper (1996), 'Autoerotic asphyxiation: Three case reports', *J. Sexual & Marital Therapy*, 22, 47–53.

50. R. Hazelwood, P. Dietz, A. Burgess (1981), 'The investigation of autoerotic fatalities', *J. Police Sci. Adm.*, 9, 404–11.

51. R. Byard, S. Hucker, R. Hazelwood (1990), 'A comparison of typical death scene features in cases of male and female autoerotic asphyxia with a review of literature', *Forensic Sci. Int.*, 48, 113–21.

52. B. R. Burg (1987), 'Masturbatory death and injury', *J. of the Royal Society of Health*, 107 (2), 60–1.

53. C. Brych (1992), 'Verdrängte Schwangerschaft', *Die Hebamme*, 5, 124–5.

54. K. M. Beier (2000), 'Female Analogies to Perversion', *J. Sexual & Marital Therapy*, 26, 79–93.

55. M. Heap (2000), 'A legal case of a man complaining of an extraordinary sexual disorder following stage hypnosis', *Contemporary Hypnosis*, 17 (3), 143–9.

CHAPTER 5: THE DELUSION OF LOVE

1. R. L. Goldstein (1987), 'More forensic romances: De Clérambault's syndrome in men', *Bulletin American Academy Psychiatry Law*, 15, 267–74.

2. A. R. Roberts, S. F. Dziegielewski (1996), 'Assessment typology and intervention with the survivors of stalking', *Aggression & Violent Behavior*, 1 (4) 359–68.

3. G. B. Leong (1994), 'De Clérambault syndrome (erotomania) in the criminal justice system', *J. Forensic Science*, 39, 378–85.

4. J. T. Meloy (1996), 'Stalking obsessional following: A review of some preliminary studies', *Aggression & Violent Behavior*, 1, 147–62.

5. J. R. Meloy (1997), 'The clinical risk management of stalking: "Someone is watching over me . . ."', *Am. J. Psychotherapy*, 51, 174–84.

6. J. R. Meloy (1996), 'Stalking (obsessional following): A review of some preliminary studies', *Aggression & Violent Behavior*, 1, 147–62.

7. W. J. Fremouw, D. Westrup, J. Pennypacker (1997), 'Stalking on campus: The prevalence and strategies for coping with stalking', *J. Forensic Sciences*, 42, 666–9.

8. J. R. Meloy (1989), 'Unrequited love and the wish to kill. Diagnosis and treatment of borderline erotomania', *Bulletin Menninger Clinic*, 53, 476–92.

9. P. E. Mullen, M. Pathe (1994), 'The pathological extensions of love', *Br. J. Psychiatry*, 165, 614–23.

10. J. W. Droust, H. S. Christie (1978), 'The pathology of love: Some clinical variants of de Clérambault's syndrome', *Soc. Sci. Med.*, 12, 99–106.

11. D. L. Evans, L. L. Jeckell, N. E. Slott (1982), 'Erotomania: A variant of pathological mourning', *Bulletin Menninger Clin.*, 46, 507–20.

12. C. G. de Clérambault (1921), 'Les psychoses passionelles', in *Oeuvre Psychiatrique* [1942] (Presses de France, Paris).

13. C. G. de Clérambault (1942), 'Les psychoses passionelles: The "passionate psychoses"', in *Oeuvres Psychiatriques* [315–22] (Presses Universitaires de France, Paris).

14. F. R. Farnham, D. V. James (1997), 'The pathology of love', *Lancet*, 350, 710.

15. B. D. Kelly, N. Kennedy, D. Shanley (2000), 'Delusion and desire: Erotomania Revisited', *Acta Psychiatr. Scand.*, 102, 74–6.

16. R. A. Collacott, E. M. Napier (1991), 'Erotomania and Fregoli-like state in Down's syndrome: Dynamic and developmental aspects', *J. Mental Deficiency Research*, 35 (5), 481–6.

17. J. Noone, L. Cockhill (1987), 'Erotomania: The delusion of being loved', *Am. J. Forensic Psychiatry*, 8, 23–31.

18. J. H. Segal (1989), 'Erotomania revisited: From Kraepelin to DSM–III–R', *Am. J. Psychiatry*, 146, 1261–2.

19. M. D. Enoch, W. H. Trethowan, J. C. Barker (1967), *Some Uncommon Psychotic Syndromes* (John Wright, Bristol).

20. J. A. Wright, A. G. Burgess, A. W. Burgess, A. T. Laszlo, G. O. McCrary, J. E. Douglas, (1996), 'A typology of interpersonal stalking', *J. Interpersonal Violence*, 11, 487–502.

21. R. B. Harmon, R. Rosner, H. Owens (1995), 'Obsessional harassment and erotomania in a criminal court population', *J. Forensic Sciences*, 40, 188–96.

22. K. R. Thomas (1993), 'How to stop the stalker: State anti-stalking laws', *Criminal Law Bulletin*, 29, 124–36.

23. D. E. Raskin, K. E. Sullivan (1974), 'Erotomania', *Am. J. Psychiatry*, 131, 1033–5.

24. R. P. D. Menzies, J. P. Fedoroff, C. M. Green, K. Isaacson (1995), 'Prediction of dangerous behaviour in male erotomania', *Br. J. Psychiatry*, 166, 529–36.

25. S. G. Noffsinger, F. M. Saleh (2000), 'Ideas of reference about newscasters', *Psychiatric Services*, 51, 679.

26. K. Wadeson, W. T. Carpenter (1976), 'Television in the hospital: Programming patients' delusions', *Am. J. Orthopsychiatry*, 46, 434–8.

27. R. L. Binder, D. E. McNeil (1996), 'Application of the Tarasoff ruling and its effect on the victim and the therapeutic relationship', *Psychiatric Services*, 47, 1212–15.

28. D. E. McNeil, R. L. Binder, F. M. Fulton (1998), 'Management of threats of violence under California's duty-to-protect statute', *Am. J. Psychiatry*, 155, 1097–1101.

29. M. Rudden, M. Gilmore, A. Frances (1980), 'Erotomania: A separate entity', *Am. J. Psychiatry*, 137, 1262–3.

30. A. M. Munro (1985), 'De Clérambault's syndrome: a nosological entity' [letter], *Br. J. Psychiatry*, 146, 561.

31. W. R. Cupach, B. H. Spitzberg (eds) (1994), *The Dark Side of Interpersonal Communication* (Erlbaum, Hillsdale, NJ).

32. M. Schachter (1977), 'Erotomania or the delusional conviction of being loved: Contribution to the psychopathology of the love life', [French], *Ann. Med. Psychol.*, 1, 729–47.

33. P. Taylor, G. Mahendra, J. Gunn (1983), 'Erotomania in males', *Psychol. Med.* 13, 645–50.

34. M. O. Enoch (1991), 'De Clérambault's syndrome, in M. O. Enoch, W. H. Trethowan (eds), *Uncommon Psychiatric Syndromes*, 3rd edn [24–60] (Butterworth-Heinemann, Cambridge).

35. M. A. Zona, K. K. Sharma, J. Lane (1993), 'A comparative study of erotomanic and obsessional subjects in a forensic sample', *J. Forensic Sci.*, 38, 894–903.

36. A. J. Giannini, A. E. Slaby, T. O. Robb (1991), 'De Clérambault's syndrome in sexually experienced women', *J. Clin. Psychiatry*, 52, 84–6.

37. N. Retterstol, S. Opjordsmoen (1991), 'Erotomania: Erotic self-reference psychosis in old maids, a long-term follow-up', *Psychopathology*, 24, 388–97.

38. J. H. Segal (1989), 'Erotomania revisited: From Kraepelin to DSM-III-R' [review], *Am. J. Psychiatry*, 146, 1261–6.

39. C. A. Anderson, J. Camp, C. M. Filley (1998), 'Erotomania after aneurysmal subarachnoid hemorrhage: Case report and literature review', *J. Neuropsychiatry Clin. Neurosci.*, 10, 330–7.

40. S. John, F. Ovsiew (1996), 'Erotomania in a brain-damaged male', *J. Intellect Disabil. Res.*, 40, 279–83.

41. E. Balduzzi (1956), 'Un caso di erotomania passionale pura secondu Clerambault [A case of pure passionate erotomania after Clérambault]', *Riu Sperim di Freniatria*, 80, 407–26.

42. D. Murray, P. Harwood, E. Eapen (1990), 'Erotomania in relation to childbirth', *Br. J. Psychiatry*, 156, 896–8.

43. W. C. Drevets, E. H. Rubin (1987), 'Erotomania and senile dementia of Alzheimer type', *Br. J. Psychiatry*, 151, 400–2.

44. J. Heinik, J. Aharon-Peretz, J. P. Hes, 'De Clérambault's syndrome in multi-infarct dementia', *Psychiatria Fennica*, 22, 23–6.

45. L. Carrier (1990), 'Erotomania and senile dementia', [letter], *Am. J. Psychiatry*, 147, 1092.

46. B. H. Price, M-M. Mesulam (1985), 'Psychiatric manifestations of right hemisphere infarctions', *J. Nerv. Ment. Dis.*, 173, 610–14.

47. S. S. Signer, J. L. Cummings (1987), 'Erotomania and cerebral dysfunction' [letter], *Br. J. Psychiatry*, 151, 275.

48. P. E. Mullen, M. Pathé, R. Purcell (2000), *Stalkers and Their Victim* (Cambridge University Press, Cambridge).

49. P. E. Mullen, M. Pathé, R. Purcell (2000), *Stalkers and Their Victim* (Cambridge University Press, Cambridge).

50. R. B. Harmon, R. Rosner, H. Owens (1995), 'Obsessional harassment and erotomania in a criminal court population', *J. Forensic Sciences*, 40, 188–96.

51. K. K. Kienlen, D. L. Birmingham, K. B. Solberg, J. T. O'Regan, J. R. Meloy (1997), 'A comparative study of psychotic and nonpsychotic stalking', *J. Am. Academy Psychiatry Law*, 25, 317–34.

52. M. A. Zona, K. K. Sharma, J. Lane (1993), 'A comparative study of erotomania and obsessional subjects in a forensic sample', *J. Forensic Sciences*, 38, 894–903.

53. L. E. Walker, J. R. Meloy (1998), 'Stalking and domestic violence', in J. R. Meloy (ed.), *The Psychology of Stalking* [139–66] (Academic Press, New York).

54. M. Pathé, P. E. Mullen (1997), 'The impact of stalkers on their victims', *Br. J. Psychiatry*, 170, 12–17.

55. J. R. Urbach, C. Khalily, P. P. Mitchell (1992), 'Erotomania in an adolescent: Clinical and theoretical considerations', *J. of Adolescence*, 15, 231–40.

56. P. E. Dietz, D. B. Matthews, C. Van Duyne, D. A. Martell, C. D. H. Parry, T. Stewart, J. Warren, J. D. Crowder (1991b), 'Threatening and otherwise inappropriate letters to Hollywood celebrities', *J. Forensic Sciences*, 36, 185–209.

57. P. E. Dietz, D. B. Matthews, D. A. Martell, T. M. Stewart, D. R. Hrouda, J. Warren (1991a), 'Threatening and otherwise inappropriate letters to members of the United States Congress', *J. Forensic Sciences*, 36, 1445–68.

58. K. G. McAnaney, L. A. Curliss, C. E. Abeyta-Price (1993), 'From imprudence to crime: Anti-stalking laws', *Notre Dame Law Review*, 68, 819–909.

59. C. Draucker (1999), 'Living in hell', *Issues in Mental Health Nursing*, 20, 473–84.

60. M. Pathé, P. E. Mullen (1997), 'The impact of stalkers on their victims', *Br. J. Psychiatry*, 170, 12–17.

61. D. M. Hall (1998), 'The victims of stalking', in J. R. Meloy (ed.), *The Psychology of Stalking* [113–37] (Academic Press, New York).

62. P. Tjaden, N. Thoennes (1998), 'Stalking in America: Findings from the National Violence Against Women Survey', Department of Justice, Washington, DC.

63. S. F. Dziegielewski, A. R. Roberts (1995), 'Stalking victims and survivors: Identification, legal remedies, and crisis treatment', in A. R. Roberts (ed.), *Crisis Intervention and Time-limited Cognitive Treatment* [73–90] (Sage, Thousand Oaks, CA).

64. J. R. Meloy (1997), 'The clinical risk management of stalking: "Someone is watching over me"', *Am. J. Psychotherapy*, 51, 174–84.

65. F. L. Coleman (1997), 'Stalking behavior and the cycle of domestic violence', *J. Interpersonal Violence*, 12, 420–32.

66. W. J. Fremouw, D. Westrup, J. Pennypacker (1997), 'Stalking on campus: The prevalence and strategies for coping with stalking', *J. Forensic Sciences*, 42, 666–9.

67. P. Mullen, M. Pathé (1994), 'The pathological extensions of love', *Br. J. Psychiatry* 165, 614–23.

68. P. E. Mullen, M. Pathé, R. Purcell, G. W. Stuart (1999), 'A Study of Stalkers', *Am. J. Psychiatry*, 156, 1244–9.

69. D. M. Hall (1998), 'The victims of stalking', in J. R. Meloy (ed.), *The Psychology of Stalking* [113–37] (Academic Press, New York).

70. M. J. Gilligan (1992), 'Stalking the stalker: Developing new laws to thwart those who terrorize others', *Georgia Law Review*, 27, 285–342.

71. P. E. Mullen, M. Pathé, R. Purcell (2000), *Stalkers and Their Victim* (Cambridge University Press, Cambridge).

CHAPTER 6: DELUSIONS OF THE BODY

1. P. M. Yap (1965), 'Koro, a culture-bound depersonalisation syndrome', *Br. J. Psychiatry*, 111, 43–50.
2. R. A. Adeniran, J. R. Jones (1994), 'Koro: Culture-bound disorder or universal symptoms?', *Br. J. Psychiatry*, 164, 559–61.
3. S. T. Cheng (1996), 'A critical review of Chinese koro', *Cult. Med. Psychiatry*, 20, 67–82.
4. R. L. Bernstein, A. C. Gaw (1990), 'Koro: Proposed classification for DSM-IV', *Am. J. Psychiatry*, 147, 1670–4.
5. W. S. Tseng, K. M. Mo, J. Hsu (1988), 'A sociocultural study of koro epidemics in Guandong, China', *Am. J. Psychiatry*, 145, 12.
6. W. S. Tseng, K. M. Mo, J. Hsu, *et al* (1988), 'A sociocultural study of koro epidemics in Guangdong, China', *Am. J. Psychiatry*, 145, 1538–43.
7. G. S. Devan, O. S. Hong (1987), 'Koro and schizophrenia in Singapore', *Br. J. Psychiatry*, 150, 106–7.
8. D. Dutta (1983), 'Koro epidemic in Assam', *Br. J. Psychiatry*, 143, 309–10.
9. A. N. Chowdhury (1996), 'The definition and classification of koro', *Cult. Med. Psychiatry*, 20, 41 65.
10. I. Modai, H. Munitz, D. Aizenberg (1986), 'Koro in an Israeli male', *Br. J. Psychiatry* 149, 503–5.
11. C. Malinick, J. A. Flaherty, T. Jobe (1985), 'Koro: How culturally specific?', *Int. J. Soc. Psychiatry*, 31, 67–73.
12. D. A. Fishbain, S. Barsky, M. Goldberg (1989), '"Koro" (genital retraction syndrome): Psychotherapeutic interventions', *Am. J. Psychother.*, 43, 87–91.
13. E. Witztum, Y. Bersudsky, H. Mayodovnik, M. Kotler (1998), 'Koro-like syndrome in a Bedouin man', *Psychopathology*, 31, 174–7.
14. B. F. Musallam (1983), *Sex and Society in Islam. (Birth Control before the Nineteenth Century)*, (Cambridge University Press, Cambridge).
15. A. N. Chowdhury, K. C. Rajbhandari (1995), 'Koro with depression in Nepal', *Transcult. Psychiatr. Res. Rev.*, 32, 87–90.
16. P. M. Yap (1965), 'Koro in a Briton', *Br. J. Psychiatry*, 111, 774–5.
17. A. L. Gwee (1963), 'Koro – a cultural disease', *Singapore Med. J.*, 4, 119–22.
18. C. T. Mun (1968), 'Epidemic koro in Singapore', *Br. Med. J.*, 1, 640–1.

19. K. L. Goetz, T. R. P. Price (1994), 'A case of koro: Treatment response and implications for diagnostic classification', *J. Nerv. Ment. Dis.*, 182 (10), 590–1.

20. P. C. Ang, M. P. I. Weller (1984), 'Koro and psychosis', *Br. J. Psychiatry*, 245, 335.

21. A. Cremona (1981), 'Another case of koro in a Briton', *Br. J. Psychiatry*, 138, 180–1.

22. S. Attila Kovács, T. H. Péter Osváth (1998), 'Genital retraction syndrome in a Korean woman: A case of koro in Hungary', *Psychopathology*, 31, 220–4.

23. I. Modai, A. Munitz, D. Aizenberg (1986), 'Koro in an Israeli male', *Br. J. Psychiatry*, 149, 503–5.

24. J. Westermeyer (1989), 'A case of koro in a refugee family: Association with depression and a *folie à deux*', *J. Clin. Psychiatry*, 50, 181–3.

25. G. E. Berrios, S. J. Morley (1984), Koro-like symptoms in a non-Chinese subject', *Br. J. Psychiatry*, 145, 331–4.

26. R. Durst, P. Rosca-Rebaudengo (1988), 'Koro secondary to a tumour of the corpus callosum', *Br. J. Psychiatry*, 153, 251–4.

27. D. N. Anderson (1990), 'Koro: The genital retraction symptom after stroke', *Br. J. Psychiatry*, 157, 142–4.

28. A. F. Bogaert, S. Hershberger (1999), 'The relation between sexual orientation and penile size', *Archives of Sexual Behaviour*, 28 (3), 213–21.

29. S. M. Martin, J. T. Manning, C. F. Dowick (1999), 'Fluctuating asymmetry, relative digit length and depression in men', *Evolution & Human Behaviour*, 20, 203–14.

30. Lukianowitz (1967), '"Body image" disturbances in psychiatry disorders', *Br. J. Psychiatry*, 113, 31–47.

31. J. Tuchel (1954), 'Wahnhafter ungezieferbefall und psychische Induktion', *Psychiat. Med. Psychol. Neurol.*, 6, 220–5.

32. M. L. Hatch (1997), 'Conceptualization and treatment of bowel obsessions: Two case reports', *Behavior Research & Therapy*, 35 (3), 253–7.

33. N. Bers, K. Conrad (1954), 'Die chroniche taktile Halluzinose', *Fortschr. Neurol. Psychiatr.*, 22, 254–70.

34. L. Perrin (1896), 'Des Nevrodermies parasitophobiques', *Annales de Dermatologie et Syphilographie* [Paris], 7, 129–38.

35. H. Mester (1975), 'Induzierter "Dermatozoenwahn"', *Psychiat. Clin.*, 8, 339–48.

36. A. Cossidente, M. Sarti (1984), 'Psychiatric syndromes with dermatologic expression', *Clin. Dermatol.*, 2, 201–19.

37. H. Ganner, E. Lorenzi (1975), 'Der Dermatozoenwahn', *Psychiatria. Clinica.*, 8, 31–44.

38. E. R. Bishop (1983), 'Monsosymptomatic hypochondriacal syndromes in dermatology', *J. Am. Acad. Dermatol.*, 9, 152–8.

39. V. Magnon, M. Saury (1889), 'Trois caves de cocainisme chronique comptes rendus: Séances et mémoire', Comptes rendus hebdomadaires des séances et mémoires de la Société de biologie et de ses filiales, 41, 60–3.

40. N. P. Sheppard, A. O'Loughlin, J. P. Malone (1986), 'Psychogenic skin disease: A review of 35 cases', *Br. J. Psychiatry*, 149, 636–43.

41. E. Sobanski, M. H. Schmidt (2000), '"Everybody looks at my pubic bone": A case report of an adolescent patient with body dysmorphic disorder', *Acta Psychiatr. Scand.*, 101, 80–2.

42. E. Andrews, J. Bellard, W. Walter-Ryan, *et al* (1986), 'Monosymptomatic hypochondriacal psychosis manifesting as delusions of infestation: Case studies of treatment with haloperidol', *J. Clin. Psychiatry*, 47, 188–90.

43. D. J. Stein, L. Le Roux, C. Bouwer, B. Van Heerden (1998), 'Is Olfactory Reference Syndrome an Obsessive-Compulsive Spectrum Disorder?' [Two Cases and a Discussion], *J. Neuropsychiatry Clin. Neurosci.*, 10, 96–9, *Australian & New Zealand J. Psychiatry*, 35 (1), 133–4.

44. E. H. Ellingwood (1967), 'Amphetamine psychosis: Description of the individuals and process', *J. Nerv. Ment. Dis.*, 44, 273–83.

45. M. Musalek, E. Kutzer (1990), 'The frequency of shared delusions in delusions of infestation', *Psychiatry & Neurological Sciences*, 239, 263–6.

46. J. de Leon, G. Simpson (1992), Delusion of parasitosis or chronic tactile hallucinosis: Hypothesis about their brain physiopathology', *Compr. Psychiatry*, 33, 25–33.

47. M. Driscol, M. Rothe, J. Grant-Kels, *et al* (1993), 'Delusional parasitosis: A dermatologic, psychiatric, and pharmacologic approach', *J. Am. Acad. Dermatol.*, 29, 1023–33.

48. W. May, M. Terpenning (1991), 'Delusional parasitosis in geriatric patients', *Psychosomatics*, 32, 88–93.

49. A. Lyell (1983), 'Delusions of parasitosis', *Br. J. Dermatol*, 108, 485–99.

50. G. Hopkinson (1970), 'Delusions of infestation', *Acta Psychiatr. Scand.*, 46, 111–19.

51. K. Zanol, J. Slaughter, R. Hall (1998), 'An approach to the treatment of psychogenic parasitosis', *Int. J. Dermatol.*, 37, 56–63.

52. M. L. Bourgeois, P. Duhamel, H. Verdoux (1992), 'Delusional parasitosis: *Folie à deux* and attempted murder of a family doctor', *Br. J. Psychiatry*, 161, 709–11.

CHAPTER 7: DANGER TO SELF

1. A. R. Favazza (1998), 'The coming age of self-mutilation', *J. Nervous & Mental Disease*, 186, 259–68.
2. S. Scheftel, A. S. Nathan, A. M. Razin, P. Mezan (1986), 'A case of radical facial self-mutilation: An unprecedented event and its impact', *Bulletin of Menninger Clinic*, 50 (6), 525–40.
3. T. Thompson, T. Hackenberg, D. Cerutti, D. Baker, S. Axtell (1994), 'Opiod antagonist effects on self injury in adults with mental retardation: Response from and location as determinants of medication effects', *Am. J. Mental Retardation*, 99, 85–102.
4. K. N. Chengappa, T. Ebeling, J. S. Kang, J. Levine, H. Parepally (1999), 'Clozapine reduces severe self-mutilation and aggression in psychotic patients with borderline personality disorder', *J. Clinical Psychiatry*, 60, 477–84.
5. R. A. Dulit, M. R. Fyer, A. C. Leon, B. S. Brodsky, A. J. Frances (1994), 'Clinical correlates of self-mutilation in borderline personality disorder', *Am. J. Psychiatry*, 151, 1305–11.
6. K. N. Chengappa, T. Ebeling, J. S. Kang, J. Levine, H. Parepally (1999), 'Clozapine reduces severe self-mutilation and aggression in psychotic patients with borderline personality disorder', *J. Clinical Psychiatry*, 60, 477–84.
7. D. Shore (1979), 'Self-mutilation and schizophrenia', *Compr. Psychiatry*, 20, 384–7.
8. B. S. Arons (1981), 'Self-mutilation: Clinical examples and reflections', *Am. J. Psychotherapy*, 35, 550–8.
9. K. L. Suyemotoa (1988), 'The functions of self-mutilation', *Clin. Psychology Review*, 18 (5), 531–54.
10. K. Menninger (1935), 'A psychoanalytic study of significance of self-mutilation', *Psychoanalytic Quarterly*, 4, 408.
11. S. S. Asch (1988), 'The analytic concepts of masochism: A re-evaluation', in R. A. Glick, D. I. Meyers (eds), *Masochism: Current Psychoanalytic Perspectives* (Analytic Press, Hillsdale, New Jersey).
12. S. Bharath, M. Neupane, S. Chatterjee (1999), 'Terminator: An unusual form of self-mutilation', *Psychopathology*, 32, 184–6.
13. R. M. Cavanaugh (2000), 'Self-induced carving and scarification of the forearms as a manifestation of sexual abuse in a 14-year-old adolescent girl', *J. Pediatric & Adolescent Gynecology*, 13 (2), 97–8.

14. L. W. Cross (1993), 'Body and self in feminine development: Implications for eating disorders and delicate self-mutilation', *Bulletin Menninger Clinic*, 57, 41–68.

15. M. A. Darche (1990), 'Psychological factors differentiating self-mutilating and non-self-mutilating adolescent in-patient females', *The Psychiatric Hospital*, 21, 31–5.

16. S. L. Ettinger (1992), 'Transforming psychic pain: The meaning and function of self-injury in women's lives' (unpublished master's thesis, Smith College School for Social Work, Northampton, MA).

17. A. R. Favazza (1989), 'Why patients mutilate themselves', *Hospital & Community Psychiatry*, 40, 137–245.

18. O. D. Ratnoff (1989), 'Psychogenic purpura (autoerythrocyte sensitization): An unsolved dilemma', *Am. J. Medicine*, 87, 16–21.

19. W. T. Hanna, R. Fitzpatrick, S. Krauss, *et al* (1981), 'Psychogenic purpura (autoerythrocyte sensitization)', *Southern Medical J.*, 74, 538–42.

20. Y. Baak Yücel, K. Emre, A. Melih (2000), 'Dissociative identity disorder presenting with psychogenic purpura', *Psychosomatics*, 41, 279–81.

21. G. Akyüz, O. Dogan, V. ar, *et al* (1999), 'Frequency of dissociative identity disorder in the general population in Turkey', *Compr. Psychiatry*, 40, 151–9.

22. C. S. North, J. Ryall, D. A. Ricci, *et al* (1993), *Multiple Personalities, Multiple Disorders* (Oxford University Press, New York).

23. F. Putnam (1989), *Diagnosis and Treatment of Multiple Personality Disorder* (Guilford, New York).

24. F. Miller, E. A. Bashkin (1974), 'Depersonalization and self-mutilation', *Psychoanalytic Quarterly*, 43, 638–49.

25. J. Kahan, E. M. Pattison (1984), 'Proposal for a distinctive diagnosis: the deliberate self-harm syndrome', *Suicide & Life-Threatening Behavior*, 14, 17–35.

26. D. E. Lee (1987), 'The self-deception of the self-destructive', *Perceptual & Motor Skills*, 65, 975–89.

27. S. H. Nelson, H. Grunebaum (1971), 'A follow-up study of wrist slashers', *Am. J. Psychiatry*, 127, 1345–9.

28. J. D. Noshpitz (1994), 'Self-destructiveness in adolescence', *Am. J. Psychotherapy*, 48, 330–46.

29. W. J. B. Raine (1982), 'Self mutilation', *J. Adolescence*, 5, 1–13.

30. R. J. Rosenthal, C. Rinzler, R. Wallsh, E. Klausner (1972), 'Wrist-cutting syndrome: The meaning of a gesture', *Am. J. Psychiatry*, 128, 47–52.

31. A. R. Favazza (1992), 'Repetitive self-mutilation', *Psychiatric Annals*, 22 (2), 60–3.

32. A. R. Favazza, K. Conterio (1988), 'The plight of chronic self-mutilators', *Community Mental Health*, 24, 22–30.

33. H. L. Field, S. Waldfogel (1995), 'Severe ocular self-injury', *Gen. Hosp. Psychiatry*, 17, 224–7.

34. D. H. Rosen, A. M. Hoffman (1972), 'Focal suicide: Self-enucleation by two psychotic individuals', *Am. J. Psychiatry*, 128, 123–6.

35. D. P. Kraft, H. M. Bibigian (1972), 'Somatic delusion or self-mutilation in a schizophrenic woman: A psychiatric emergency-room case report', *Am. J. Psychiatry*, 128, 893–5.

36. I. Bennum (1984), 'Psychological models of self-mutilation', *Suicide & Life-Threatening Behavior*, 14, 166–86.

37. A. M. Ghadirian (1997), 'Bulimic purging through blood donation', *Am. J. of Psychiatry*, 154, 435–6.

CHAPTER 8: YOU ARE WHAT YOU EAT

1. G. G. Marquez (1991), *One Hundred Years of Solitude* (Harper & Row, New York).
2. R. D. Goldman, P. Schacter, M. Katz, R. Bilik, I. Avigad (1998), 'A bizarre bezoar: Case report and review of the literature', *Pediatric Surgery International*, 14 (3), 218–19.
3. D. Barltrop (1966), 'The prevalence of pica', *Am. J. Diseases of Children*, 112, 116–20.
4. H. Beange, A. McElduff, W. Baker (1995), 'Medical disorders of adults with mental retardation: A population study', *Am. J. Mental Retardation*, 99 (6), 595–604.
5. Z. Ali (2001), 'Pica in people with intellectual disability: A literature review of aetiology, epidemiology and complications', *J. Intellectual & Developmental Disability*, 26 (2), 205–15.
6. C. C. Piazza, G. P. Hanley, W. W. Fisher (1996), 'Functional analysis and treatment of cigarette Pica', *J. Applied Behavior Analysis*, 29 (4), 437–50.
7. P. Accardo, B. Whitman, J. Caul, U. Rolfe (1988), 'Autism and plumbism: A possible association', *Clinical Pediatrics*, 27 (1), 41–4.
8. B. McMahon, M. Cataldo, M. Collier, R. Haggerty (1986), 'Health applications of smokeless tobacco', *J. Am. Med. Assoc.*, 255, 1045–8.
9. G. O'Brien, A. M. Whitehouse (1990), 'A psychiatric study of deviant eating behaviour among mentally handicapped adults', *Br. J. Psychiatry*, 157, 281–4.
10. I. J. McLoughlin (1987), 'The picas: A study of their aetiology', *Br. J. Hospital Medicine*, 37, 286.
11. C. Solyom, L. Solyom, R. J. Freeman (1991), 'An unusual case of pica', *Canadian J. Psychiatry*, 36 (1), 50–3.
12. B. J. Blinder, S. L. Goodman, P. Henderson (1988), 'Pica: A critical review of diagnosis and treatment', in B. J. Blinder, B. F. Chaitlin, R. Goldstein, *et al* (eds), *The Eating Disorders – Medical and Psychological Basis for Diagnosis and Treatment* (PMA, New York).
13. B. Parry-Jones, W. L. Parry-Jones (1992), 'Pica: symptoms or eating disorder? A historical assessment', *Br. J. Psychiatry*, 160, 341–54.
14. D. Benoit (1993), 'Phenomenology and treatment of failure to thrive', *Child Adolescent Psychiatry Clinic North America*, 2, 61–73.

15. C. H. Morris, C. G. Fairburn (1989), 'Eating habits in dementia', *Br. J. Psychiatry,* 154, 801–6.

16. R. M. Reid (1992), 'Cultural and medical perspectives in geophagia', *Medical Anthropology,* 13 (4), 337–51.

17. N. Beecroft, L. Bach, N. Tunstall, R. Howard (1998), 'An unusual case of pica', *Int J. Geriatric Psychiatry,* 13 (9), 638–41.

18. L. C. Bogart, W. C. Piersel, E. J. Gross (1995), 'The long-term treatment of life-threatening pica: A case study of a woman with profound mental retardation living in an applied setting', *J. Developmental & Physical Disabilities,* 7 (1), 39–50.

19. P. J. Donovick, R. G. Burright (1992), 'Lead poisoning, toxocariasis, and pica: Links to neurobehavioral disorders', in R. L. J. K. F. Isaacson (ed.), *The Vulnerable Brain and Environmental Risks:* vol. 1 (Plenum Press, New York).

20. M. Goldstein (1998), 'Adult pica: A clinical nexus of physiology and psychodynamics', *Psychosomatics* 39, 465–9.

21. M. F. Gutelius, F. K. Millican, G. J. Cohen, C. D. Dublin (1962), 'Nutritional studies of children with pica ii. Treatment of pica with iron given IM', *Pediatrics,* 29, 1018–23.

22. D. Danford, A. Huber (1981), 'Eating dysfunction in an institutionalized mentally retarded population', *Appetite,* 2, 281.

23. E. A. Arbiter, D. Black (1991), 'Pica and iron-deficiency anaemia', *Child: Care, Health & Development,* 17 (4), 231–4.

24. F. C. Mace, D. Knight (1986), 'Functional analysis and treatment of severe pica', *J. Applied Behavior Analysis,* 19 (4), 411–16.

25. C. McAlpine, N. N. Singh (1986), 'Pica in institutionalised mentally retarded persons', *J. Mental Deficiency,* 30, 171–8.

26. J. K. Luiselli (1996), 'Pica as obsessive–compulsive disorder', *J. Behavioural Therapy & Experimental Psychiatry,* 27 (2), 195–6.

27. C. Bugle, H. B. Rubin (1993), 'Effects of a nutritional supplement on coprophagia: A study of three cases', *Research in Developmental Disabilities,* 14 (6), 445–56.

28. R. M. Foxx, E. D. Martin (1975), 'Treatment of scavenging behaviour (coprophagy and pica) by overcorrection', *Behaviour Research & Therapy,* 13, 153–62.

29. S. B. Zeitlin, J. Polivy (1995), 'Coprophagia as a manifestation of obsessive-compulsive disorder: A case report', *J. Behavior Therapy & Experimental Psychiatry,* 26 (1), 57–63.

30. G. M. Gould, W. L. Pyle (1898), *Anomalies and Curiosities of Medicine* (Rebman Publishing, London).

31. M. Regard, T. Landis (1997), '"Gourmand Syndrome": Eating passion associated with right anterior lesions', *Neurology*, 48 (5), 1185–90.

32. M. A. Hoon, E. Adler, J. Lindemeier, J. F. Battey, N. J. Ryba, C. S. Zuker (1999), 'Putative mammalian taste receptors', *Cell*, 96 (4), 541–5.

33. G. Nelson, J. Chandrasheka, M. A. Hoon, L. Feng, G. Zhao, N. J. Ryba, C. S. Zuker (2002), 'An amnio-taste receptor', *Nature*, 416 (6877), 199–202.

34. M. A. Hoon, E. Adler, J. Lindemeier, J. F. Battey, N. J. Ryba, C. S. Zuker (1999), 'Putative mammalian taste receptors', *Cell*, 96 (4), 541–5.

35. J. Chandrasheka, K. L. Mueller, M. A. Hoon, E. Adler, L. Feng, W. Guo, C. S. Zuker, N. J. Ryba (2000), 'T2Rs function as bitter taste receptors', *Cell*, 100 (6), 703–11.

36. G. Nelson, J. Chandrasheka, J. Zhang, N. J. Ryba, C. S. Zuker (2001), 'Mammalian sweet taste receptors', *Cell*, 106 (3), 381–90.

37. E. Adler, M. A. Hoon, K. L. Mueller, J. Chandrashekar, N. J. Ryba, C. S. Zuker (2000), 'A novel family of mammalian taste receptors', *Cell*, 100 (6), 693–702.

Chapter 9: A Load of Old Rubbish

1. R. O. Frost, R. C. Gross (1993), 'The hoarding of possessions', *Behaviour Research & Therapy*, 31, 367–81.
2. R. O. Frost, H. J. Kim, C. Morris, C. Bloss, M. Murray-Close, G. Steketee (1998), 'Hoarding, compulsive buying and reasons for saving', *Behaviour Research & Therapy*, 36, 657–64.
3. A. N. G. Clark, G. D. Mankikar, I. Gray (1975), 'Diogenes syndrome: A clinical study of gross self-neglect in old age', *Lancet*, 1, 366–8.
4. L. M. Drummond, B. Turner, S. Reid (1997), 'Diogenes syndrome – a load of old rubbish?' *Irish J. Psychiatric Medicine*, 14, 99–102.
5. G. A. Jackson (1977), 'Diogenes Syndrome – How should we manage it?', *J. Mental Health*, 6 (2), 113–16.
6. D. MacMillan, P. Shaw (1966), 'Senile breakdown in standards of personal and environmental cleanliness', *Br. Medical J.*, 2, 1032–7.
7. T. Whitehead (1975), 'Diogenes syndrome', *Lancet*, 1, 627–8.
8. J. Snowdon (1997), 'Squalor syndrome', *J. Am. Geriatrics Society*, 45, 1539–40.
9. D. MacMillan, P. Shaw (1966), 'Senile breakdown in standards of personal and environmental cleanliness', *Br. Medical J.*, II, 1032–7.
10. M. Gannon, J. O'Boyle (1992), 'Diogenes syndrome', *Irish Medical J.*, 85, 124.
11. E. Cybulska, I. Rucinski (1986), 'Gross self-neglect in old age', *Br. J. Hospital Medicine*, 36, 21–5.
12. B. V. Reifler (1996), 'Diogenes syndrome: Of omelettes and soufflés', *J. Am. Geriatrics Society*, 44, 1484–5.
13. M. Wrigley, C. Cooney (1992), 'Diogenes syndrome – an Irish series', *Int. J. Psychol. Med.*, 9, 37–41.
14. J. Snowdon (1987), 'Uncleanliness among persons seen by community health workers', *Hospital Community Psychiatry*, 38, 491–4.
15. G. Halliday, S. Banerjee, M. Philpot, A. Macdonald (2000), 'Community study of people who live in squalor', *Lancet*, 355, 882–6.
16. W. Lauder (1999a), 'A survey of self-neglect in patients living in the community', *J. Clinical Nursing*, 8, 95–102.
17. J. Johnson, J. Adams (1996), 'Self-neglect in later life', *Health & Social Care in the Community*, 4, 226–33.
18. R. Moore (1989), 'Diogenes syndrome', *Nursing Times*, 85, 46–8.

19. G. S. Ungvari, P. M. Hantz (1991), 'Social breakdown in the elderly: 1', *Case Studies & Management*, 32, 440–4.

20. G. Halliday, S. Banerjee, M. Philpot, A. Macdonald (2000), 'Community study of people who live in squalor', *Lancet*, 355, 882–6.

21. M. W. Orrell, B. J. Sahakian, K. Bergmann (1989), 'Self-neglect and frontal lobe function', *Br. J. Psychiatry*, 155, 101–5.

22. T. L. Hartl, R. O. Frost (1999), 'Cognitive-behavioral treatment of compulsive hoarding: A multiple baseline experimental case study', *Behaviour Research & Therapy*, 37 (5), 451–61.

23. R. O. Frost, G. Steketee, V. R. Youngren, G. K. Mallya (1996), 'The threat of the housing inspector: A case of hoarding', *Harvard Rev. Psychiatry*, 6, 270–8.

24. R. O. Frost, T. L. Hartl, R. Christian, N. Williams (1995), 'The value of possessions in compulsive hoarding: Patterns of use and attachment', *Behaviour Research & Therapy*, 33, 897–902.

25. E. Richartz, H. Wormstall (2001), 'A case of paranoia with severe consequences; from a historical approach to a multidimensional understanding of chronic delusional disorder', *Psychopathology*, 34, 104–8.

26. K. Jaspers (1973), *Allgemeine Psychophatologie* (Springer, Berlin).

27. E. Gabriel (1987), 'Continental viewpoints on the concept of reactive psychoses', *Psychopathology*, 20, 87–91.

28. P. Berner (1972), 'Paranoide Syndrome', in K. P. Kisker, H. Lauter, J. E. Meyer, C. Müller, E. Strömgren (eds), *Klinische Psychiatrie 1, Psychiatrie der Gegenwart* [153–82] (Springer, Berlin).

29. R. O. Frost, T. L. Hartl (1996), 'A cognitive-behavioral model of compulsive hoarding', *Behaviour Research & Therapy*, 34, 341–50.

30. S. G. Ball, L. Baer, M. W. Otto (1996), 'Symptom subtypes of obsessive-compulsive disorder in behavioral treatment studies: A quantitative review', *Behaviour Research & Therapy*, 34, 47–51.

31. R. O. Frost, D. L. Shows (1993), 'The nature and measure of compulsive indecisiveness', *Behaviour Research & Therapy*, 31, 683–92.

32. T. E. Joiner, N. Sachs-Ericsson (2001), 'Territoriality and obsessive-compulsive symptoms', *J. Anxiety Disorders*, 15 (6), 471–99.

33. F. Frankenburg (1984), 'Hoarding in anorexia nervosa', *Br. J. Medical Psychology*, 57, 57–60.

34. D. Greenberg (1987), 'Compulsive hoarding', *Am. J. Psychotherapy*, XLI, 409–16.

35. M. Basoglu, T. Lax, Y. Kasvikis, I. M. Marks (1988), 'Predictors of improvement in obsessive-compulsive disorder', *J. Anxiety Disorders*, 2, 299–317.

36. M. J. Kozak, E. B. Foa (1997), 'Mastery of obsessive-compulsive disorder: A cognitive-behavioral approach' [Therapist Guide] (Graywind Publications, Albany, New York).

37. R. Shafran, R. Tallis (1996), 'Obsessive-compulsive hoarding: A cognitive-behavioural approach', *Behavioural & Cognitive Psychotherapy*, 24, 209–21.

38. I. M. Lane, M. D. Wesolowski, W. H. Burke (1989), 'Teaching socially appropriate behavior to eliminate hoarding in a brain-injured adult', *J. Behavior Therapy & Experimental Psychiatry*, 20, 79–82.

39. D. Greenberg, E. Witztum, A. Levy (1990), 'Hoarding as a psychiatric symptom', *J. Clinical Psychiatry*, 51, 417–21.

40. M. Pato, J. Zohar (eds) (1991), *Current Treatments of Obsessive Compulsive Disorder* (American Psychiatric Press, Washington, DC).

41. W. K. Goodman, L. H. Price, S. A. Rasmussen, C. Mazure, R. L. Fleischmann, C. L. Hill, G. R. Heninger, D. S. Charney (1989), 'The Yale-Brown Obsessive-Compulsive Scale I: Development, use and reliability', *Archives General Psychiatry*, 46, 1006–11.

Chapter 10: Obsession

1. C. Fear, D. Healy (1995), 'Obsessive compulsive disorders and delusional disorders: Notes on their history, nosology and interface', *J. Serotonin Research*, 1(1), 1–13.
2. World Health Organization (1992), 'International classification of diseases and related health problems: Tenth revision (ICD-10)', (World Health Organization, Geneva).
3. T. R. Insel, H. S. Akiskal (1986), 'Obsessive-compulsive disorder with psychotic features: A phenomenologic analysis', *Am. J. Psychiatry*, 143, 1527–33.
4. A. O'Dwyer, I. Marks [Inst. of Psych. and Maudsley Hosp., London] (2000), 'Obsessive-compulsive disorder and delusions revisited', *Br. J. Psychiatry*, 176, 281–4.
5. L. Solyom, V. F. Di Nicoal, *et al* (1985), 'Is there an obsessive psychosis? Aetiological and prognostic factors of an atypical form of obsessive-compulsive neurosis', *Canadian J. Psychiatry*, 30, 372–9.
6. P. Lelliott, H. F. Noshirvani, M. Basoglu, *et al* (1988), 'Obsessive-compulsive beliefs and treatment outcome', *Psychological Medicine*, 18, 697–702.
7. K. A. Phillips, J. M. Kim, J. I. Hudson (1995), 'Body image disturbance in body dysmorphic disorder and eating disorders – obsessions or delusions?', *Psychiatric Clinics of North America*, 18, 317–34.
8. K. Eisen, S. A. Rasmussen (1993), 'Obsessive compulsive disorder with psychotic features', *J. Clinical Psychiatry*, 54, 373–9.
9. I. Rosen (1957), 'The clinical significance of obsessions in schizophrenia', *Journal of Mental Science*, 103, 773–85.
10. H. Tei, M. Iwata, Y. Miura (1998), 'Paroxysmal compulsion to handle keys in a computer operator due to meningioma in the left supplementary motor area', *Behavioural Neurology*, 11, 93–6.
11. M. L. Berthier, J. Kulisevsky, A. Gironell, J. A. Heras (1996), 'Obsessive-compulsive disorder associated with brain lesions: Clinical phenomenology, cognitive function, and anatomic correlates', *Neurology*, 47, 353–61.
12. J. M. Orgogozo, B. Larsen (1979), 'Activation of the supplementary motor area during voluntary movement in man suggests it works as a supramotor area', *Science*, 206, 847–50.

13. H. H. Morris, D. S. Dinner, H. Luders, E. Wyllie, R. Kramer (1988), 'Supplementary motor seizures: Clinical and electroencephalographic findings', *Neurology*, 38, 1075–82.

14. B. Levin, M. Duchowny (1991), 'Childhood obsessive-compulsive disorder and cingulate epilepsy', *Biological Psychiatry*, 30, 1049–55.

15. M. Frankel, J. L. Cummings, M. M. Robertson, *et al* (1986), 'Obsessions and compulsions in Gilles de la Tourette's syndrome', *Neurology*, 36, 378.

16. D. E. Comings, J. A. Himes, B. G. Comings (1990), 'An epidemiologic study of Tourette's syndrome in a single school district', *J. Clinical Psychiatry*, 51, 288.

17. J. Itard (1825), 'Mémoire sur quelques fonctions involontaires des appareils de la locomotion de la préhension et de la voix', *Arch. Gen. Med.*, 8, 385.

18. G. Gilles de la Tourette (1885), 'Étude sur une affection nerveuse caracterisée par de l'incoordination motrice accompagnée d'écholalie et de copralalie', *Arch. Neurol.*, 9, 158.

19. R. Brunn, C. Budman (1992), 'The natural history of Tourette's syndrome', in T. N. Chase, A. J. Friedhoff, D. J. Cohen (eds), *Gilles de la Tourette Syndrome. Advances in Neurology*, vol. 58 (Raven Press, New York).

20. J. Jankovic (1997), 'Phenomenology and classification of tics', *Neurol. Clin.*, 15, 267.

21. B. Coffey, K. Park (1997), 'Behavioral and emotional aspects of Tourette's syndrome', *Neurol. Clin.*, 15, 277.

22. M. Robertson (1989), 'Gilles de la Tourette Syndrome: The current status', *Br. J. Psychiatry*, 154, 147–69.

23. M. M. Robertson (1989), 'The Gilles de la Tourette syndrome: The current status', *Br. J. Psychiatry*, 154, 147–69.

24. J. Jankovic, H. Rohaidy (1987), 'Motor, behavioral and pharmacologic findings in Tourette's syndrome', *Canadian J. Neurol. Science*, 14 (3), 541.

25. J. Serra-Mestres, M. M. Robertson, T. Shetty (1998), 'Palicoprolalia: An unusual variant of palilalia in Gilles de la Tourette's syndrome', *J. Neuropsychiatry & Clinical Neuroscience*, 10, 117–18.

26. C. L. Templeman, S. Paige Hertweck (2000), 'An unusual presentation of Tourette's syndrome', *J. Pediatric & Adolescent Gynecology*, 13 (1), 33–6.

27. F. Boller, M. Albert, F. Denes (1975), 'Palilalia', *Br. J. Disorders of Communication*, 10, 92–7.

28. S. Dulaney, A. P. Fiske (1994), 'Cultural rituals and obsessive-compulsive disorder: Is there a common psychological mechanism?', *Ethos*, 22, 243–83.

29. F. J. Jarrett (1979), 'Locophobia: A case report', *Psychiatric Quarterly*, 44 (4), 607–12.

30. P. Gilbert (1993), 'Defence and safety: Their function in social behaviour and psychopathology', *Br. J. Clinical Psychology*, 2, 131–53.

31. H. L. Leonard, E. L. Goldberger, J. L. Rapoport, D. L. Cheslow, S. E. Swedo (1990), 'Childhood rituals: Normal development or obsessive-compulsive symptoms?', *J. Am. Academy of Child & Adolescent Psychiatry*, 29, 17–23.

32. S. Rachman, P. De Silva (1978), 'Abnormal and normal obsessions', *Behavioural Research & Therapy*, 16, 233–48.

33. J. Rapoport, A. Fiske (1998), 'The new biology of obsessive-compulsive disorder: Implications for evolutionary psychology', *Perspectives in Biology & Medicine*, 41, 159–79.

34. J. Briscoe (1996), 'A case of glenophobia', *Irish J. Psychological Medicine*, 13 (3), 114–15.

35. S. Rachman, R. Shafran (1998), 'Cognitive and behavioural features of obsessive-compulsive disorder', in R. P. Swinson, M. M. Antony, S. Rachman, M. A. Richter (eds), *Obsessive-compulsive Disorder: Theory, Research and Treatment* (Guilford Press, New York).

36. D. J. Stein, J. L. Rapoport (1996), 'Cross-cultural studies and obsessive-compulsive disorder', *CNS Spectrums*, 1, 42–6.

37. J. F. Lipinski, H. G. Pope (1994), 'Do "flashbacks" represent obsessional imagery?' *Comprehensive Psychiatry*, 35, 245–7.

CHAPTER 11: MUNCHAUSEN SYNDROME

1. M. D. Feldman, C. V. Ford, T. Reinhold (1994), *Patient or Pretender: Inside the Strange World of Factitious Disorders* (Wiley & Sons, New York).

2. A. B. Jones, L. J. Llewellyn (1917), *Malingering or the Simulation of Disease* (J. Blackistons, Philadelphia, PA).

3. G. G. Hay (1983), 'Feigned psychosis: A review of the simulation of mental illness', *Br. J. Psychiatry*, 143, 8–10.

4. P. Fink (1993), 'Admission patterns of persistent somatization patients', *Gen. Hosp. Psychiatry*, 15, 211–18.

5. D. G. Cornell, G. L. Hawk (1989), 'Clinical presentation of malingerers diagnosed by experienced forensic psychologists', *Law & Human Behaviour*, 13, 357–83.

6. G. Cizza, L. K. Nieman, J. L. Doppman, *et al* (1996), 'Factitious Cushing syndrome', *J. Clinical Endocrinol Metab.*, 81, 3573–7.

7. R. Asher (1951), 'Munchausen syndrome', *Lancet*, 1, 339–41.

8. P. Van Heerden, B. Power, I. R. Jenkins (1993), 'The baron and sepsis: A clinical model of self-induced endotoxemia', *Anesth. Intensive Care*, 21, 447–9.

9. L. G. Anderson (1994), 'Munchausen syndrome: Hospital Hobo of the 1990s', *Plastic Surg. Nurs.*, 14, 220–4.

10. C. E. Baker, E. Major (1994), 'Munchausen's syndrome. A case presenting as asthma requiring ventilation', *Anesthesia*, 49, 1050–1.

11. L. Pankratz, J. Jackson (1994), 'Habitually wandering patients', *New England J. Medicine*, 331, 1752–5.

12. H. G. Pope, *et al* (1982), 'Factitious psychosis: phenomenology, family history, and the long-term outcome of nine patients', *Am. J. Psychiatry*, 139, 1480–3.

13. E. C. O. Edi-Osagie, J. Patrick (1997), 'Munchausen syndrome: Gynaecological trauma with Stanley-knife blades', *Int. J. Gynaecology & Obstetrics*, 59, 65–6.

14. G. E. Gordon, H. Lyons, C. Muniz, B. Most (1973), 'The migratory disabled veteran', *J. Fla. Med. Assoc.*, 60, 27–30.

15. R. Powell, N. Boast (1993), 'The millon-dollar man: Resource implications for chronic Munchausen's syndrome' (Royal College of Psychiatrists, England), *Br. J. Psychiatry*, 162, 253–6.

16. A. D. Bruns, P. A. Fishkin, E. A. Johnson, *et al* (1994), 'Munchausen's syndrome and cancer', *J. Surg. Oncol.*, 56, 136–8.

17. B. Wright, D. Bhugra, S. J. Booth (1996), 'Computers, communication and confidentiality: Tales of Baron Munchausen', *J. Accident & Emerg. Med.*, 13, 18–20.

18. R. Yassa (1978), 'Munchausen syndrome: A successfully treated case', *Psychosomatics* 19, 242–3.

19. R. E. Gordon, S. Webb (1975), 'The orbiting psychiatric patient', *J. Fla. Med. Assoc.*, 62, 21–5.

20. L. Pankratz, J. Jackson (1994), 'Habitually wandering patients', *New England J. Medicine*, 331, 1752–5.

21. L. Pankratz, D. H. Hickam, S. Toth (1989), 'The identification and management of drug-seeking behavior in a medical center', *Drug Alcohol Depend.*, 24, 115–18.

22. L. Pankratz, J. Lipkin (1978), 'The transient patient in a psychiatric ward: Summering in Oregon', *J. Operation Psychiatry*, 9 (1), 42–7.

23. C. R. Victor, J. Connelly, P. Roderick, C. Cohen (1989), 'Use of hospital services by homeless families in an inner London health district', *Br. Medical J.*, 299, 725–7.

24. H. A. Schreier, J. A. Libow (1994), 'Munchausen by proxy syndrome: A modern pediatric challenge', *J. Pediatr.*, 125, S110–S115.

25. V. B. Ossipov (1944), 'Malingering: The Simulation of Psychosis', *Bulletin Menninger Clinic*, 8, 39–42.

26. P. H. Pollock, *et al* (1997), 'Feigned mental disorder in prisoners referred to forensic mental health services', *J. Psychiatric & Mental Health Nursing*, 4, 9–15.

27. P. J. Resnick (1994), 'Malingering', in R. Rosner (ed.), *Principles and Practice of Forensic Psychiatry* (Chapman & Hall, New York).

28. D. L. Rosenhan (1973), 'On being sane in insane places', *Science*, 179, 250–358.

29. N. Broughton, P. Chesterman (2001), 'Malingered psychosis', *J. Forensic Psychiatry*, 12, 407–22.

30. D. Chiswick, E. Dooley (1995), 'Psychiatry in Prisons', in D. Chiswick, R. Cope (eds), *Seminars in Practical Forensic Psychiatry* [243–71] (Gaskell, London).

31. E. W. Anderson, W. H. Trethowan, J. C. Kenna (1959), 'An experimental investigation of simulation and pseudo-dementia', *Acta Psychiatrica et Neurologica Scandinavica*, 132, 5–42.

32. H. Miller, N. Cartlidge (1972), 'Simulation and malingering after injuries to the brain and spinal cord', *Lancet* 1, 580–5.

33. L. Andreyev (1902), 'The dilemma', in L. Hamalian, V. von Wiren-Garczynski (eds), *Seven Russian Short Novel Masterpieces* (Popular Library, New York).
34. S. R. Schwartz, S. M. Goldfinger (1981), 'The new chronic patient: Clinical characteristics of an emerging subgroup', *Hospital Community Psychiatry*, 32, 470–4.
35. R. C. Surles, M. C. McGurrin (1987), 'Increased use of psychiatric emergency services by young chronic mentally ill patients', *Hospital Community Psychiatry* 38, 401–5.

CHAPTER 12: BORN INTO THE WRONG BODY

1. G. Catalano, M. Morejon, V. A. Alberts, M. C. Catalano (1996), 'Report of a case of male genital self–mutilation and review of the literature, with special emphasis on the effects of the media', *J. Sexual Marital Therapists*, 22, 35–46.

2. A. Shimizu, I. Mizuta (1995), 'Male genital self–mutilation: A case report', *Br. J. Med. Psychology*, 68, 187–9.

3. N. Eke (2000), 'Genital self-mutilation: There is no method in this madness', *Br. J. Urology*, 85 (3), 295–8.

4. D. C. Hall, B. Z. Lawson, L. G. Wilson (1981), 'Command hallucinations and self-amputation of the penis and hand during a first psychotic break', *J. Clin. Psychiatry*, 42, 322–4.

5. R. Mendez, W. F. Kiely, J. W. Morrow (1972), 'Self-emasculation', *J. Urology*, 107, 981–5.

6. D. Reardon (1994), 'Psychological reactions reported after abortion', *Post-Abortion Review*, 2 (3), 4–8.

7. A. W. Kushner (1967), 'Two cases of auto-castration due to religious delusions', *Br. J. Medical Psychology*, 40, 293–8.

8. S. C. Evins, T. Whittle, S. N. Rous (1977), 'Self-emasculation: Review of the literature, report of a case and outline of the objectives of management', *J. of Urology*, 118, 775–6.

9. C. S. Romilly, M. T. Isaac (1996), 'Male genital self-mutilation', *Brit. J. Hosp. Medicine*, 55, 427–31.

10. M. Nakaya (1996), 'On background factors of male genital self-mutilation', *Psychopathology*, 29, 242–8.

11. M. J. Gleeson, J. Connolly, R. Grainger (1993), 'Self-castration as treatment for alopecia', *Brit. J. Urology*, 71, 614–15.

12. S. P. Wan, D. W. Soderdahl, E. Blight Jr. (1985), 'Nonpsychotic genital self-mutilation', *Urology*, 26, 286–7.

13. K. H. Blacker, N. Wong (1963), 'Four cases of autocastration', *Archives Genital Psychiatry*, 8, 169–76.

14. A. Anumonye (1973), 'Self-inflicted amputation of the penis in two Nigerian males', *Nigerian Med. J.*, 3, 51–2.

15. G. N. Conacher, D. Villeneuve, G. Kane (1991), 'Penile self-mutilation presenting as rational attempted suicide', *Canadian J. Psychiatry*, 36, 682–5.

16. M. D. Goldfield, I. D. Glick (1970), 'Self-mutilation of the female genitalia', *Dis. Nerv. Syst.*, 31, 843–5.

17. E. Koops, K. Puschel (1990), 'Self-mutilation and autophagia', *Arch. Für Kriminologie*, 186, 29–36.

18. R. Kenyon, R. M. Hyman (1953), 'Total auto-emasculation', (report of three cases), *J. Am. Med. Assoc.*, 151, 207–10.

19. A. C. Waugh (1986), 'Autocastration and biblical delusions in schizophrenia', *Br. J. Psychiatry*, 149, 656–8.

20. C. C. Abbou, M. Servant, F. Bonnet, *et al* (1979), 'Reimplantation of the penis and both testicles after complete auto-castration', [author's translation], *Chirurgie*, 105, 354–7.

21. L. M. Beilin, J. Grueneberg (1948), 'Genital self-mutilations by mental patients', *J. Urology*, 59, 635–41.

22. R. A. Clark (1981), 'Self-mutilation accompanying religious delusions: A case report and review', *J. Clin. Psychiatry*, 42, 243–5.

23. M. A. Simpson (1973), 'Female genital self-mutilation', *Archives Genital Psychiatry*, 29, 808–10.

24. S. Sweeney, K. Zameknic (1981), 'Predictors of self-mutilation in patients with schizophrenia', *Am. J. Psychiatry*, 138, 1086–9.

25. D. Ames (1987), 'Autocastration and biblical delusions in schizophrenia', *Br. J. Psychiatry*, 150, 407.

26. I. Schweitzer (1990), 'Genital self-amputation and the Klingsor syndrome', *Aust. & New Zealand J. Psychiatry*, 24, 566–9.

27. L. Weiss Roberts, M. Hollifield, T. McCarthy (1998), 'Psychiatric Evaluation of a "Monk" requesting castration: A patient's fable, with morals', *Am. J. Psychiatry*, 155, 415–20.

28. R. J. Lifton (1956), *Thought Reform and the Psychology of Totalism* (W. W. Norton, New York).

29. M. Galanter (1990), 'Cults and zealous self-help movements: A psychiatric perspective', *Am. J. Psychiatry*, 147, 543–51.

30. 'Did cultists castrate themselves?' (1997), *Albuquerque Tribune*, A8.

31. T. McCarthy, L. W. Roberts, K. Hendrickson (1996), 'Urologic sequelae of childhood genitourinary trauma and abuse in men: Principles of recognition with fifteen case illustrations', *Urology*, 47, 617–21.

32. T. N. Wise, R. C. Kalyanam, M. Hirschfeld (1948), *Sexual Anomalies* (Emerson, New York).

33. J. Godlewski, M. Szalankiewicz (1987), 'Apotemnophilia', *Psychiatrica Poliska*, 21, 141–4.

34. J. Money (1984), 'Paraphilias: Phenomenology and classification', *Am. J. Psychotherapy*, 38, 164–79.

35. R. V. Krafft-Ebing (1953), *Psychopathia Sexualis* (Pioneer Publications, New York).

36. L. S. London, F. S. Caprio (1950), *Sexual Deviation* (Linacre Press, Washington, DC).

37. J. Money, R. Jobaris, G. Furth (1977), 'Apotemnophilia: Two cases of self-demand amputation as a paraphilia', *J. Sex Research*, 13, 115–25.
38. B. Taylor (1976), 'Amputee fetishism: An exclusive journal interview with Dr John Money of Johns Hopkins', *Maryland State Medical J.*, 35–9.
39. T. N. Wise, R. Chandran Kalyanam (2000), 'Amputee fetishism and genital mutilation: Case report and literature review', *J. Sex & Marital Therapy*, 26, 339–44.
40. W. Everaerd (1983), 'A case of apotemnophilia: A handicap as sexual preference', *Am. J. Psychotherapy*, 37, 285–93.
41. T. N. Wise, J. K. Meyer (1980), 'Transvestism: Previous findings and new areas for inquiry', *J. Sex & Marital Therapy*, 6, 116–28.
42. R. J. Stoller (1974), 'The Samuel Novey Lecture: Does sexual perversion exist?', *Johns Hopkins Med. J.*, 134, 43–57.
43. G. R. Brown (1990), 'A review of clinical approaches to gender dysphoria', *J. Clinical Psychiatry*, 51, 57–64.
44. Harry Benjamin International Gender Dysphoria Association (1998), 'Standards of Care', *Int. J. Transgender*, vol. 1.
45. E. Person, L. Ovesey (1974), 'The transsexual syndrome in males', *Am. J. Psychotherapy*, 28, 4–20, 174–93.
46. L. Roberto (1983), 'Issues in diagnosis and treatment of transsexualism', *Archives Sexual Behaviour*, 12, 445–73.
47. J. M. Dixen, H. Maddever, J. Van-Massdam, P. W. Edwards, (1984), 'Psychosocial characteristics of applicants evaluated for surgical gender reassignment', *Archives Sexual Behaviour*, 13, 269–76.
48. L. Ovesey, E. Person (1976), 'Transvestism: A disorder of the sense of self', *Int. J. Psychoanal Psychother.*, 4, 219–35.
49. L. Gooren (1990), 'The endocrinology of transsexualism: A review and commentary', *Psychoneuroendocrinology*, 15, 3–14.
50. J. K. Meyer (1974), 'Clinical variants among applicants for sex reassignment surgery', *Archives Sexual Behaviour*, 3, 527–58.
51. H. Bower (1998), 'The differential diagnosis of transsexualism', in W. A. W. Walters, M. W. Ross (eds), *Transsexualism and Sex Reassignment* (Oxford University Press, Oxford).
52. D. Barlow, G. Abel, E. Blanchard (1977), 'Gender identity change in a transsexual: An exorcism', *Archives Sexual Behaviour*, 6, 387–95.
53. E. R. Shore (1984), 'The former transsexual: A case study', *Archives Sexual Behaviour*, 3, 277–85.

54. I. M. Marks, D. Mataix-Cols (1997), 'Four-year remission of transsexualism after comorbid obsessive-compulsive disorder improved with self-exposure therapy', *Br. J. Psychiatry*, 171, 389–90.

55. C. Commander, C. Dean (1990), 'Symptomatic transsexualism', *Br. J. Psychiatry*, 156, 894–6.

56. J. Modestin, G. Ebner (1995), 'Multiple personality disorder manifesting itself under the mask of transsexualism', *Psychopathology*, 28 (6), 317–21.

57. D. Barlow, G. Abel, E. Blanchard (1979), 'Gender identity change in transsexuals', *Archives General Psychiatry*, 36, 1001–7.

CHAPTER 13: TWO'S COMPANY, THREE'S A CROWD

1. C. Thigpen, H. M. Cleckley (1957), *The Three Faces of Eve* (Secker & Warburg, London).
2. C. Thigpen, H. M. Cleckley (1954), 'A case of multiple personality', *J. Abnormal and Social Psychology*, 49, 135–51.
3. G. Sliker (1992), *Multiple Mind: Healing the Split in Psyche and World* (Shambhala, Boston).
4. M. Boden (1994), 'Multiple personality and computational models', in A. Phillips Griffiths (ed.), *Philosophy, Psychology and Psychiatry* (Cambridge University Press, Cambridge).
5. I. Brenner (1999), 'Deconstructing DID', *Am. J. Psychotherapy*, 53, 344–60.
6. F. W. Putnam (1991), 'Recent research on multiple personality disorder', *Psychiatr. Clin. North Am.*, 14, 489–502.
7. A. M. Ludwig, J. M. Brandsma, C. B. Wilbur, F. Benfeldt, D. H. Jameson (1972), 'The objective study of a multiple personality', *Archives General Psychiatry*, 26, 298–310.
8. E. L. Bliss (1980), 'Multiple personalities. A report of 14 cases with implications for schizophrenia and hysteria', *Archives General Psychiatry* 37, 1388–97.
9. C. L. Anderson, P. C. Alexander (1996), 'The relationship between attachment and dissociation in adult survivors of incest', *Psychiatry* 59, 240–54.
10. J. H. Krystal, A. L. Bennett, J. D. Bremner, S. M. Southwick, D. S. Charney (1995), 'Towards a cognitive neuroscience of dissociation and altered memory function in post-traumatic stress disorder', in M. J. Friedman, D. S. Charney, A. Y. Deutch (eds), *Neurobiological and Clinical Consequences of Stress: From Normal Adaptation to Post-traumatic Stress Disorder* (Lippincott-Raven, Philadelphia).
11. J. H. Krystal, J. D. Bremner, S. M. Southwick, D. S. Charney (1998), 'The emerging neurobiology of dissociation: Implications for treatment of posttraumatic stress disorder', in J. D. Bremner, C. R. Marmar (eds), *Trauma, Memory, and Dissociation* [321–63] (American Psychiatric Press, Washington, DC).
12. B. Cutler, J. Reed (1975), 'Multiple personality: A single case study with a 15-year follow-up', *Psychological Medicine*, 5, 18–26.
13. G. Bower (1994), 'Temporary emotional states act like multiple personality', in R. M. Klein, B. K. Doane (eds), *Psychological Concepts and Dissociative Disorder* [207–234] (Erlbaum, Hillsdale).

14. M. Dick-Barnes (1987), 'Behavioral measures of multiple personality: The case of Margaret', *J. Behavioral Therapy & Experimental Psychiatry*, 18, 229–39.

15. A. Herzog (1985), 'On multiple personality: comments on diagnosis, etiology, and treatment', *Int. J. Clinical & Experimental Hypnosis*, 32, 210–21.

16. E. R. Hilgard (1992), 'Divided consciousness and dissociation', *Consciousness & Cognition*, 1, 16–31.

17. J. F. Kihlstrom, D. J. Tataryn, I. P. Hoyt (1993), 'Dissociative Disorders', in P. B. Sutker, H. E. Adams (eds), *Comprehensive Handbook of Psychopathology* [203–34] (Plenum Press, New York).

18. A. M. Ludwig, J. M. Brandsma, C. B. Wilbur, F. Benfeldt, D. H. Jameson (1972), 'The objective study of a multiple personality', *Archives General Psychiatry*, 26, 298–310.

19. H. Merskey (1992), 'Manufacture of multiple personality disorder', *Br. J. Psychiatry*, 160, 327–40.

20. H. Merskey (1995), 'Multiple personality and false memory syndrome', *Br. J. Psychiatry*, 166 (3), 281–3.

21. D. Cohen (1995), 'Now we are one, or two, or three', *New Scientist*, 146 (1982), 14–15.

22. F. W. Putnam, J. J. Guroff, E. K. Silberman, L. Barban, R. M. Post (1986), 'The clinical phenomenology of multiple personality disorder: A review of 100 recent cases', *J. Clinical Psychiatry*, 47, 285–93.

23. M. J. Nissen, J. L. Ross, D. B. Willingham, T. B. Mackenzie, D. L. Schacter (1988), 'Memory and awareness in a patient with multiple personality disorder', *Brain & Cognition*, 8, 117–34.

24. W. S. Taylor, M. F. Martin (1944), 'Multiple personality', *J. Abnormal & Social Psychology*, 39, 281–300.

25. A. D. Macleod (1999), 'Posttraumatic stress disorder, dissociative fugue and a locator beacon', *Australian & New Zealand J. Psychiatry*, 33, 102–4.

26. H. J. Markowitsch, A. Thiel, M. Reinkemeier, J. Kessler, A. Koyuncu, H. Wolf-Dieter (2000), 'Right amygdalar and temporofrontal activation during autobiographic, but not during fictitious memory retrieval', *Behavioural Neurology*, 12 (4), 181–90.

27. W. F. Prince (1917), 'The Doris case of quintuple personality', *J. Abnormal Psychology*, 11, 73–122.

28. British Psychological Society, 1995. Recovered Memories: The Report of the Working Party of the British Psychological Society.

29. Australian Psychological Association, 1994. Guidelines Relating to the Reporting of Recovered Memories. Australian Psychological Association, Sydney, NSW.

30. American Psychological Association, 1994. Interim Report of the APA Working Group on Investigation of Memories of Childhood Abuse. American Psychological Association, Washington, DC.

31. E. Loftus (1996), Data presented at the Southwestern Psychological Association Meeting, Houston, Texas, summarized in False Memory Syndrome Foundation Newsletter (1996).

32. H. J. Markowitsch, A. Thiel, M. Reinkemeier, J. Kessler, A. Koyuncu, H. Wolf-Dieter (2000), 'Right amygdalar and temporofrontal activation during autobiographic, but not during fictitious memory retrieval', *Behavioural Neurology*, 12 (4), 181–90.

33. W. F. Prince (1917), 'The Doris case of quintuple personality', *J. Abnormal Psychology*, 11, 73–122.

34. D. E. Jacome (2001), 'Transitional Interpersonality Thunderclap Headache', *Headache: J. of Head & Face Pain*, 41 (3), 317–20.

35. R. C. Packard, F. Brown (1986), 'Multiple headaches in a case of multiple personality disorder', *Headache*, 26, 99–102.

36. R. C. Packard (1986), 'Multiple headaches in multiple personality disorder', in C. S. Adler, S. Adler, R. C. Packard (eds), *Psychiatric Aspects of Headache* (Williams & Wilkins, Baltimore).

37. A. Cantagallo, L. Grassi, S. Della Sala (1999), 'Dissociative disorder after traumatic brain injury', *Brain Injury*, 13 (4), 219–28.

38. J. R. Fann (1997), 'Traumatic brain injury and psychiatry', *J. Psychosomatic Research*, 43, 335–43.

39. Y. Uchinuma, Y. Sekine (2000), 'Dissociative identity disorder (DID) in Japan: A forensic case report and the recent increase in reports of DID', *Int. J. Psych. Clin. Pract.*, 4, 155–60.

40. E. Loftus (1996), Data presented at the Southwestern Psychological Association Meeting, Houston, Texas, summarized in False Memory Syndrome Foundation Newsletter (1 May 1996).

41. D. Spiegel, E. J. Frischholz, J. Spira (1993), 'Functional disorders of memory', *Review of Psychiatry*, 12, 747–82.

42. C. A. Ross (1989), *Multiple Personality Disorder: Diagnosis, Clinical Features and Treatment* (Wiley, New York).

43. G. E. Tsai, D. Condie, M-T. Wu, I-W. Chang (1999), 'Functional magnetic resonance imaging of personality switches in a woman with Dissociative Identity Disorder', *Harvard Review Psychiatry*, 7, 119.

44. J. P. Rosenfeld, J. Ellwanger, J. Sweet (1995), 'Detecting simulated amnesia with event-related brain potentials', *Int. J. Psychophysiology*, 19, 1–11.

45. H. F. Ellenberger (1970), *The Discovery of the Unconscious* (Basic Books, New York).

46. E. R. Hilgard (1977), *Divided Consciousness: Multiple Controls in Human Thought and Action* (Wiley, New York).

47. E. K. Silberman, F. W. Putnam, H. Weingartner, B. G. Braun, R. M. Post (1985), 'Dissociative states in multiple personality disorder', *Psychiatry Research*, 15, 153–60.

48. N. P. Spanos (1994), 'Multiple identity enactments and multiple personality disorder: A sociocognitive perspective', *Psycological Bulletin*, 116, 143–65.

49. S. E. Braude (1991), *First Person Plural: Multiple Personality and the Philosophy of Mind* (Routledge, London).

1. H. D. Ellis, A. W. Young (1990), 'Accounting for delusional misidentifications', *Br. J. Psychiatry*, 157, 239–48.

2. N. Breen *et al* (2000), 'Models of face recognition and delusional misidentification: A critical review', *Cognit. Neuropsychol.*, 17, 55–71.

3. M. Coltheart, *et al* (1997), 'Misidentification syndromes and cognitive neuropsychiatry', *Trends Cognit. Sci.*, 1, 157–8.

4. K. Stern, D. MacNaughton (1945), 'Capgras syndrome, a peculiar illusionary phenomenon, considered with special reference to the Rorschach findings', *Psychiat. Quarterly*, 19, 139–63.

5. H. D. Ellis, *et al* (1994), 'Delusional misidentification: The three original papers on Capgras, Frégoli and intermetamorphosis delusions', *Hist. Psychiatry*, 5, 117–46.

6. J. Capgras, J. Reboul-Lachaux (1923), 'L'illusion des sosies dans un délire systématise chronique', *Bulletin Soc. Clin. Med. Ment.*, 11, 6–16.

7. H. D. Ellis (1998), 'Cognitive neuropsychiatry and delusional misidentification syndromes: An exemplary vindication of the new discipline', *Cognit. Neuropsychiatry*, 3, 81–90.

8. G. N. Christodoulou (1991), 'The delusional misidentification syndromes', *Br. J. Psychiatry*, 159 (14), 65–9.

9. S. M. Coleman (1933), 'Misidentification and nonrecognition', *J. Ment. Sci.*, 79, 42–51.

10. H. D. Ellis, M. B. Lewis (2001), 'Capgras delusion: A window on face recognition trends', *Cognitive Sciences*, 5 (4), 149–56.

11. H. D. Ellis, J. W. Shepherd (1992), 'Face memory-theory and practice', in M. Gruneberg, *et al* (eds), *Aspects of Memory* (Routledge, London).

12. *The Independent* (4 March 1998).

13. H. D. Ellis, A. W. Young (1990), 'Accounting for delusional misidentification', *Br. J. Psychiatry*, 157, 239–48.

14. N. M. J. Edelstyn, F. Oyebode, M. J. Riddoch, R. Soppitt, H. Moselhy, M. George (1997), 'A neuropsychological perspective on three schizophrenic patients with midline structural defects', *Br. J. Psychiat.*, 170, 416–21.

15. H. Forstl (1990), 'Capgras delusion: An example of coalescent psychoanalytic and organic factors', *Comp. Psychiat.*, 31 (5), 447–9.

16. R. O'Reilly, L. Malhotra (1987), 'Capgras Syndrome: An unusual case and discussion of psychoanalytic factors', *Br. J. Psychiatry*, 151, 263–5.

17. A. I. Goldfard, N. B. Weiner (1977), 'The Capgras phenomenon as an adaptional manoeuvre in old age', *Am. J. Psychiatry*, 134, 1433–6.

18. E. Koritar, W. Steiner (1988), 'Capgras' syndrome: A synthesis of various viewpoints, *Can. J. Psychiatry*, 33, 62–6.

19. E. L. Merrin, P. M. Silberfarb (1976), 'The Capgras phenomenon', *Arch. Gen. Psychiatry*, 33, 965–8.

20. J. Arturo Silva, G. Leong, T. O'Reilly (1990), 'An unusual case of Capgras syndrome: The psychiatric ward as a stage', *Psychiatric J. University of Ottawa*, 5 (1).

21. T. Wenzel, I. Sibitz, W. Kieffer, R. Strobl (1999), 'Capgras Syndrome and Functional Psychosis in 2 Survivors of Torture', *Psychopathology*, 32, 203–6.

22. D. Tranel, A. R. Damasio (1985), 'Knowledge without awareness: An autonomic index of facial recognition by prosopagnosics', Science (Washington), 228, 1453–4.

23. W. Hirstein, V. Ramachandran (1997), 'Capgras syndrome: A novel probe for understanding the neural representation of the identity and familiarity of persons', *Proc. Roy. Soc. Lond. Biol. Sci.*, 264 (1380), 437–44.

24. J. Sergent, *et al* (1992), 'Functional neuroanatomy of face and object processing', *Brain*, 115, 15–36.

25. M. L. Paillere-Martinot, M. H. Dao-Castellana, M. C. Masure, *et al* (1994), 'Delusional misidentification: A clinical, neuropsychological and brain-imaging case study', *Psychopathology* 27 (3–5), 200–10.

26. H. D. Ellis, *et al* (1997), 'Reduced autonomic responses to faces in Capgras delusion', *Proc. Roy. Soc. London: Ser. B.*, 264, 1085–92.

27. H. D. Ellis, K. dePauw (1994), 'Origins of Capgras delusion', in A. S. David, J. C. Cutting (eds), *The Neuropsychology of Schizophrenia* (Oxford University Press, Oxford).

28. H. D. Ellis, K. W. dePauw, G. N. Christodoulou, A. J-P. Luaute, E. Bidault, T. K. Szulecka (1992), 'Recognition memory in psychotic patients', *Behav. Neurol.*, 5, 23–6.

29. S. C. Rastogi (1990), 'A variant of Capgras syndrome with substitution of inanimate objects', *Br. J. Psychiat.*, 156, 883–4.

30. T. Murai, M. Toichi, H. Yamagishi, A. Sengoku (1998), 'What is meant by "misidentification" in delusional misidentification syndromes? Comparison between Capgras' syndromes and "clonal pluralization of a person" ', *Psychopathology*, 31, 313–17.

31. M. P. Alexander, D. T. Stuss, D. F. Benson (1979), 'Capgras syndrome: A reduplicative phenomenon', *Neurol.*, 29, 334–9.

32. N. M. J. Edelstyn, F. Oyebode (1999), 'A review of the phenomenology and cognitive neuropsychological origins of the Capgras Syndrome', *Int. J. Geriat. Psychiatry*, 14, 48–59.

CHAPTER 15: STRANGER THAN FICTION?

1. H. Ay, F. S. Buonanno, B. H. Price, D. A. Le, W. J. Koroschetz (1998), 'Sensory alien hand syndrome: Case report and review of the literature', *J. Neurology, Neurosurgery & Psychiatry*, 65 (3), 366–9.
2. G. Berlucchi, S. Aglioti (1999), 'Interhemispheric disconnection syndromes', in G. Denes, L. Pizzamiglio (eds), *et al*, *Handbook of Clinical and Experimental Neuropsychology* [1108] (Psychology Press/Erlbaum, Hove).
3. T. E. Feinberg, R. J. Schindler, N. G. Flanagan, *et al* (1992), 'Two alien hand syndromes', *Neurology*, 42, 19–24.
4. G. Goldberg, K. K. Bloom (1990), 'The alien hand sign: Localization, lateralization and recovery', *Am. J. Phys. Med. Rehab.*, 69, 228–38.
5. D. H. Geshwind, M. Iacoboni, M. S. Mega, *et al* (1995), 'Alien hand syndrome: Interhemispheric motor disconnection due to a lesion of the midbody of the corpus callosum', *Neurology*, 45, 802–8.
6. J. L. Chan, E. D. Ross (1977), 'Alien hand syndrome: Influence of neglect on the clinical presentation of frontal and callosal variants', *Cortex*, 33, 287–99.
7. M. G. Ventura, S. Goldman, J. Hildebrand (1995), 'Alien hand syndrome without a corpus callosum lesion', *J. Neurol. Neurosurg. Psychiatry*, 58, 735–7.
8. S. Della Sala, C. Marchietti, H. Spinnler (1991), 'Right-sided anarchic (alien) hand: A longitudinal study', *Neuropsychologia*, 29, 1113–27.
9. A. N. Meltzoff (1995), 'Understanding the intentions of others', Re-enactment of intended acts by 18-month-old children', *Developmental Psychology*, 31, 838–50.
10. A. N. Meltzoff, M. K. Moore (1983), 'Newborn infants imitate adult facial gestures', *Child Development*, 54, 702–9.
11. J. Decety, J. Grezes, Costes, *et al* (1997), 'Brain activity during observation of action. Influence of action content and subject's strategy', *Brain*, 120, 1763–77.
12. A. N. Meltzoff, M. K. Moore (1977), 'Imitation of facial and manual gestures by human neonates', *Science*, 198, 74–8.
13. G. Berlucchi, S. Aglioti (1997), 'The body and the brain: Neural basis of corporeal awareness', *Trends in Neuroscience*, 20, 560–4.
14. E. Daprati, N. Franck, N. Georgieff, J. Proust, E. Pacherie, J. Dalery, M. Jeannerod (1997), 'Looking for the agent: An investigation into consciousness of action and self-consciousness in schizophrenic patients', *Cognition*, 65 (1), 71–86.

15. C. D. Frith (1987), 'The positive and negative symptoms of schizophrenia reflect impairments in the perception and initiation of action', *Psychological Medicine*, 17, 631–48.

16. C. D. Frith (1995), 'Consciousness is for other people', *Behavioural & Brain Sciences*, 18, 682–3.

17. C. Frith (1996), 'The role of the prefrontal cortex in self-consciousness: The case of auditory hallucinations', *Philosophical Transactions Royal Society London*, 351, 1505–12.

18. C. D. Frith, D. J. Done (1989), 'Experiences of alien control in schizophrenia reflect a disorder in the central monitoring of action', *Psychological Medicine*, 19, 359–63.

19. C. D. Frith (1992), *The Cognitive Neuropsychology of Schizophrenia* (Erlbaum, Hove).

20. P. K. McGuire, D. A. Silbersweig, I. Wright, R. M. Murray, R. S. J. Frackowiak, C. D. Frith (1996), 'The neural correlates of inner speech and auditory verbal imagery in schizophrenia: Relationship to auditory verbal hallucinations', *Brit. J. Psychiatry*, 169, 148–59.

21. O. Creutzfeldt, G. Ojeman, E. Lettich (1989), 'Neuronal activity in the human lateral temporal lobe: II. Responses to own voice', *Experimental Brain Research*, 77, 475–89.

22. C. Marchetti, S. Della Sala (1998), 'Disentangling the alien and anarchic hand', *Cognitive Neuropsychiatry*, 3 (3), 191–207.

23. S. A. Spence (2000), 'Between will and action', *J. Neurology, Neurosurgery & Psychiatry*, 69 (5), 702.

24. R. Hanninen, T. Makinen (1997), 'Failure of bodily meta control: Three hands and three legs or only half a body. A longitudinal study', *Int. J. Psychophysiology*, 25, 44.

25. J. Gerstman (1942), 'Problem of imperception of disease and impaired body territories with organic lesions', *Archives Neurology & Psychiatry*, 48, 890–913.

26. R. Inzelberg, P. Nisipeanu, S. C. Blumen, R. L. Carasso (2000), 'Alien hand sign in Creutzfeldt-Jakob disease', *J. Neurology, Neurosurgery & Psychiatry*, 68 (1), 103–4.

27. T. M. Lewis, M. McClain, A. Pittenger (1997), 'Alien hand syndrome and ataxia: A case study of a unique presentation of the disorder', *Archives Clin. Neuropsychology*, 14 (4), 357–8.

28. H. Ay, F. S. Buonanno, B. H. Price, D. A. Le, W. J. Koroschetz (1998), 'Sensory alien hand syndrome: Case report and review of the literature', *J. Neurology, Neurosurgery & Psychiatry*, 65 (3), 366–9.

29. A. L. Wigan (1844), *A View of Insanity: The Duality of the Mind* (Longman, London).

30. J. E. Bogen (1993), 'The callosal syndromes', in K. M. Heilman, E. Valenstein (eds), *Clinical Neuropsychology*: 3rd edn [337–407] (Oxford University Press, New York).

31. K. Baynes, M. J. Tramo, A. G. Reeves, M. S. Gazzaniga (1997), 'Isolation of a right hemisphere cognitive system in a patient with anarchic (alien) hand sign', *Neuropsychologia*, 35 (8), 1159–73.

32. A. Parkin (1996), 'The alien hand in method and madness: Case studies', in P. W. Halligan, J. C. Marshall (eds), *Cognitive Neuropsychiatry* (Psychology Press, Erlbaum).

33. R. Smith Doody (1993), 'Alien hand', in C. A. Molgaard (ed.), *et al*, *Neuroepidemiology: Theory and Method* [181–93] (Academic Press, San Diego, CA).

34. A. J. Parkin, C. Barry (1991), 'Alien hand sign and other cognitive deficits following ruptured aneurysm of the anterior communicating artery', *Behavioural Neurology*, 4 (3), 167–79.

35. G. Rizzolatti, L. Fadiga, Matelli, *et al* (1996a), 'Localisation of grasp representations in humans by PET 1: Observation versus execution', *Experimental Brain Research*, 111, 246–52.

36. G. Rizzolatti, L. Fadiga, V. Gallese, L. Fogassi (1996b), 'Premotor cortex and the recognition of motor actions', *Cognitive Brain Research*, 3, 131–41.

37. S. A. Spence, D. J. Brooks, S. R. Hirsch, P. F. Liddle, J. Meehan, P. M. Grasby (1997), 'A PET study of voluntary movement in schizophrenic patients experiencing passivity phenomena (delusions of alien control)', *Brain*, 120, 1997–2011.

38. J. Decety, J. Grèzes, N. Costes, D. Perani, M. Jeannerod, E. Procyk, F. Grassi, F. Fazio (1997), 'Brain activity during observation of actions. Influence of action content and subject's strategy', *Brain*, 120, 1763–77.

39. J. Decety, D. Perani, M. Jeannerod, V. Bettinardi, B. Tadary, R. Woods, J. Mazziotta, C. Fazio (1994), 'Mapping motor representations with PET', *Nature*, 371, 600–2.

40. G. Di Pellegrino, L. Fadiga, L. Fogassi, V. Gallese, G. Rizzolatti (1992), 'Understanding motor events: A neurophysiological study', *Experimental Brain Research*, 91, 176–80.

41. S. A. Spence, D. J. Brooks, S. R. Hirsch, P. F. Liddle, J. Meehan, P. M. Grasby (1997), 'A PET study of voluntary movement in schizophrenic patients experiencing passivity phenomena (delusions of alien control)', *Brain*, 120, 1997–2011.

42. T. I. Nielsen (1963), 'Volition: A new experimental approach', *Scandinavian J. Psychology*, 4, 225–30.

43. C. D. Frith, K. J. Friston, P. F. Liddle, R. S. J. Frackowiak (1991), 'Willed action and the prefrontal cortex in man: A study with PET', *Proceedings Royal Society, London*, 244, 241–6.
44. A. S. David (1994), 'The neuropsychological origin of auditory hallucinations', in A. S. David, J. C. Cutting (eds), *The Neuropsychology of Schizophrenia* [269–313] (Erlbaum, Hove).
45. G. Goldberg (1987), 'From intent to action: Evolution and function of the premotor systems of the frontal lobe', in E. Perecman (ed.), *et al, The Frontal Lobes Revisited* [273–306] (The Iron Press, New York).
46. P. Chadwick, M. Birchwood (1994), 'The omnipotence of voices. A cognitive approach to auditory hallucinations', *Brit. J. Psychiatry*, 164, 190–201.
47. S. H. Ahmed (1978), 'Cultural influences on delusion', *Psychiatr. Clin.*, (Basel) 11, 1–9.
48. G. E. Berrios (1996), *The History of Mental Symptoms: Descriptive Psychopathology Since the Nineteenth Century* (Cambridge University Press, Cambridge).
49. F. S. Klaf, J. G. Hamilton (1961), 'Schizophrenia: A hundred years ago and today', *J. Ment. Sci.*, 107, 819–27.
50. G. Catalano, M. C. Catalano, C. S. Embi, R. L. Frankel (1999), 'Delusions about the Internet', *South Med. J.*, 92, 609–10.
51. A. P. Shubsachs, A. Young (1988), 'Dangerous delusions and the Hollywood phenomenon', *Br. J. Psychiatry*, 152, 722b.
52. A. R. Tomison, W. M. Donovan (1998), 'Dangerous delusions: The Hollywood phenomenon', *Brit. J. Psychiatry*, 153, 404–5.
53. R. Forsyth, R. Harland, T. Edwards (2001), 'Computer game delusions', *J. Royal Soc. Med.*, 94, 184–5.
54. S. A. Spence (1993), 'Nintendo hallucinations: A new phenomenological entity', *Irish J. Psychol. Med.*, 10, 98–9.
55. S. A. Spence (Academic Dept. of Psychiatry, University of Sheffield) (2001), 'Computer game delusions', *J. Royal Soc. Med.*, 94, 369.
56. A. Ichimura, I. Nakajima, H. Juzoji (2001), 'Investigation and analysis of a reported incident resulting in an actual airline hijacking due to a fanatical and engrossed VR state', *CyberPsychology & Behavior*, 4 (3).
57. Y. Bar-El, R. Durst, G. Katz, *et al* (2000), 'Jerusalem syndrome', *Br. J. Psychiatry*, 176, 86–90.
58. J. S. E. Hellewell, P. M. Haddad (2000), 'Further comments on Jerusalem syndrome', *Br. J. Psychiatry*, 176, 594a–594.

59. J. Séglas (1887), Melancholie anxieuse avec délire de négations', *Progr. Med.*, 46, 417–19.

60. J. Cotard (1880), 'Du délire hypocondriaque dans une forme grave de mélancolie anxieuse', *Ann. Med. Psychol.*, 4, 168–74.

61. G. E. Berrios, R. Luque (1995), 'Cotard's syndrome: Analysis of 100 cases', *Acta Psychiatr. Scand.*, 91, 185–8.

62. M. D. Enoch, W. H. Trethowan (1979), *Uncommon Psychiatric Syndromes* (John Wright, Bristol).

63. R. Descartes, translated by John Cottingham (1986), *Meditations on First Philosophy With Selections from the Objections and Replies* (Cambridge University Press, Cambridge).

64. A. W. Young, I. H. Robertson, D. J. Hellawell, W. de Pauw, B. Pentland (1922), 'Cotard delusion after brain injury', *Psychol. Med.*, 22, 799–804.

65. A. B. Joseph (1986), 'Cotard's syndrome with coexistent Capgras' syndrome, syndrome of subjective doubles and palinopsia', *J. Clin. Psychiatry*, 47, 605–6.

CHAPTER 16: WOULD YOU KNOW WHAT A DELUSION IS – EVEN IF YOU HAD ONE?

1. A. C. L. Gordon, D. R. Olson (1998), 'The relation between acquisition of a theory of mind and the capacity to hold in mind', *J. Exp. Child Psychol.*, 68, 70–83.

2. D. Freeman, P. A. Garety, E. Kuipers (2001), 'Persecutory delusions: Developing the understanding of belief maintenance and emotional distress', *Psychological Medicine*, 31, 1293–1306.

3. M. Klein (1946), 'Notes on some schizoid mechanisms', in *The Writings of Melanie Klein*, vol. 3, *Envy and Gratitude* [reprinted 1975] (Hogarth Press, London).

4. C. G. Jung (1914), 'The content of the psychoses', in *The Psychogenesis of Mental Disease: Collected works of Carl Jung*, vol. 3 [reprinted 1960] (Routledge & Kegan Paul, London).

5. J. Westermyer (1988), 'Some cross-cultural aspects of delusions', in T. O. Oltmanns, B. Maher (eds), *Delusional Beliefs* (Wiley, London).

6. L. R. Mujica-Parodi, H. A. Sackeim (2001), 'Cultural invariance and the diagnosis of delusions', *J. Neuropsychiatry Clin. Neurosci*, 13, 403–9.

7. *Ibid.*

8. *Ibid.*

9. *Ibid.*

10. *Ibid.*

11. *Ibid.*

12. *Ibid.*

13. *Ibid.*

14. *Ibid.*

15. *Ibid.*

16. R. P. Bentall (1994), 'Cognitive biases and abnormal beliefs: Towards a model of persecutory delusions', in A. S. David, J. Cutting (eds), *The Neuropsychology of Schizophrenia* (LEA, London).

17. K. C. Winters, J. M. Neal (1983), 'Delusions and delusional thinking in psychotics: A review of the literature', *Clinical Psychology Review*, 3, 227–53.

18. S. Freud (1900), *The Interpretation of Dreams* (Pelican Books, Aylesbury).

19. P. A. Garety, D. Freeman (1999), 'Cognitive approaches to delusions: A critical review of theories and evidence', *Br. J. Clinical Psychology*, 38, 113–54.

20. A. T. Beck, A. J. Rush, B. F. Shaw, G. Emery (1979), *Cognitive Therapy of Depression* (Guilford Press, New York).

21. J. E. Rhodes, S. Jakes (2000), 'Correspondence between delusions and personal goals: A qualitative analysis', *Br. J. Medical Psychology*, 73 (2), 211–25.

22. C. G. Jung (1914), 'The content of the psychoses', in *The Psychogenesis of Mental Disease: Collected Works of Carl Jung*, vol. 3 [reprinted 1960] (Routledge & Kegan Paul, London).

23. S. Freud (1900), *The Interpretation of Dreams* (Pelican Books, Aylesbury).

24. A. C. L. Gordon, D. R. Olson (1998), 'The relation between acquisition of a theory of mind and the capacity to hold in mind', *J. Exp. Child Psychol.*, 68, 70–83.

25. A. Whiten, R. W. Byrne (1997), *Machiavellian Intelligence, II: Extensions and Evaluations* (Cambridge University Press, Cambridge).

26. S. Baron-Cohen (1995), *Mindblindness: An Essay on Autism and Theory of Mind* (Bradford/MIT, Cambridge).

27. J. K. Buitelaar, M. van der Wees, H. Swaab-Barneveld, R. J. van der Gaag (1999), 'Theory of mind and emotion-recognition functioning in autistic spectrum disorders and in psychiatric control and normal children', *Dev. Psychopathol.*, 11, 39–58.

28. C. D. Frith, R. Corcoran (1996), 'Exploring "theory of mind" in people with schizophrenia', *Psychol. Med.*, 26, 521–30.

29. S. Baron-Cohen (1991), 'The theory of mind deficit in autism: How specific is it?', *Br. J. Dev. Psychol.*, 9, 301–14.

30. M. Harrow, I. Lanin-Kettering, J. G. Miller (1989), 'Impaired perspective and thought pathology in schizophrenic and psychotic disorders', *Schizophr. Bull.*, 15, 605–23.

31. R. I. M. Dunbar (1998), 'The social brain hypothesis', *Evolutionary Anthropology*, 6, 178–90.

32. R. Foley (1995), *Humans Before Humanity* (Cambridge University Press, Cambridge).

33. T. H. Joffe (1997), 'Social pressures have selected for an extended juvenile period in primates', *J. Human Evolution*, 32, 593–605.

34. D. J. Povinelli (1993), 'Reconstructing the evolution of mind', *Am. Psychology* 48, 493–509.

35. D. F. Bjorklund (1997), 'The role of immaturity in human development', *Psychol. Bull.*, 122, 153–69.

36. R. W. Byrne (1995), *The Thinking Ape: Evolutionary Origins of Intelligence* (Oxford University Press, Oxford).

37. L. Brothers (1990), 'The social brain: A project for integrating primate behavior and neurophysiology in a new domain', *Concepts Neurosci.*, 1, 27–51.

38. H. D. Ellis, A. W. Young (1990), 'Accounting for delusional misidentifications', *Br. J. Psychiatry*, 157, 239–48.

39. B. G. Charlton (1995), 'Cognitive neuropsychiatry and the future of diagnosis', *Br. J. Psychiatry*, 167, 149–53.

40. R. W. Byrne, A. Whiten (1988), *Machiavellian Intelligence: Social Expertise and the Evolution of Intellect: Monkeys, Apes and Humans* (Clarendon Press, Oxford).

41. D. S. Wilson, D. Near, R. R. Miller (1996), 'Machiavellianism: A synthesis of the evolutionary and psychological literatures', *Psychol. Bull.*, 119, 285–99.

42. A. Jolly (1966), 'Lemur social behaviour and primate intelligence', *Science*, 153, 501–6.

43. N. K. Humphrey (1976), 'The social function of intellect', in P. P. G. Bateson, R. A. Hinde (eds), *Growing Points in Ethology* (Cambridge University Press, Cambridge).

44. M. T. McGuire, A. Troisi (1998), *Darwinian Psychiatry* (Oxford University Press, Oxford).

45. L. Cosmides (1989), 'The logic of social exchange: Has natural selection shaped how humans reason?: Studies with the Wason selection task', *Cognition*, 31, 187–276.

46. F. Walston, A. S. David, B. David, B. G. Charlton (1998), 'Sex differences in the content of delusions', *Evolution & Human Behaviour*, 19 (4), 257–60.

47. M. Brüne (2001), 'Social cognition and psychopathology in an evolutionary perspective', *Psychopathology*, 34, 85–94.

48. B. A. Maher (1988), 'Anomalous experience and delusional thinking: The logic of explanation', in T. F. Oltmanns, B. A. Maher (eds), *Delusional Beliefs* (Wiley, London).

49. T. F. Oltmanns (1988), 'Approaches to the definition and study of delusions', in T. F. Oltmanns, B. Maher (eds), *Delusional Beliefs* (Wiley, London).

50. N. K. Denzin (1970), *The Research Act in Sociology* (Butterworth, London).

51. J. V. Oakhill, P. N. Johnson-Laird (1985), 'Rationality, memory and the search for counterexamples', *Cognition*, 20, 79–94.

52. R. E. D'Andrade (1992), 'Schemas and motivation', in R. G. D'Andrade, C. Strauss (eds), *Human Motives and Cultural Models* (Cambridge University Press, Cambridge).

53. A. J. Chalmers (1982), *What Is This Thing Called Science?*, 2nd edn (Open University Press, Milton Keynes).

54. J. S. Bruner, L. Postman (1949), 'On the Perception of Incongruity: A Paradigm', *J. of Personality*, 18, 206–23.

55. M. Boyle (1990), *Schizophrenia – A Scientific Delusion?* (Routledge, London).

56. J. Searle (1992), *The Rediscovery of the Mind* (MIT Press, Cambridge, MA).

57. D. C. Dennett (1992), *Consciousness Explained* (Viking, London).

58. D. Munro, J. E. Schumaker, S. C. Carr (eds) (1997), *Motivation and Culture* (Routledge, London).

59. N. Hayes (ed.) (1997), *Doing Qualitative Analysis in Psychology* (Psychology Press, Hove).

60. N. Cameron (1959), 'The paranoid pseudo community revisited', *American J. Sociology*, 65, 52–6.

61. J. Cutting, D. Murphy (1990), 'Preference for denotative as opposed to connotative meanings in schizophrenia', *Brain & Language*, 39, 459–68.

62. G. Lakoff, M. Johnson (1980), *Metaphors We Live By* (University of Chicago Press, Chicago, IL).

63. J. Searle (1992), *The Rediscovery of the Mind* (MIT Press, Cambridge, MA).

64. P. D. Slade, R. P. Bentall (1988), *Sensory Deception: A Scientific Analysis of the Hallucination* (Wiley, Chichester).

65. J. Mirowsky, C. E. Ross (1983), 'Paranoia and the structure of powerlessness', *Am. Sociological Review*, 48, 228–39.

66. R. D. Laing (1960), *The Divided Self* (Penguin, Harmondsworth).

67. D. Rosenthal (1993), 'Thinking that one thinks', in M. Davies, G. W. Humphreys (eds), *Consciousness: Psychological and Philosophical Essays* (Blackwell, Oxford).

68. J. Brett-Jones, P. Garety, D. Hemsley (1987), 'Measuring delusional experience: A method and its application', *Br. J. Clin. Psychology*, 26, 257–65.

69. P. A. Garety, D. R. Hemsley (1994), *Delusions* (Oxford University Press, Oxford).

POSTSCRIPT

1. P. A. Garety, D. R. Hemsley (1994), *Delusions* (Oxford University Press, Oxford).

2. R. Littlewood, M. Lipsedge (1982), *Aliens and Alienists* (Penguin, Harmondsworth).

3. K. C. Winters, J. M. Neal (1983), 'Delusions and delusional thinking in psychotics: A review of the literature', *Clin. Psychology Review*, 3, 227–53.

4. B. A. Maher (1988), 'Anomalous experience and delusional thinking: The logic of explanation', in T. F. Oltmanns, B. A. Maher (eds), *Delusional Beliefs* (Wiley, London).

5. J. M. Neale (1988), 'Defensive functions of manic episodes', in T. F. Oltmanns, B. Maher (eds), *Delusional Beliefs* (Wiley, London).

6. R. P. Bentall, H. F. Jackson, D. Pilgrim (1988), 'Abandoning the concept of "schizophrenia": Some implications of validity arguments for psychological research into psychotic phenomena', *Br. J. Clinical Psychology*, 27, 303–24.

7. V. M. Drury, E. J. Robinson, M. Birchwood (1998), 'Theory of mind skills during an acute episode of psychosis and following recovery', *Psychol. Med.*, 28, 1101–12.

8. P. A. Garety, D. Freeman (1999), 'Cognitive approaches to delusions: A critical review of theories and evidence', *Br. J. Clinical Psychology*, 38, 113–54.

9. R. P. Bentall, P. Kinderman, S. Kaney (1994), 'The self, attributional processes and abnormal beliefs: Towards a model of persecutory delusions', *Behav. Res. Therapy*, 32, 331–41.

10. P. A. Garety, D. Freeman (1999), 'Cognitive approaches to delusions: A critical review of theories and evidence', *Br. J. Clinical Psychology*, 38, 113–54.

INDEX

Hellewell, Dr J. S. E. 385
Herod, King 58
Herodotus 210
Hershberger, Dr Scott 196–7
highway hypnosis 335
hijacking of plane by CAWD patient
  380–2
Hill, Susanna 142–3
'Hillside Strangler' 333
Hinckley, John 119
Hirstein, Dr William 362
History (Herodotus) 210
histrionic/hysterical personality disorder
  164
Hitler, Adolf 122
hoarding, compulsive 249–64
Hollywood phenomenon 377
homelessness 289
homicide 63–4, 164, 179, 356, 357
  pact 75–7
homosexuality 41, 219, 236–7, 307,
  310, 315, 324
  fantasies 140, 141
  and penis size 196
  see also lesbianism
hormones 126
Horney, Karen 149
hospital hobo syndrome 284
Houston Community College, Texas 40
Hungary 193
Huws, Dr Rhodri 138
hyperphagia 247
hypertrichosis 31
hypnosis 153–60
hypochondria 84
hypoxiphilia 132
hysteria 46
  anxiety 89–90, 94–5
  epidemic 89–95, 94
  mass 90–5
  motor 89–90
  national 394
hysterical fugue 333, 336–7

iatrogenic disorders 334
Iceland 16
Ichimura, Dr Atsushi 379, 380
id, superego and ego 35
ideas of reference 169, 218
identity, personal 333
imaginary relationships 117
Impostor syndrome 1
impotence 190, 343
In the Realm of the Senses 142
incest 22, 192, 215

delusions of 103
incontinence, faecal 197, 198–9, 241
incubus syndrome 97, 100–4, 104
India 189
Induced Psychotic Disorder (IPD) 70, 81
Innocent VIII, Pope 101
Inova Fairfax Hospital, Virginia 317
insertion of thought 368
Institute of Neurology, London 368
Institute of Psychiatry, London 126,
  132, 252, 266, 328, 391
Institute for Sexual Medicine, Berlin 149
interaction, mental 410
internal body representation 367
International Student Organization 114
Internet 375
Iowa, University of 15
iron deficiency 31, 239
irritable bowel syndrome 197, 199
Istanbul Medical School 223
Itard, J. 271

Jackson, James 288–9
Jacome, Dr Daniel E. 338
Jaffé, Dr Philip 61
Jakes, Simon 399
James, Dr 157–8
James, William 361
Janet, Pierre 197, 261
Jankovic, Dr J. 371
Japan 30, 90–5
Jarrett, Dr F. J. 274
Jaspers, Karl 260
jealousy 105, 110–14
Jefferson, Thomas 110
Jeremiah (prophet) 4
'jerks' 93–4
Jerusalem syndrome 382–5
Joan of Arc 52
Johns Hopkins Hospital, Baltimore,
  Maryland 110, 311, 317, 326
  Psychohormonal Research Unit 312
Johnstone, Jo 138
Joiner, Dr Thomas E., Jr 261, 263
Jorgensen, Christine (George) 326
Journal of the Royal Society of Health
  148
Joyce, James 71, 142
Jung, Carl Gustav 18–19, 398, 401
Justine (de Sade) 142, 143

Kahlbaum, Karl Ludwig 352
Kalyanam, Ram Chandran 317
Keats, John 66
Keck, Dr Paul 21

485

Kent State University, Ohio, School of Nursing 177
Kfer Shaul Mental Health Centre, Jerusalem 382
Kinsey, Alfred 127
Kinsey Institute of Sex Research, Indiana University 196
Kiraly, Dr S. J. 71
Kiribati 108–9
Klingsor syndrome 305
koko 109
Korea 195
koro syndrome 188–98, 301
  in women 193–5
Kotzwara, Franz 142–3
Kourany, Dr Ronald-Frederic C. 48
Kovács, Dr Attila 193
Kraepelin, Emil 167
Krafft-Ebing, Richard 311
Kramer, Heinrich, and Sprenger, James 101
Kubrick, Stanley 365
Kuhn, Thomas 405
Kulick, Dr Aaron 26, 28
Kurten, Peter 57

The Lancet 252
Langdon Hospital, Exeter 377
Lasèque, C., and Falret, J. 68
Latin America 31
lead poisoning, and pica 234
Leafhead, Dr Kate 388
League for Sexual Reform 150
Leger, Antoine 57, 59
Lennon, John 119
Leong, Dr Gregory 105–6
lesbianism 41, 238, 328
Lewis, D. E. 109
Lewis, Dr T. M. 369
Lewis, Michael 353
libido 128
A Life of Grime 252
locophobia 274–7
Lofting, Hugh, Dr Dolittle stories 39
Loftus, Elizabeth 337
Logic of Scientific Discovery (Popper) 405
Los Angeles Police Department 187
  Database 186
Louis VII, King of France 97
love 104
  as addiction 170
  falling in 116, 161
Lucia, St 228
Lundsgaarde, Henry 108–9

Luque, R. 387
lycanthropy (werewolf disorder) 18–35, 40, 56, 66
lysergic acid diethylamide (LSD) 94

McGuire, Brian 136
Mackenzie, John 110–11
McLuhan, Marshall 95
magnetic image resonance technology 336, 348–9
Malaysia 21
Malhotra, Dr Ladi 354
malingering 154, 159–60, 283, 288, 291–7, 341
  and MPD 333
  pure and partial 296
Malleus Maleficarum, or the Witches Hammer 21, 101
manic depression 68
manic-depressive psychosis 167, 261, 375
Manning, Dr John 196
Maori 21
Mark, Gospel of 210
Markowitsch, Dr Hans 337
Marks, Professor Isaac 266, 328
marriage, delusion in 2–3
masochism 148, 312, 314, 320
mass, Catholic 58
Massachusetts General Hospital, Boston 369
masturbation
  in adolescents 127, 320, 325
  in children 104
  and doll phobia 279
  and fantasies 317
  guilt over 33, 303, 305, 307
  and koro 192
  in paraphilia 129–30, 132–3, 136–9
  and self-mutilation 219, 325
  visual aids to 313, 325
  in women 41
mathematics 387
Matthew, Gospel of 301, 303, 307
Maudsley Hospital, London 4, 15, 234, 266, 285, 405
Meadow, Dr Roy 290
mecrophagia 66
melancholia 71
Melbourne, University of, Australia 305
Meloy, Dr J. Reid 164, 165
menstruation 227
Mental Health Act (1983) 293
Messiah, self-identification as 4, 367, 401–2, 410

486

metabolic deficiency 31
metamorphosis 56
Michigan Womyn's Music Festival 328
millennium, delusions concerning 385–6,
   394
'The Million-Dollar Man' 285–6
mirrors, preoccupation with 65
miscarriage 237, 238
misidentification syndromes 351–63,
   403
Mistree, Farrokhg 114–16
mixed personality disorder 190
Modern Propensities (Vanbutchell) 143
Modestin, Dr J. 328
modification of belief 412–13
Mohammad 52
Mohandie, Dr Kris 187
Money, Dr John 311, 319, 325
monoamine oxidase inhibitors (MAOIs)
   170
mood disorders 25, 184
mood swings 15, 360
Moore, Dr Lawrence 115
morbid interpsychology 74
Morselli, Enrique 202
motherhood 149
Mowat, R. R. 107
Mujica-Parodi, Dr 395
Mullen, Dr Paul 180
multiple personality disorder (MPD; dissociative identity disorder) 46, 47,
   223, 225, 328–31, 332–50
   and amnesia 334
   and child sexual abuse 336
   and post-traumatic brain injury 339
   traumagenic and iatrogenic theories
   on 334–5
Münchausen syndrome 154, 280–91,
   312, 316
   by proxy 289–91
Münchhausen, Baron Karl von 284, 290
murder *see* homicide
Murnau, W. 55
Murray, Dr Sandra 2 3
mythology, Greek 29

The Naked Lunch (Burroughs) 142
Napoleon I, Emperor 3
narcissism 165
nasogenital reflex 110
National Health Service 4
National Institute of Dental and
   Craniofacial Research 248
National Institute of Mental Health and
   Neurosciences, Bangalore, India 32, 220

National Violence Against Women
   (NVAW) Survey 182
Neagoe, Dr Adriana 77
Nebuchadnezzar, King 21–2
necrophagia 57, 59
necrophilia 57, 59, 65, 66, 347
necrosadism 59, 65
needles, inserted into body 220
New Mexico, University of, Health
   Sciences Center, Albuquerque 306
New Scientist 336
New South Wales, University of 82
New York Psychiatric Institute 170
New York State Psychiatric Institute 395
Newberg, Dr Andrew, and d'Aquili, Dr
   Eugene 54
Newcastle upon Tyne
   Royal Victoria Infirmary 86
   University of 404
Nietzsche, Elisabeth 408
Nietzsche, Friedrich 407–8
Nintendo Game Boy 91
Nixon, Richard 124
Noffsinger, Dr Stephen G., and Saleh, Dr
   Fabian M. 168
North Carolina, University of, School of
   Medicine 75
North Central Bronx Hospital, New
   York 210
North Queensland, University of,
   Australia 91
Northcoast Behavioral Healthcare
   System, Northfield, Ohio 168
Norton, Dr Scott 108
nose, amputation of 110
nose-biting (as punishment for adultery)
   108–11
Nosferatu 55
nymphomania 166

obsessions, defined 265
Les Obsessions et la Psychoasthénie
   (Janet) 197, 261
obsessive-compulsive disorder (OCD)
   260–4, 265–79
   age pattern in 260, 263
   and bowel obsession 197
   checking rituals in 198, 265, 274
   cognitive techniques in 200–1
   and coprophagia 244
   Diogenes syndrome as 249, 253
   exposure and response prevention
   treatment of 242–3
   and gender identity disorder 328
   and paraphilias 134

stroke 368
The Structure of Scientific Revolution
405
substance abuse 184, 189, 289, 359
sudden infant death syndrome 290–1
suicide 81–2, 267, 309, 389
  attempted 27, 204, 224, 290, 293,
  301, 306, 338, 376, 386
  pacts 81–2
  and self-mutilation 219
  thoughts of 308, 322, 328, 338
Summis Desiderontis Affectibus
  (Innocent VIII) 101
Sun 123
Sun Tzu 12
superman concept 408
Sussex, University of 371
Sutcliffe, Peter 296
swearing, repeated 273–4
Sybil 332
syllogomania 249–64

taijin kyofusho 205
Tarasoff, Tanya 114–16
taste system 248
tattooing 134–6
Tei, Dr H. 269
Teikyo University School of Medicine,
  Tokyo 342
The Terminator 220
Terrel State Hospital, Texas 129
territoriality 261–4
testosterone levels 196
Texas Medical Branch, Houston 40
Texas, University of 110, 128
Thailand 110, 189
Thales 9
theory of mind 368, 402, 408
therapist–patient confidentiality 114
therianthropy (shape-shifting) 22
Thibierge, Georges 207
Thomas, Archbishop of York 96
Thomas Jefferson University Hospital,
  Philadelphia, PA 228
thought control 51
Three Bridges Regional Secure Unit,
  Middlesex 293
Three Faces of Eve 332
tics 271
tiger, delusion of being 26–8
Time magazine 91
tobacco, ingestion 233
Tokai University
  Medical Research Institute, Japan 379
  School of Medicine, Japan 379

Tokyo
  University 342
  Women's Medical College,
  Neurological Institute 269
Tomison, Dr A. R. 377
tongue, removal of 219
Toronto, University of 99, 240
Tourette, Georges Gilles de la 271
Tourette's syndrome 271
Toyohashi, Japan 92
Trafford General Hospital, Manchester
  385
transgender movement 328
transportation to another world, fear of
  268
transsexualism 301, 302, 312, 317, 319,
  326–31
  cryptic 312–13
  see also gender identity disorder
transvestism *see* cross–dressing
traumatic brain injury 341
triangulation 164–5
trichobezoars (swallowed hairballs) 232
troilism 122
The Truman Show 120, 121
truth determination 404
truth-value, preservation of 395
Tsai, Guochuan 348
Tsukuba, University of, Japan 133
Tübingen, University of 257
Tucker, Dr Landrum S. 75
Turkey 226
TV Tokyo 92
Twain, Mark 71, 110

Uchinuma, Dr Yukio 342
Uffculme Clinic, Birmingham 277
UFOs 310
  delusions involving 78
Ulysses (Joyce) 142
unintelligibility theorem 260
United States of America 334
urine, preoccupation with odour of
  205–6

vampirism 31, 55–66, 347, 389
Van Gogh, Vincent 219
Vanbutchell, Martin 143
Vanderbilt University, Nashville,
  Tennessee 48
Venetius, King 29
Verdun, Michael 29
Veterans Affairs Medical Center,
  Portland, Oregon 288
vibrators, trapped 148